Transvenous Lead Extraction

Maria Grazia Bongiorni
Editor

Transvenous Lead Extraction

From Simple Traction to Internal Transjugular Approach

Foreword by
Bruce L. Wilkoff

Springer

Editor
Maria Grazia Bongiorni
2nd Cardiovascular Department
AOUP, Santa Chiara University Hospital
Pisa, Italy

ISBN 978-88-470-5614-5 ISBN 978-88-470-1466-4 (eBook)

DOI 10.1007/978-88-470-1466-4

Springer Milan Dordrecht Heidelberg London New York

Softcover re-print of the Hardcover 1st edition 2011

9 8 7 6 5 4 3 2 1 2011 2012 2013 2014

Cover design: Simona Colombo, Milan, Italy
Typesetting: Graphostudio, Milan, Italy

Springer-Verlag Italia S.r.l. – Via Decembrio 28 – I-20137 Milan
Springer is a part of Springer Science+Business Media (www.springer.com)

Dedicated
to all patients dealing with device-related complications
and
to all doctors and nurses devoting their lives to care for them

Foreword

The evolution of the management of transvenous leads has been born out of the furnace of clinical care and the pathophysiology of lead dysfunction. Transvenous lead extraction is only one tool in the management tool chest. At first it wasn't much of a tool, just a rag tag group of ideas used by a few people trying to solve problems for patients without a solution. However, over the last 25 years and particularly with the visionary efforts of Dr. Charles Byrd and his creative collaboration with Cook Pacemaker Inc. (now Cook Vascular Inc.), transvenous lead extraction is not only a tool but an armory of techniques.

There were many steps to the elevation of these ideas to an accepted solution, practiced by many; tools continuously evolving and a community developed over years, results published, passionate teachers, minor and major complications, fatal mistakes, disparate ideas, society guidelines and all progressing due to the ongoing clinical need to solve problems. It is an important story and a one well told by Dr. Bongiorni and her colleagues. How do we teach our hard learned lessons to the next generation of physicians? Can we prevent future mistakes from being made? We must commit ourselves to recording, analysis and communication. This book on lead extraction is unique and systematic and it is my prayer that it is never left on the shelf but studied intently and built upon endlessly.

February 2011

Bruce L. Wilkoff MD
Director Cardiac Pacing and Tachyarrhythmia Devices
Department of Cardiovascular Medicine
Professor of Medicine
Cleveland Clinic Lerner College of Medicine
of Case Western Reserve University
Cleveland, Ohio

Preface

"I can do it…, I can do it..., I can do it…" This affirmation could be read on pins on jackets of many participants of the Cardiac Pacing and Arrhythmology Congress in 1989. These simple words mean that a procedure for transvenous lead extraction was now a possibility. One participant was a dear Italian friend of mine, a salesman, who showed me some tools for lead extraction that had recently been produced by an American company, Cook Pacemaker, Inc., in collaboration with a genius in the field, Dr. Charles Byrd (the father of lead extraction). At that time, there were three different opinions about lead extraction: most physicians were unbelievers; many were frightened by the idea; and some were simply curious. I was in the latter group. My interest came from the following: (1) many patients could benefit from transvenous lead extraction (at that time, I had a patient with lead-related endocarditis); (2) some years earlier, my professor began extracting transvenous leads using empirical tools (weights, pulleys, etc.) and, if not for his premature death, would have fully appreciated possibility of safe transvenous lead extraction; (3) if my clever and forward-looking friend was wearing the pin being displayed at the 1989 congress, it would have meant that, in his opinion, transvenous lead extraction was coming of age. So, my professional journey into transvenous lead extraction began like a fairy tale ("Once upon a time…"), starting with a clinical need, enhanced by intellectual curiosity, and guided by a lucky star that put the right people in the right place at the right moment.

Since that time, there has been great progress in the field, and transvenous lead extraction is becoming a widespread procedure in many arrhythmology centers, with increasing indications for its performance. Consequently, physicians feel the need for recommendations, indications, training, equipment, facilities, and other guidelines for performing transvenous lead extraction. Subsequently, the most important scientific organizations have responded to these needs. Many publications are now available regarding this subject, reflecting an obviously increasing interest in solving cardiac pacing and defibrillation lead-related complications. This book is the result of 20 years of personal experience in this field, and it is addressed to young cardiologists and arrhythmologists, as well as to nurses and technicians, who want to learn about lead extraction. Lead extraction is a true team procedure. All participants must know – and keep in mind – the interaction between the lead and the cardiovascular structure, removal indications, patient preparation, extraction tools and techniques, and complication management in order to achieve the best possible outcomes. This volume describes, in particular, an innovative approach to transvenous lead extraction – the internal jugular vein approach – which is used to extract leads otherwise difficult to remove from the venous entry site or via the femoral vein.

This is the first edition of this book, the authors having been selected from the Pisa School in order to provide cohesive information while avoiding redundancies and contradictions. In future additions, advances in this increasingly important field of medicine will be described. I thank the many people who contributed to the realization of this book. First, sincere thanks to my great professor Carlo Contini for teaching me about arrhythmology but especially for teaching me to care about my patients. Next, heartfelt thanks to my coworkers, all of whom devoted much time to this book. A special thanks to "tireless" Dr. Ezio Soldati for his constant support and ability to graphically reproduce ideas and actions, and to Dr. Raffaele De Lucia for the book's arrangement. Transvenous lead extraction demands a team effort, so thank you to my long-devoted and passionate nurses, Giampietro Ercoli, Michela Favaro, Cristina Giannessi, and Mascia Sarti, and to Guglielmo Liva e Susy Bardelli, who recently joined our team. My thanks also to the University Hospital cardiac surgeon and anesthesia team for their invaluable support, and thanks to all cardiologists and nurses who care for these fragile patients during preparation for surgery and postoperatively. Finally, a sweet thought to my parents, Teresa and Ernesto, who – through great sacrifice – made my studies and my wonderful profession possible.

Pisa, February 2011 *Maria Grazia Bongiorni, MD*

Contents

Contributors

Maria Stella Baccillieri Interventional Electrophysiology Unit, Cardiovascular Department, P. Cosma Hospital, Camposampiero (PD), Italy

Francesco Bandera 2nd Cardiovascular Department AOUP, Santa Chiara University Hospital, Pisa, Italy

Maria Grazia Bongiorni 2nd Cardiovascular Department AOUP, Santa Chiara University Hospital, Pisa, Italy

Giovanni Coluccia 2nd Cardiovascular Department AOUP, Santa Chiara University Hospital, Pisa, Italy

Raffaele De Lucia 2nd Cardiovascular Department AOUP, Santa Chiara University Hospital, Pisa, Italy

Andrea Di Cori 2nd Cardiovascular Department AOUP, Santa Chiara University Hospital, Pisa, Italy

Pier Giorgio Golzio Cardiology Division, Department of Internal Medicine AOU, Molinette San Giovanni Battista Hospital, Turin, Italy

Luca Paperini 2nd Cardiovascular Department AOUP, Santa Chiara University Hospital, Pisa, Italy

Elisa Pelissero Faculty of Medicine, University of Turin, Turin, Italy

Luca Segreti 2nd Cardiovascular Department AOUP, Santa Chiara University Hospital, Pisa, Italy

Gianluca Solarino 2nd Cardiovascular Department AOUP, Santa Chiara University Hospital, Pisa, Italy

Ezio Soldati 2nd Cardiovascular Department AOUP, Santa Chiara University Hospital, Pisa, Italy

Pietro Turrini Interventional Electrophysiology Unit, Cardiovascular Department P. Cosma Hospital, Camposampiero (PD), Italy

Roberto Verlato Interventional Electrophysiology Unit, Cardiovascular Department P. Cosma Hospital, Camposampiero (PD), Italy

Stefano Viani 2nd Cardiovascular Department AOUP, Santa Chiara University Hospital, Pisa, Italy

Melissa Vinci Faculty of Medicine, University of Turin, Turin, Italy

Giulio Zucchelli 2nd Cardiovascular Department AOUP, Santa Chiara University Hospital, Pisa, Italy

Importance of Knowing Lead and Patient Interaction

1

Raffaele De Lucia, Giovanni Coluccia, Stefano Viani and Luca Paperini

1.1 Structure, Function, and Clinical Aspects of Pacemaker and Defibrillator Leads

The implantable cardiac pacemaker (PM)/defibrillator is a technically sophisticated system composed of a generator connected to one or more leads. Pacemaker/defibrillator leads play a pivotal role for system function, delivering the output pulse or the endocardial shock from the generator to the myocardium and acquiring spontaneous intracardiac electrogram from the heart to the device. Leads are also the most frequently involved component in case of system malfunction, and when a generator-pocket infection is present, their extraction – always necessary to guarantee complete resolution – is a challenge. The success of lead extraction is highly influenced by lead characteristics; for that reason, this chapter is dedicated to lead technology, i.e., polarity, electrodes, fixation mechanisms, electrode–tissue interaction, conductors, insulators, and connectors, with particular attention to aspects that may interfere with the extraction procedure. We discuss separately cardiac PM and defibrillator leads to emphasize their different technology.

R. De Lucia (✉)
2nd Cardiovascular Department AOUP, Santa Chiara University Hospital, Pisa, Italy

M. G. Bongiorni (Ed.), *Transvenous Lead Extraction*.

1.1.1 Pacemaker Leads

1.1.1.1 Lead Polarity

Transvenous lead polarity simply indicates the number of electrodes in contact with the heart. A unipolar lead has only one electrode, the cathode, on his tip. In this configuration, the PM case serves as the anode of the circuit (Fig. 1.1). A bipolar lead has two electrodes at the distal end separated by a short distance. The tip electrode is the cathode, and the proximal ring electrode serves as the anode (Fig. 1.2). In this configuration, the PM case is not involved in the electrical circuit. The distance between tip and ring electrode varies with manufacturer and design.

In the VDD-pacing lead, there are two bipolar systems. The distal one is used to pace and sense the ventricle chamber, whereas the proximal, floating one in the atrial chamber, with no contact with the endocardial surface, is only used to sense spontaneous atrial signals. These leads are called quadripolar, and distances from the four electrodes vary among manufacturer and lead design (Fig. 1.3). Bipolar may be superior to unipolar pacing/sensing because it is less prone to cause extracardiac stimulation at the pulse generator or to detect myopotentials, far-field signals, and electromagnetic interference. Moreover a bipolar lead can function in the unipolar mode, whereas the converse is obviously not possible. Historically, unipolar had a smaller external diameter than bipolar leads due to the presence of only one conductor and were therefore easier to manipulate during implantation than their counterpart. Otherwise, in a lead extraction procedure, the advantages of this

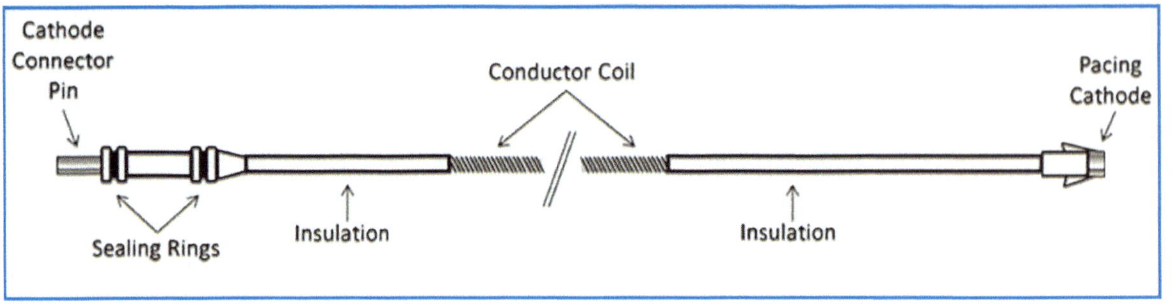

Fig. 1.1 Typical unipolar, straight, passive-fixation lead

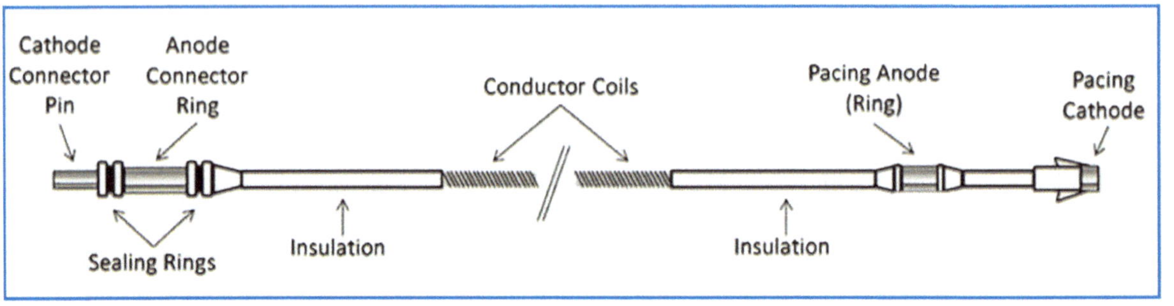

Fig. 1.2 Typical bipolar, straight, passive-fixation lead

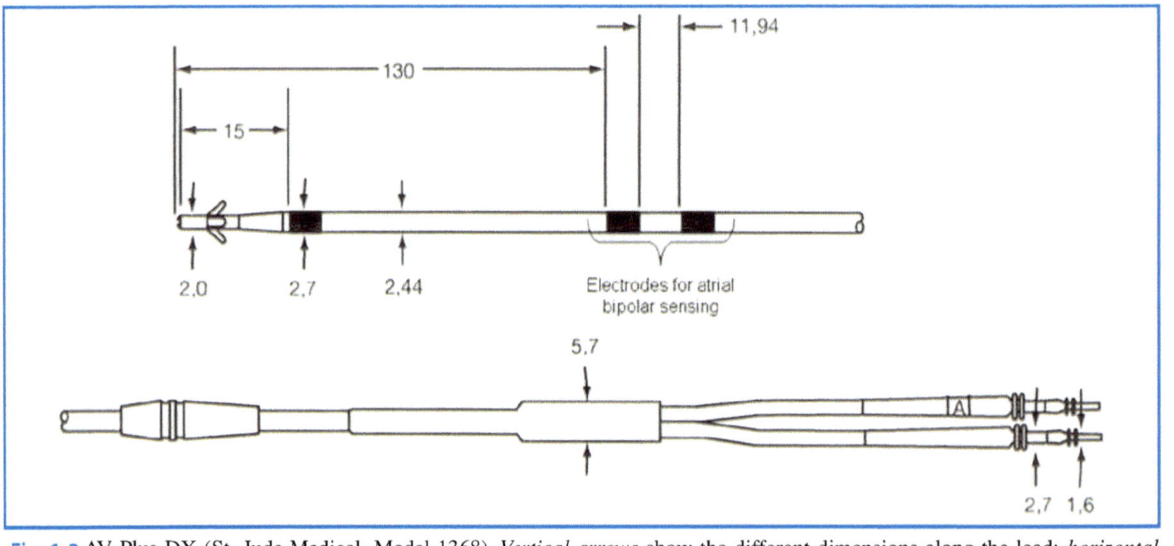

Fig. 1.3 AV Plus DX (St. Jude Medical, Model 1368). *Vertical arrows* show the different dimensions along the lead; *horizontal arrows* show the distance between the four electrodes. Measurements in millimeters (courtesy of St. Jude Medical)

design could be disadvantages: unipolar leads are smaller and usually more fragile than bipolar leads (with two or more conductors) because they are not as stiff.

1.1.1.2 Pacing Electrodes

The electrode is the portion of a pacing lead that acts as a long-term interface between the lead and the heart tissue providing functions of pacing and sensing, and these functions are influenced by the electrode's surface area. To describe pacing, we use the following analogy from Ken Stokes (former Medtronic senior research fellow): "The battery of the PM is like a bucket of water. There is a hole in the bucket, and that represents the current drain through the pacing system electrode. If the hole (electrode) is larger, the water (or current) drains out quickly. But if we can make the hole small, then it will drain more slowly". In the same manner, in a pacing lead system, if we reduce the electrode size (the bucket's hole), we increase the pacing impedance and deliver energy more efficiently.

The earliest transvenous pacing leads had a stimulating electrode surface area greater than 100 mm^2. Such a broad area was associated with a very low pacing impedance and, consequently, excessive current drain which influenced negatively battery longevity. So, from the 1960s to the 1990s, the cathode area of most pacing leads had been reduced from 8 to 1.2 mm^2 (Figs. 1.4 and 1.5) [1]. Unfortunately, continued reduction of electrode size is undesirable because it increases the polarization phenomenon. But what is polarization?

When there is no voltage difference between the cathode (tip) and the electrode (ring), ions are distributed randomly, but when the pacing pulse begins, ions move, which results in current flow from the electrode to the myocardium. As the current pulse continues, a charged layer surrounds the electrode tip and produces capacitive effect, which is the buildup of charge layers on the electrode, called polarization. When polarization is excessive, a substantial amount of lead current must be used to overcome it, which means that less current is available to stimulate the myocardium. As a consequence, output voltage must be increased, and more lead current is required to maintain adequate electrode-tip voltage and a safety margin. Nevertheless, if electrode size is reduced, sensing capability is also reduced, because decreasing the stimulation surface area, the area available for sensing is also reduced (Fig. 1.6).

To guarantee a small geometric electrode radius maintaining a large surface area, the porous electrode was developed. By altering the surface structure to be more porous, the geometric surface area

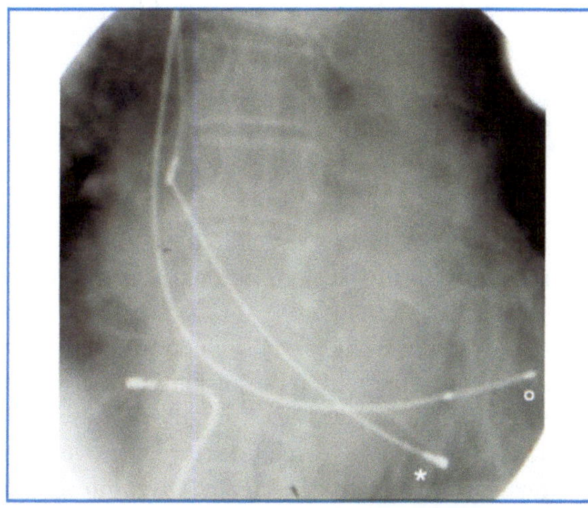

Fig 1.5 This patient was referred to our institution for lead extraction using the internal transjugular venous approach. The fractured lead (*) was implanted in 1975. Note that the old lead has an electrode with a broader stimulating electrode surface area. Temporary pacing lead (°)

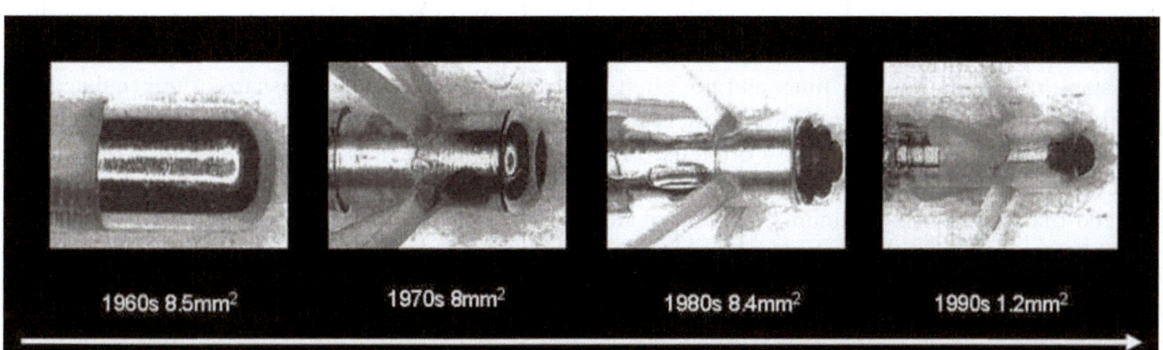

Fig. 1.4 Progressive variation in stimulating electrode surface area over the years (from [1], chap. 8 p. 69 (courtesy of Medtronic)

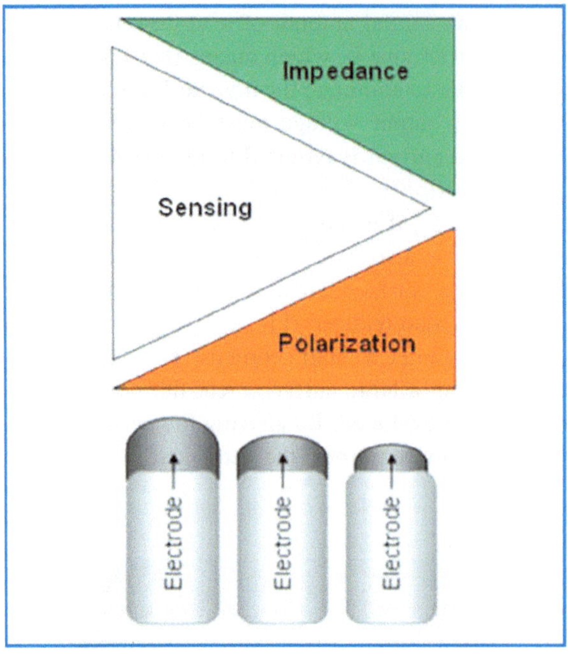

Fig 1.6 Correlation between stimulating surface area, impedance, polarization, and sensing

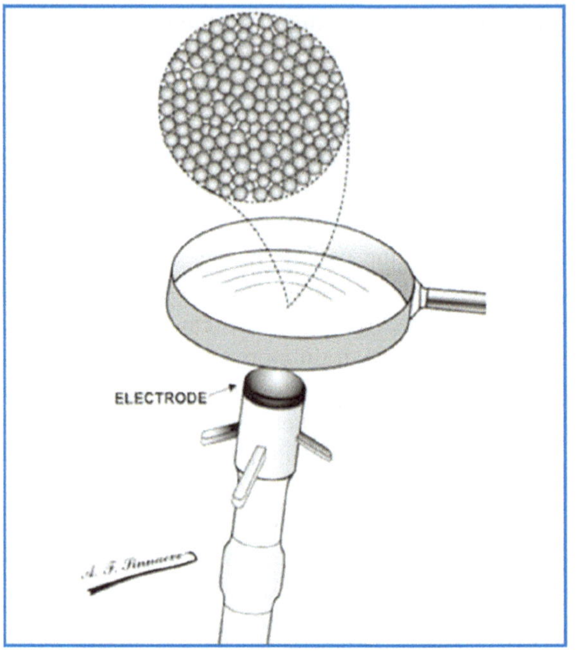

Fig. 1.7 Porous-surface electrodes (from [2], p. 38)

of the electrode increases and therefore lowers polarization. In this design, internal spaces within the electrode pores increase the surface area with the same radius. The porous electrodes initially consisted of a fine wire mesh of platinum–iridium fibers and were referred to as totally porous electrodes. Subsequently, manufactures moved to porous-surface electrodes created by sintering a metal powder or microspheres onto a solid metal substrate (Fig. 1.7) [2]. Summarizing, porous electrodes show lower stimulation threshold, better sensing properties, lower current drainage (higher impedance), and lower polarization [3–5]. Relatively few conductive materials have proven to be satisfactory for use in pacing electrodes.

Ideal material should be biologically inert, resistant to degradation over time, and not elicit a marked tissue reaction at the electrode–myocardium interface. Today, materials most often used for electrode building are platinum–iridium, platinized-titanium-coated platinum, iridium oxide, and platinum. Carbon electrodes finally seem to be the least susceptible to corrosion. To increase their surface area, they can be treated with a process called activation, which roughens the lead surface. Carbon electrodes elicit only minimal tissue reaction compared with the reaction surrounding platinum–iridium electrodes [6–8].

1.1.1.3 Lead Fixation and Electrode-Tissue Interaction

Lead Fixation

Lead fixation provides lead-tip stabilization during the hours immediately following the procedure. Fixation may be passive or active. Passive means that no part of the lead itself is actually embedded in the endocardium. After first experiences with flanged or helicoidal-shaped tips, endocardial leads now incorporate different numbers and kinds of tines at the tip that ensnare in trabeculated tissue of the right atrium or ventricle, providing stabilization (Fig. 1.8) [2]. Active fixation means that part of the lead actually embeds in the heart tissue for fixation. These leads utilize screw-based mechanisms to adhere to the myocardium to provide lead stability. Some leads incorporate screws that are electrically active, whereas others are inactive. Therefore, some screws are extendable and retractable from the lead tip and others are fixed on

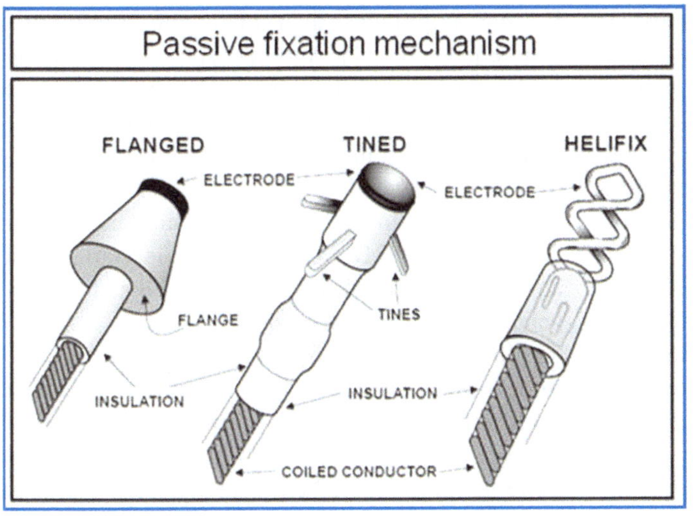

Fig. 1.8 Types of passive fixation leads (from [2], p. 36)

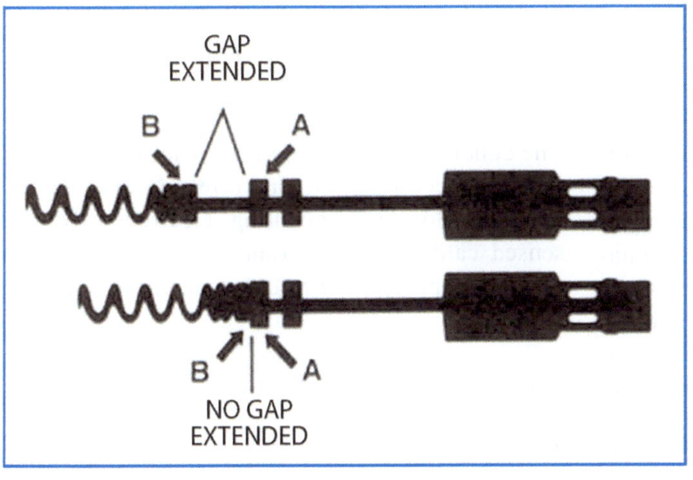

Fig. 1.9 Extendable/retractable screw-in lead at fluoroscopy (courtesy of Medtronic)

the tip. In the latter case, screws are covered with a material that dissolves in the blood stream in a time period sufficient for lead positioning in the heart. Mannitol compounds, for example, have been used for this purpose. While covering the screw, mannitol prevents it from catching on tissue and allows easier lead advancement in the venous system. Fixing these leads is possible by rotating the entire lead. In this case, the helix is always out. Otherwise, in an extendable/ retractable design, is possible to activate the screw by applying a tool to the connector pin and rotating the inner conductor. In these leads, is possible to determine when the screw is out by apposite fluoroscopy markers, as shown in Fig. 1.9.

Passive and active fixation mechanisms have both advantages and disadvantages. The clinical situation and operator preference dictate which kind of lead is chosen. Active fixation leads are preferred in cases of distorted anatomy (postsurgical or congenital heart disease), high right-sided pressure, after lead extraction procedure, or when an alternative site of pacing [i.e., atrial septum, right ventricular (RV) outflow tract] is deemed necessary.

Electrode–Tissue Interaction

After lead implantation, an inflammatory process develops at the electrode–tissue interface. This process causes an acute rise in stimulation threshold, but when the inflammatory process subsides and a fibrous capsule is formed, the stimulation threshold progressively falls to a chronic plateau level, which is reached about 4–6 months after implantation. Fibrous reaction and tissue ingrowth over tines and into porous and grooved electrodes consistently improve mechanical stability and intimate electrode–tissue contact but may also negatively influence chronic stimulation threshold.

The electric field strength at the cathode increases with current density but decreases as a function of the square of the distance between the electrode surface and the tissue, In the case of a thick, fibrous capsule developing at the tip of the electrode, the stimulation threshold inevitably increases, and sometimes it may be impossible to obtain myocardial electrical activation (exit block). For this reason, inflammation after lead implantation is the crucial factor that must be controlled to achieve a chronic, low-stimulation threshold.

The mechanical lead configuration can influence inflammatory reaction: for example, a lead design that allows excessive pressure to the distal electrode or an excessive lead stiffness can traumatize the endocardium resulting in accelerated inflammatory response, myocardial ischemia or even ventricular perforation [9]. To prevent traumatic contact at the electrode–tissue interface, softer forms of silicone or polyurethane may be used for the distal portion of the lead. Local pharmacologic agents were developed some years ago to reduce inflammatory reaction at the lead tip. Today, only glucocorticoids are used for this purpose. Dexamethasone sodium phosphate demonstrated the best performance compared with other glucocorticoids. The original design of drug-eluting leads was composed of a platinum-coated titanium electrode with an internal chamber behind it containing a plug of silicone rubber soaked with 1 mg or less of dexamethasone sodium phosphate; the internal chamber communicates with the outer electrode surface through a porous channel. The plug is referred to as a monolithic controlled release device (MCRD). This kind of electrode has demonstrated both acute and chronic very low stimulation thresholds, with elimination of the early postoperative peak. Steroid-eluting electrodes also show higher acute and long-term R- or P-wave amplitudes than their non-drug-eluting counterpart [10, 11]. Another type of drug-eluting lead is designed with a porous ceramic or silicone collar soaked with dexamethasone sodium phosphate positioned immediately proximal to tip electrode. This system is used in steroid-eluting, active fixation screw-in leads and shows similar performance as the MCRD. Steroid elution is available on atrial and ventricular leads and as well as coronary venous and epicardial leads.

Obviously, fixation mechanisms and electrode–tissue interaction have crucial implications for lead extraction also. Encasement of the tines of a passive fixation lead by fibrous reaction may make transvenous lead removal more difficult than that of an active-fixation isodiametric leads.

1.1.1.4 Pacing Conductors: Materials and Designs

The conductor of a pacing lead is basically a wire that conducts the electrical current from the pulse generator to the stimulating electrode and the sensed cardiac signals from the electrode to the sensing amplifier of the pulse generator.

Materials

The early conductor for unipolar pacing leads, developed by Elema-Schönander and Ericsson, consisted of four thin bands of stainless steel wound around a core of polyester braid (Fig. 1.10) [1]. This design was later abandoned because of possible corrosion. The same problem happened later with another conductor made with a drawn-brazed-strand (DBS) technique and insulated with polyurethane. In this design the silver occupies the central core and the spaces between the nickel alloy wires and also forms a thin coating around the wires. These leads had a high rate of insulation failure caused by internal oxidation from the DBS. Another early type of electrical conductor was the tinsel wire, but this design also showed later to be less than optimal. Separated from a central textile core (created to provide a high tensile strength), the individual strands or ribbons were relatively fragile (Fig. 1.11) [1]. Alloys such as MP35N

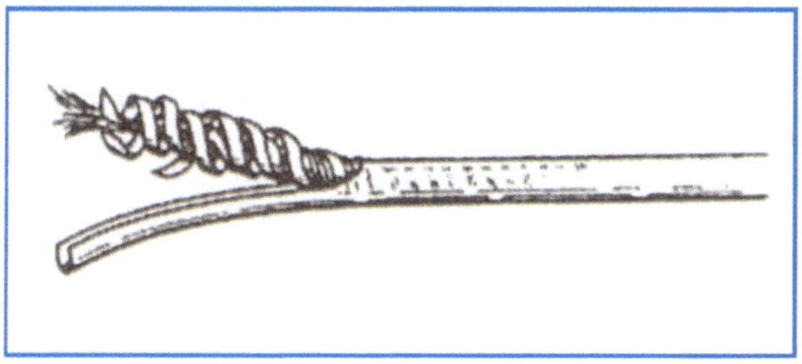

Fig. 1.10 Elema–Schönander unipolar lead with conductor made of stainless steel bands. (from [1], Chap. 9, p. 1) (courtesy of Medtronic)

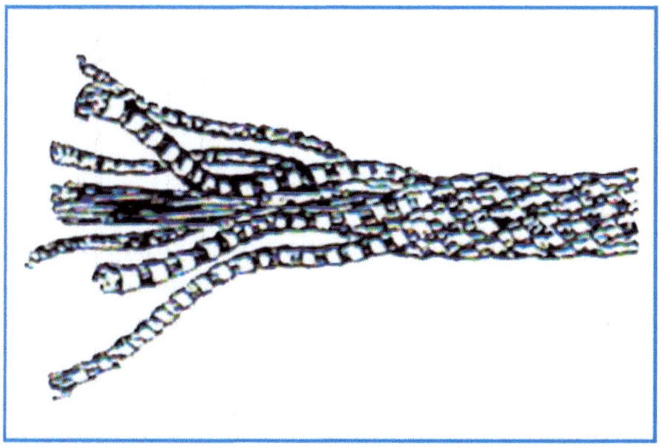

Fig. 1.11 Platinum/iridium ribbons intertwined around polyester yarn (from [1], Chap. 9, p. 76) (courtesy of Medtronic)

(35% cobalt, 35% nickel, 20% chromium, and 10% molybdenum) and nickel–silver are the most frequently used materials for modern lead conductors. It is corrosion resistant, flexible and durable, and offers a low resistance to allow efficient transfer of energy from the PM to the lead tip. When the MP35N conductor is silver-cored, it also offers enhanced conductivity.

Designs

Conductor coils are commonly of a multifilament or cable structure instead of unifilar to make them more flexible and resistant to fracture. Unifilar conductor is a single wire wound spirally around a central axis (Fig. 1.12), whereas a multifilar cable consists of two or more wires wound together in parallel spirally around a central axis (Fig. 1.13) [1]. In a multifilar coil, each conductor strand is individually coated with a thin layer of insulator, and the entire helical coil is then insulated again with a thicker conventional insulator (Fig. 1.13) [1].

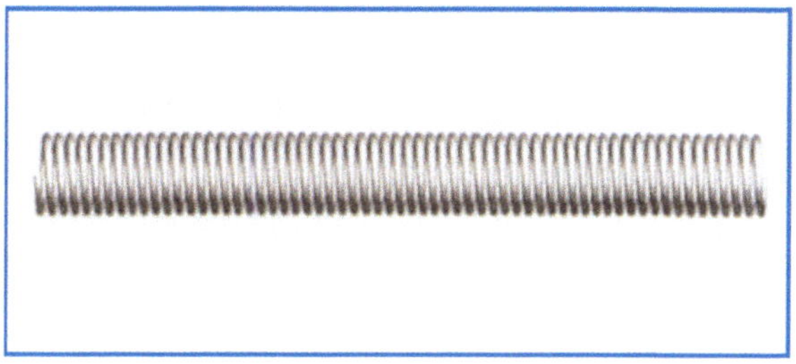

Fig. 1.12 Unifilar conductor: a single wire coil is wound around a central axis in a spiral (from [1], Chap. 9, p. 37) (courtesy of Medtronic)

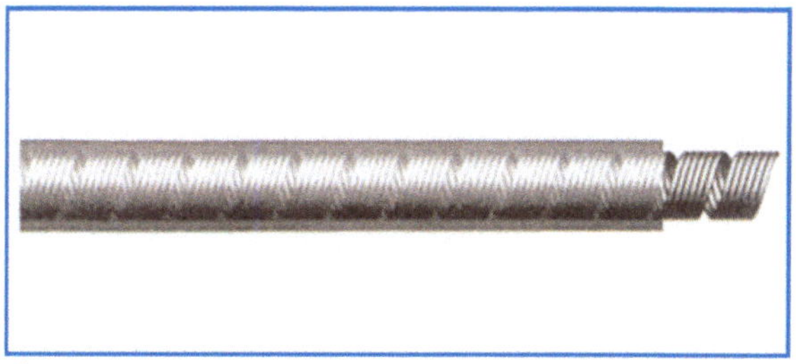

Fig. 1.13 Multifilar conductor: each conductor strand is individually coated with a thin layer of insulator, and the entire helical coil is insulated again with a thicker conventional insulator (from [1], Chap. 9, p. 79) (courtesy of Medtronic)

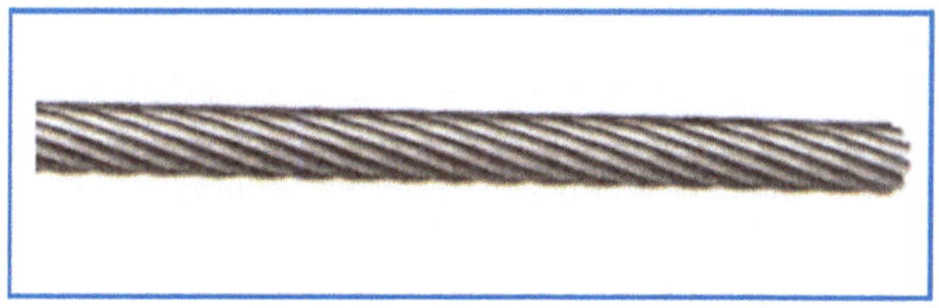

Fig. 1.14 Cable conductor: two or more wires twisted together as a strand and then bundled with other strands around each other like a rope (from [1], Chap. 9, p. 78) (courtesy of Medtronic)

This design reduces pacing impedance and the redundancy prevents pacing failure if a filar breaks. A third design is the cable. A cable conductor is obtained by two or more wires twisted together as a strand and then bundled with other strands around each other as a rope. Cable-leads have lower electrical resistance but are less prone to crush failure and smaller than coils (Fig. 1.14) [1].

Unipolar leads obviously have only one conductor coil, whereas bipolar leads require two – one for the proximal and the other for the tip electrode. Bipolar leads may have a coaxial, a co-radial or parallel wound, and a parallel or multiluminal design. Coaxial bipolar leads, standard in treating

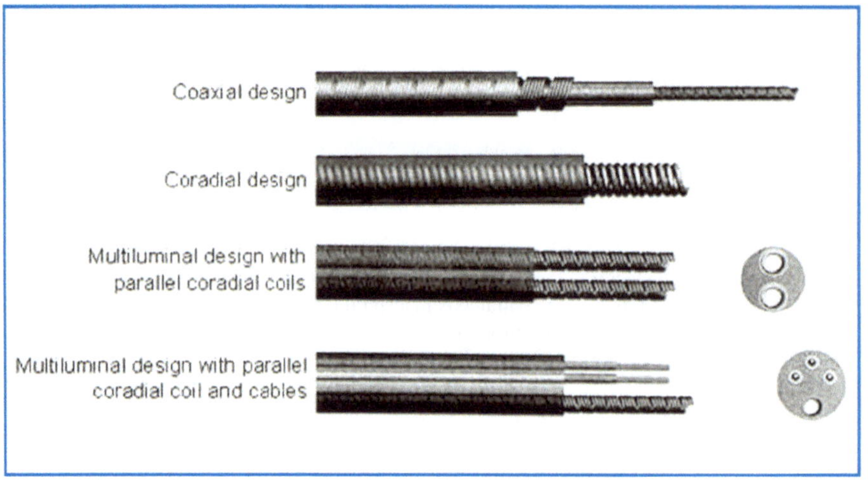

Fig. 1.15 Many kinds of conductor designs (from [1], Chap. 9, pp. 79, 80) (courtesy of Medtronic)

bradyarrhythmias, have an inner coil extending to the cathode and an outer coil terminating at the proximal electrode (anode). The inner coil is insulated from the outer coil by his own insulator. Coradial bipolar leads have two or more individually insulated coils wound next to each other in a single coil and a common outer insulation. With this configuration, the outside diameter of the polar lead is as small as that of a unipolar lead. Multiluminal leads, the standard for treating tachyarrhythmias, have conductor coils and cables parallel to each other, and are again separated by insulating materials. Coaxial, co-radial, and multiluminal designs are shown in Fig. 1.15 [1].

1.1.1.5 Lead Insulation

Insulation is a nonconducting material that prevents electrical current from leaving the lead and entering the surrounding tissue. Usually, lead insulation extends from the lead connector to the cathode tip and, in bipolar leads, is interrupted by the anode ring. Insulation also prevents tissue stimulation, except at the electrode–myocardial interface, and protects the conductor from corrosion due to body fluids and exposure to tissue.

Insulation Materials

The story of insulation materials started in 1958 with polyethylene and silicone rubber, going through many changes – from polyurethane 80A to 55D – and is still in evolution, with emerging biomaterials such as fluoropolymer and copolymer. The most commonly used insulation materials in pacing leads are silicone and polyurethane, the advantages and disadvantages of which are shown in Table 1.1 and Fig. 1.16.

Silicone rubber that was introduced as insulating material for pacing leads in 1958, is flexible, soft and continues to be used today. It is a reliable substance but has some disadvantages: it is relatively fragile and susceptible to abrasion and has low tear strength. To avoid this problem, it must be thick. This is acceptable in a unipolar lead in which there is only a conductor coil to insulate, but in bipolar leads, thickness increases the external diameter. For this reason, it has been recently upgraded to platinum-cured silicone rubber that, even though thinner, allows better mechanical performance. Silicone rubber also has a high coefficient of friction in blood, especially when two leads are implanted in the same vein. One method recently developed to avoid this problem is to use an insulating system with lubricious coatings.

Polyurethane is a stiffer and firmer material than silicone introduced in 1977 for its better tear strength and low coefficient of friction. Due to documented cases of stress cracking discovered a few years after implantation, some processing changes were made, increasing performance satisfaction. Compared with silicone, it allows for a thinner lead body and when moist is slippery. This represents an advantage in cases in which two

Table 1.1 Lead insulation: comparison of silicone rubber and polyurethane

Silicone rubber (first use in 1958)	Polyurethane (first use in 1977 as 80A and 1978 as 55D)
Advantages	
Excellent biostability (structure and material remain relatively unchanged in vivo)	Biocompatible (with no injurious or toxic effects, and inherently less thrombogenic and fibrotic because the slippery surface reduces platelet adhesion)
Inert (structural composition chemically inactive)	Low friction coefficient in blood (get very slippery in blood by adsorbing proteins out of the blood)
Flexibility	High tear strength (more resistant to damage by abrasion, high cuts, and surface nicks)
Biocompatible (no toxic or injurious effects) Performance record > 30 years	Superior compressive properties Allows for thinner lead-body diameter
Disadvantages	
High friction coefficient in blood (silicone is not inherently slippery and can make venous insertion difficult)	More susceptible to cautery heat damage
More thrombogenic	Relatively stiff (55D)
Abrades, tears, and cuts easily; attention to handling is imperative	Potential for environmental stress cracking (Fig. 1.16b), which is an oxidative condition that takes place on the surface of polyurethane leads (true for P80A)
Subject to cold flow failure	Potential for metal ion oxidation (Fig. 1.16a), an oxidative degradation of polyurethane insulation, true for both kinds (80A and 55D)
Because silicone has less tear strength, some types of leads with this insulation tend to be larger in diameter than polyurethane leads	

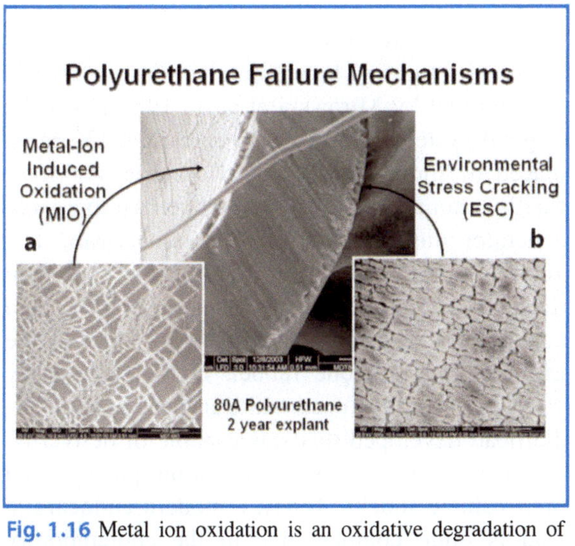

Fig. 1.16 Metal ion oxidation is an oxidative degradation of polyurethane insulation, true for both kinds of polyurethane (80A and 55D) (**a**). Environmental stress cracking is an oxidative condition that takes place on the surface of polyurethane leads (true for 80A) (**b**)

leads are implanted in the same vein. Polyurethane is available in a softer and more flexible version, known as Pellethane (P) 80A, and a stiffer version, known as P55D. Most polyurethane leads now used in clinical practice have the P55D polymer insulation, which is far less prone to degradation than the P80A version.

Some currently used bipolar coaxial leads use both silicone (inner insulation) and polyurethane (outer insulation) coating, incorporating the durability of silicone with the ease of handling of polyurethane while maintaining a thinner external lead diameter.

Fluoropolymers are polytetrafluoroethylene (PTFE) and ethylene tetrafluoroethylene (ETFE). They can assist as redundant insulation and are primarily used as a coating to defend conductor wires from corrosion. The advantages of those materials are their inert and biocompatible behavior and high tensile strength. Otherwise, their stiffness, creep, and trend to metal ion oxidation during manufacturing represent important disadvantages.

Finally, new insulators for cardiac leads have recently been developed that are silicone rubber–polyurethane copolymer to combine the advantages of both materials [12]. The possibility of matching the biocompatibility and biostability of silicone with the processability and resistance of polyurethane is an appealing step toward a nearly ideal biomaterial. The first copolymer used on cardiac leads was the Optim™, which was actually used only on St. Jude Medical, Inc. pacing leads. As indicated by St. Jude Medical, Optim should have the following characteristics: improved flexibility and lubricity, increased abrasion resistance, and excellent biostability. Obviously insulator characteristics and integrity not only influence the reliability/failure of pacing leads (sometimes the indication for lead extraction) but deeply influence the transvenous lead extraction procedure. A low resistance to tear or traction may predispose to insulator fracture during attempts at lead removal, with potentially dangerous direct exposure of the bare metal coil to the venous system.

1.1.1.6 Connectors

The connector electrically binds the lead to the PM. Many types of connectors have been developed in the past, and this created considerable confusion among physicians and, in some cases, a potential hazard to the patient. Historically, unipolar leads were 5 or 6 mm in diameter, and bipolar leads required a bifurcated design with similar 5- or 6-mm sizes. Only after some years a bipolar, in-line design with a 3.2-mm diameter was developed.

In 1986, a voluntary standard for lead connectors and pulse-generator-connector cavities was established. This voluntary standard, known as VS-1, incorporates sealing rings on 3.2-mm unipolar and bipolar in-line lead connectors [13]. Unfortunately, intercompany rivalry resulted in three variations of VS-1 lead connector and connector cavity standard: the VS-1, VS-1A, and VS-1B, which were not completely interchangeable. Subsequently, a manufacturer agreement was reached on an international standard configuration known as International Standard 1, or IS-1 UNI/BI, in which lead connectors are 3.2-mm in diameter, have sealing rings, and have a short (0.508-cm) connector pin. To prevent damage to a unipolar IS-1 lead from the anode set-screw of a bipolar PM connector, IS-1 unipolar leads have an electrically inactive ring electrode.

Coronary venous lead connectors were initially developed to accommodate patients with heart failure who were previously implanted for other reasons and were considered eligible for an upgrade to biventricular pacing. For these patients, the ventricular output of the PM generator was divided via a Y connector from one bipolar output to two separate outputs – one for the previously implanted RV lead and the other for the new left ventricular (LV) lead.

Currently, LV leads are connected to the PM independently. Also, coronary venous leads have an IS-1 standard; only Guidant, now Boston Scientific, continued to maintain, until few time ago, a different connector for its leads – the LV-1.

Very recently a tetrapolar LV lead has been developed: the St. Jude Medical Quartet 1458Q lead with a four electrode configurating that allows ten different pacing vectors.

1.1.2 Implantable Cardioverter–Defibrillator Leads

Implantable cardioverter–defibrillator (ICD) leads began with the first human implant of a defibrillator, reported by Mirowski et al. in 1980 [14]. The original system comprised an epicardial LV patch placed by thoracotomy and an intravascular free-floating, nonpacing shock coil tunnelized to a large generator implanted in the abdominal wall. The 100-cm, 12-F, 6.55-cm^2 coil anode was placed in the right atrium or superior vena cava (SVC), the conductor was a silver-cored tinsel wire and the insulator was silicone rubber. Only in the early 1990s was a fully functional transvenous endocardial lead developed that was capable of delivering antitachycardia pacing, bradycardia pacing, and high-voltage shocks. Today, a modern endocardial lead is quite complex due to the contemporary necessity of working as a standard pacing lead as well as delivering short-cycle-length sequences for antitachycardia pacing and high-voltage discharges from the ICD to the heart. As with pacing leads, ICD leads have multiple components: pacing and sensing electrodes, a lead fixation system, exposed high-voltage coils in contact with the endocardium, conductors, insulators, and a connector linking the lead to the high-voltage generator.

1.1.2.1 ICD Lead Electrodes and Fixation Mechanisms

Before describing ICD lead electrodes, it must be underscored that for ICD lead sensing function, two kind of bipolar configurations have been developed. The first is the integrated bipolar configuration in which sensing is done between the tip electrode and the RV distal shock coil placed about 1–1.5 cm from the tip. The second is the dedicated or true bipolar configuration in which a conventional ring electrode (anode) is placed again 1–1.5 cm proximal to the tip. In case of a true bipolar configuration, an extra conductor is obviously necessary for the anodal ring (Fig. 1.17). However, true bipolar configuration probably reduces the risk of oversensing of far-field signals, which could happen with integrated bipolar configuration, especially if a portion of the distal coil extends back across the tricuspid valve into the right atrium. Integrated bipolar configuration could guarantee, in principle, superior defibrillation performance because of the shorter distance between the RV shock coil and the RV apex (pullback distance).

As with pacing leads, the ICD lead cathode is a platinum, iridium, and titanium combination; the electrode structure depends on whether fixation mechanism is passive with tines or active with a screw. In an active-fixation lead, the platinum–iridium screw is usually electrically active, but there are also models with both electrically active collar and helix or others with electrically silent helix and active carbon cathode collar. A platinum–iridium anode lies immediately behind the cathode in a true bipolar system. All models now elute steroids to reduce chronic threshold and prevent pacing threshold rise or exit block.

1.1.2.2 ICD Lead Defibrillation Coils

A high-voltage shock coil is the unique feature that distinguished ICD leads from pacing leads. At least one distal RV coil, about 5- to 6-cm long, is always present in ICD leads immediately behind the pacing/sensing electrode(s). In double-coiled leads, a proximal defibrillation coil of 7–8 cm is located over the lead at the level of the SVC or high right atrium. Defibrillation coil material is platinum–iridium or platinum alloy-clad tantalum, occasionally with an iridium oxide (IROX) coating that reduces shock-induced polarization.

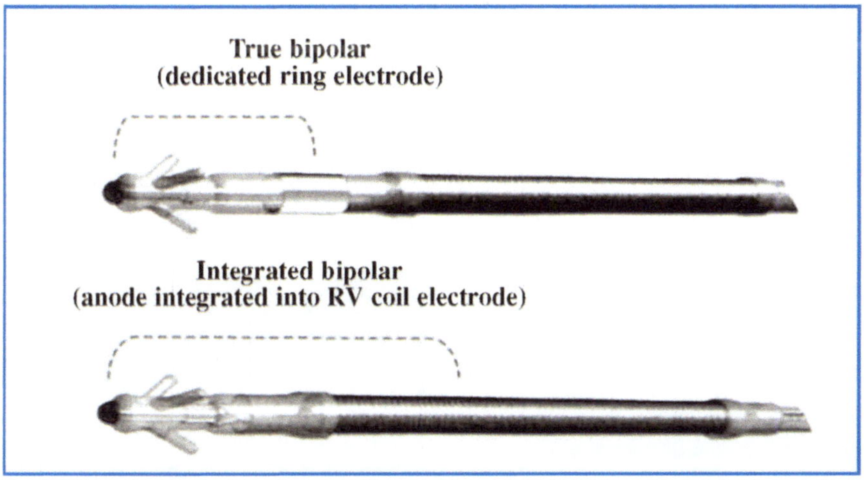

Fig. 1.17 True bipolar (*top*) and integrated bipolar (*bottom*) leads. The true bipolar lead senses between the distal tip and the proximal ring, which are dedicated for pacing and sensing. In contrast, integrated bipolar leads pace and sense between the tip and the distal coil. The distal coil is used for sensing, pacing, and defibrillation. Integrated bipolar leads also contain a second, proximal coil, increasing the lead surface area for defibrillation (from [1], Chap. 4, p. 42) (courtesy of Medtronic)

To increase electrical efficiency of coils, many kinds of connection have been proposed, and recently low-resistance core materials within the wire have been developed (Fig. 1.18).

Shock coils have a large surface structure that is directly in contact with blood, vascular tissue, and endocardium, and their presence in the venous system elicits a vigorous fibrotic reaction that tightly encapsulates the lead body after implantation (Fig. 1.19a,b) [15]. At the level where the coil wires are in contact with the endocardium or the endothelial tissue, fibrous tissue proliferation develops in the interstices between helical turns of the coiled wire anchoring the lead to the venous system, the endocardial wall, or the tricuspid valve. This fibrous reaction could make any attempt at lead extraction quite difficult and potentially dangerous. For this reason, ICD manufacturers have developed many solutions. In some leads, the spaces between helical turns of the coiled wire are backfilled with silicone rubber (Fig. 1.20). This backfilling is necessarily incomplete because of the necessity to leave a bare high surface area (for voltage interface) with the tissues to enable high current delivery. Otherwise, wires can still be subjected to fibrous ingrowths. Flat-wire technology is a potential solution to this problem (Fig. 1.21). A third solution is the deployment of a thin, porous, electrically conductive fluoropolymer jacket over the coils to prevent tissue ingrowths. The material developed for this purpose is expanded PTFE (ePTFE), or Gore-Tex. The ultra structure of this material does not allow cellular migration and therefore tissue proliferation between helical turns of the coils (Fig. 1.22). Extraction of this kind of lead seems easier compared with bare-metal coils [16–18].

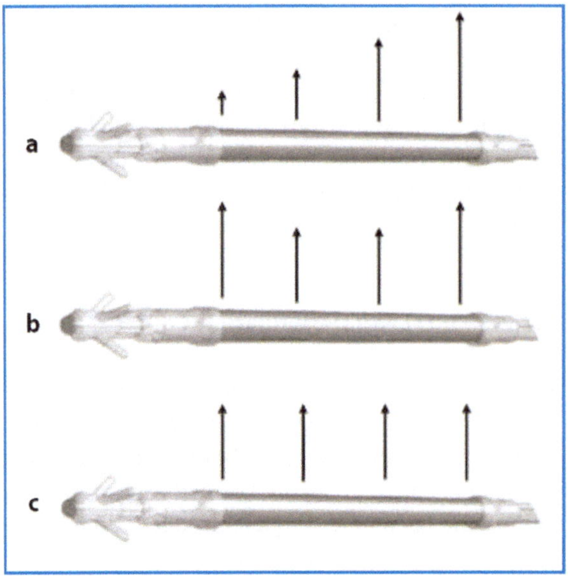

Fig. 1.18a-c Proximal connection of coil electrode (**a**): in this case, the spread of energy decreases from the proximal connection to the distal end of the coil; dual connection (proximal and distal) of the coil electrode (**b**): this design allows better current distribution during the shock; dual connection of the coil electrode designed with low-resistance core material (**c**): in this case, current distribution is more uniform

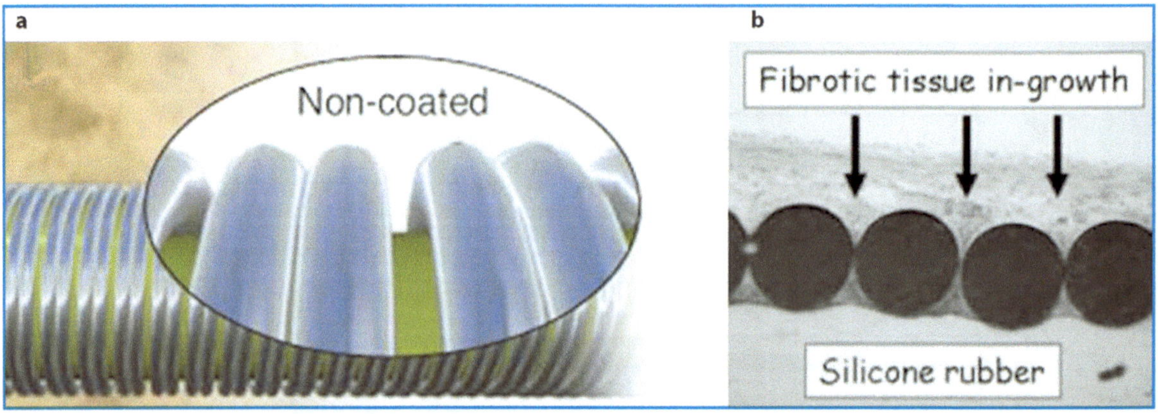

Fig. 1.19 Noncoated defibrillation electrodes (**a**): in this type of lead, coils are loose, and the extraction procedure can be more difficult. Histological cross-section of an implanted cardioverter–defibrillator (ICD) lead at the level of the bare shock coils in the heart (**b**). Fibrous tissue ingrowth in interstices between coils (*arrows*), which fixes the ICD lead to the heart wall (from [13], and courtesy of St. Jude Medical)

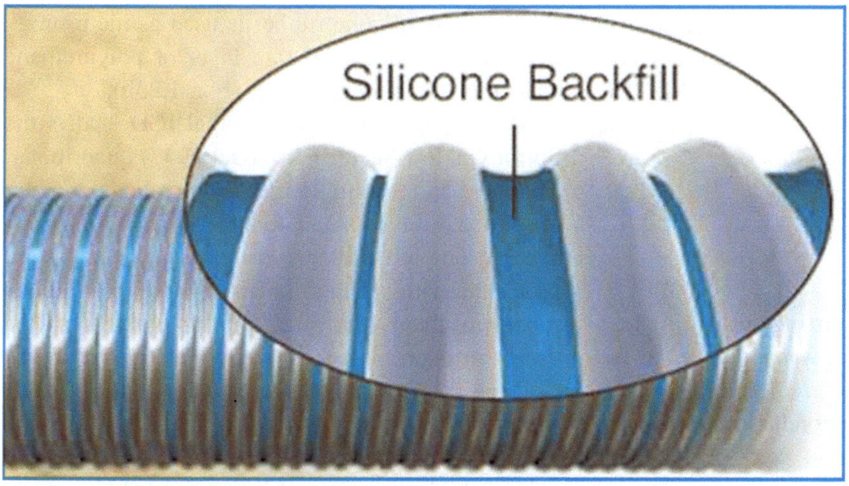

Fig. 1.20 Example of leads in which the coiled wires are back-filled with silicone rubber

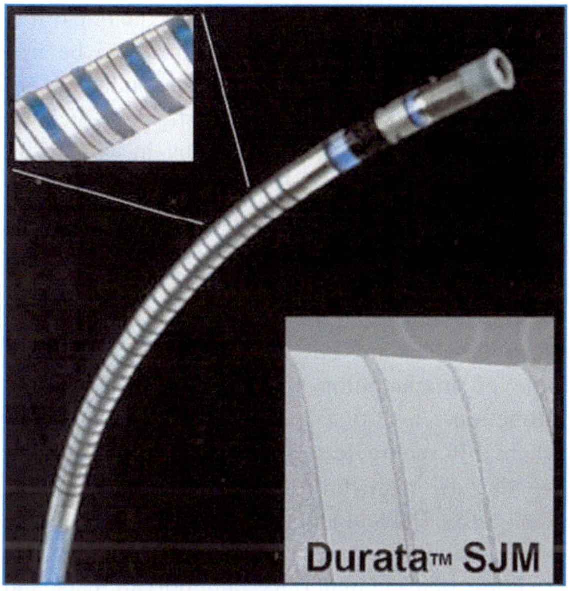

Fig. 1.21 Durata™, St. Jude Medical. This tachy lead has a flat-wire technology for defibrillating coils. Note the wire on electron microscope (courtesy of St. Jude Medical)

1.1.2.3 ICD Lead Conductors and Insulation Materials

Materials

ICD lead conductors must be constructed with low-resistance materials to minimize voltage drops and heat losses during high-voltage shocks. The MP35N alloy, developed for pacing lead conductors, shows low susceptibility to corrosion and stress damage; however, because of its relatively high resistance, it requires special modifications to maintain high-voltage defibrillation capacity. This may be accomplished creating a mesh with low-resistance metals such as silver, which can be incorporated with MP35N in a composite wire conductor. Despite its high resistance to fracture, conductor damage may occur as a consequence of fatigue or subclavian crush. It has been recently discovered that inclusions of titanium contaminant in MP35N conduc-

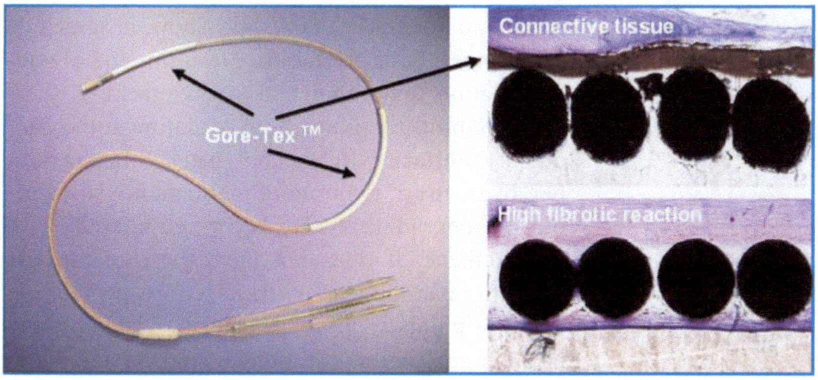

Fig. 1.22 Boston Scientific Endotak quadripolar Reliance G implantable cardioverter–defibrillator lead. Two expanded polytetrafluoroethylene (ePTFE; or Gore-Tex) jackets (*black arrows*) cover the shock coils to prevent tissue ingrowth (courtesy of Boston Scientific)

tors may predispose them to fracture at vulnerable positions. For this reason, some manufacturers have developed low-titanium MP35N alloy [19]. ICD conductors may be designed as coils or as a cable according to their specific role.

Design

The first conductor design, starting with a PM-lead platform and now abandoned, was a coaxial or triaxial structure in which a layered arrangement of tip, anode, and high-voltage conductors, individually separated by an insulator, were coiled over each other and coated with a common external insulation. As for pacing leads, the innermost conductor for the tip electrode contained a lumen that allowed passage of a stylet to facilitate lead positioning into the RV (Fig. 1.23a). This design was replaced in the late 1990s due to excessive stiffness, too large a diameter, and high failure rate.

Modern ICD lead body design is multiluminal: separated lumens contain, in parallel, single cable or coil conductors according to their role. The tip (cathode) electrode conductor is coiled to allow insertion of a stylet and attachment of a screw fixation mechanism, whereas anode-electrode and defibrillation coil conductors are cabled. All conductors are coated with a Teflon-like fluoropolymer

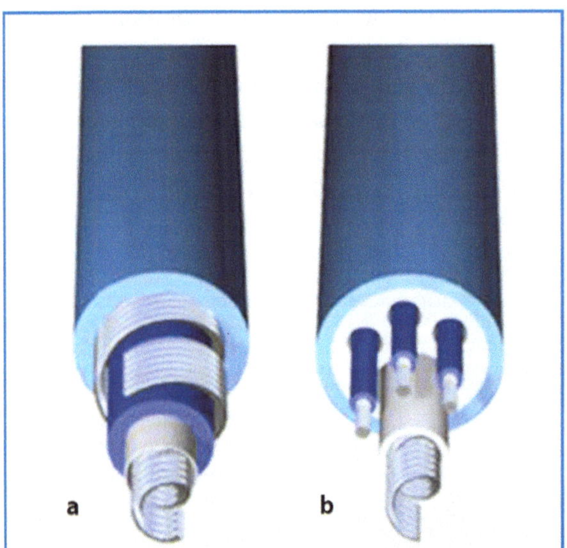

Fig. 1.23 Two implantable cardioverter–defibrillator lead-body designs. Coaxial (a); multiluminal (b)

(ETFE), and silicone rubber is used as the primary insulator; an additional thin layer of polyurethane coats the soft silicone rubber (Fig. 1.23b).

An example of a multiluminal ICD lead is the Sprint Quattro Secure^{TM} (model 6947) quadripolar. This lead has the single multifilar cathode conductor coil and three cabled conductors: two high-voltage and one low-voltage anode. All conductors are protected with a fluoropolymer, and the silicone rubber insulator is covered with polyurethane. Two decompression passages are present (Fig. 1.24). Coil position with respect to the cables varies according to the manufacturer: some leads have a concentric design in which the coil is in the central axis of the lead body and is surrounded by cables; others have an asymmetrical lead body, with the coil located on one side and the cables on the other. It is not completely clear which design could be less prone to damage (Fig. 1.24). Cabled conductors are far more resistant to mechanical stress than coiled conductors. This is the reason why in case of an ICD lead failure caused by disruption of the pace-sense coil conductor, the cabled high-voltage conductors may still remain intact.

Multiluminal design has allowed ICD leads to be more resistant, reliable, and thinner, and these characteristics are obviously very useful at the time of implantation but also in case of lead extraction. A critical point in lead structure is where different materials are crimped or connected together as conductors to electrodes or defibrillation coils. Detachment at this level is possible while attempting lead extraction.

For insulation materials, both polyurethane and silicone have been used. Polyurethane has an excellent tensile strength and abrasion resistance, allowing creation of smaller-diameter leads with good handling capability; unfortunately polyurethane, particularly P80A, may show, in some circumstances, poor biostability, resulting in polymer degradation (environmental stress cracking, thermal instability, and metal ion oxidation at the conductor interface with the polymer). Silicone rubber, by contrast, is far more inert and not susceptible to degradation. However, compared with polyurethane, it does not have the same tensile strength, can be easily damaged (especially at pressure points such as beneath the clavicle), and has a high friction coefficient, making implanta-

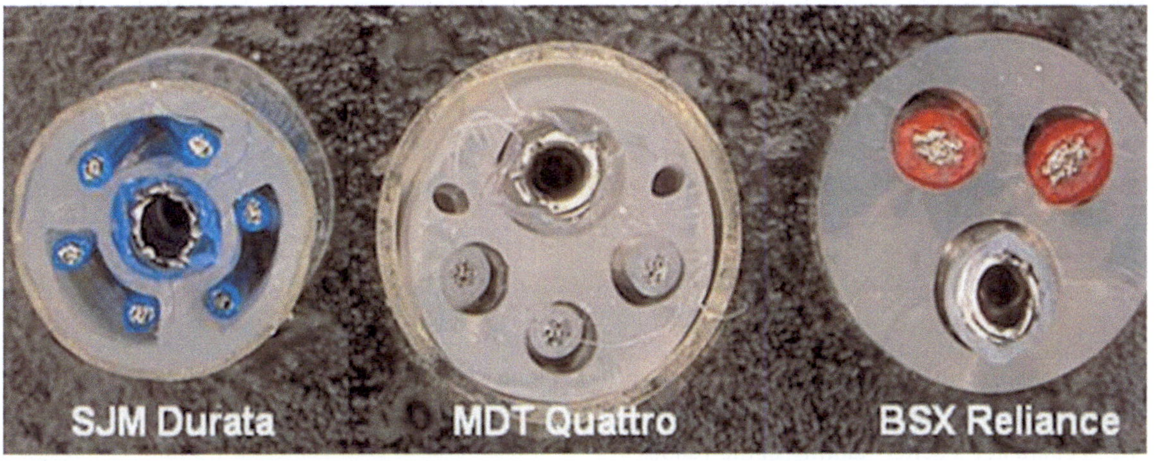

Fig. 1.24 Guidant Reliance and Medtronic Quattro™ implantable cardioverter–defibrillator (ICD) leads have asymmetrical body designs, with the cables located on one side and the coiled conductor on the other. New models of St. Jude ICD leads have a concentric design (SJM Durata). In this case, the coil is in the body's central axis, equally surrounded by six protective cables (courtesy of St. Jude Medical, Boston Scientific, and Medtronic)

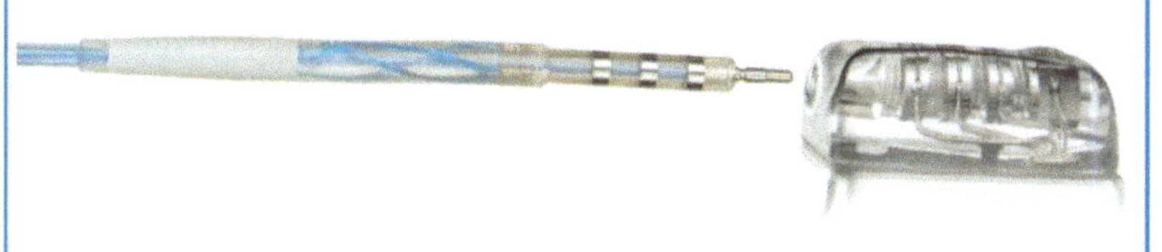

Fig. 1.25 New standard DF-4 implantable cardioverter–defibrillator connector with a single, four-pole lead connector (courtesy of St. Jude Medical)

tion of two leads through the same vein entry quite difficult.

In practice, manufacturers have tried to combine the best characteristics of all insulating materials by using silicone for the lead body, with each cable and coil conductor coated with a fluoropolymer and a thin polyurethane layer to cover the entire lead. In this way, is possible to improve abrasion resistance and handling performance. Recently developed copolymer obtained by mixing silicone rubber and polyurethane can also be used for the outer layer.

1.1.2.4 ICD Lead Connectors

After an initial period characterized by nonstandard lead connectors, the modern ICD system was standardized, with the pacing/sensing portion of the lead using a bipolar IS-1 connector. Every shock coil also has a standard lead connector, called DF-1. These lead connectors emerge as tails from a trifurcated yoke (in case of double-coiled ICD leads). This kind of lead connector system is cumbersome, difficult to adapt to the subcutaneous or subpectoral pocket and exposed to insulation or conductor fractures. Moreover, during lead extraction, débridement of all tails up to the yoke may be time consuming. For those reasons, a newer standard has been developed known as the DF-4 quadripolar lead connector. This design allows two high-voltage conductors to be incorporated into the one-connector pin together with the bipolar IS-1 pace-sense component (Fig. 1.25). Despite obvious advantages of this system, clinical studies are necessary to confirm the reliability of this new connector.

1.1.3 Lead Shapes

Increasing knowledge about cardiac pacing has led over the years to the development of morphologically specific construction leads for specific use in the different cardiac chambers. For example atrial pacing leads with a broad terminal hook (J form) were developed (Fig. 1.26) that are ideal for implantation and stabilization inside the right atrial appendage. Moreover, whereas RV pacing leads retain their conventional linear form, LV epicardial leads in which the distal end is characterized by different shapes (corner, S, corkscrew, etc) (Fig. 1.27) guarantee a better stability in the venous system. The development of different shapes at the distal end of linear leads due to the specific needs to change stimulation characteristics, creates an additional obstacle in the extraction procedure, such as, for example, advancement of a mechanical sheath over the body of an atrial bipolar J lead, which can be difficult in the region of the proximal electrode, thus carrying the risk of wire rupture and the consequent complication of the extraction procedure.

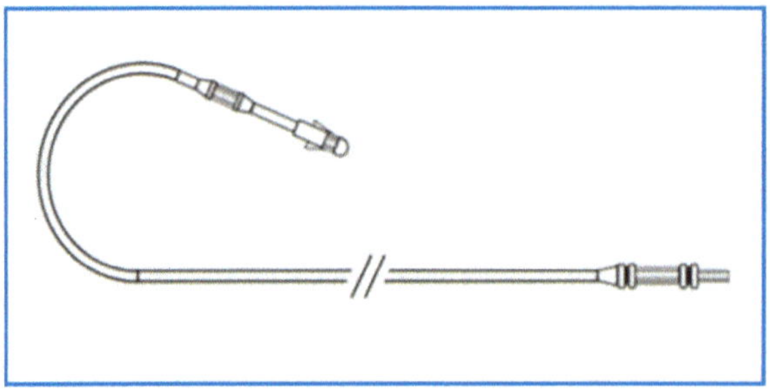

Fig. 1.26 Bipolar J-shape passive fixation lead

1.1.4 Special Leads

This definition includes leads in which structural characteristics have seen a significant innovation in the context of cardiac stimulation. For example, leads covered with polyurethane-based material instead of silicon; leads with pre-formed ends for better stability in the different cardiac chambers (for example, the J lead for atrial pacing); the most recent leads with the system of "fixing" through tines opening from the outside through a sheath that slides over the lead body (Medtronic Starfix for coronary sinus pacing, Fig. 1.28); fixing systems with similar mechanism to a stent; or defibrillation leads with linear pins (Fig. 1.25). It should also be remembered that these technological advances often represent, along with the undeniable progress, a source of new issues to be overcome.

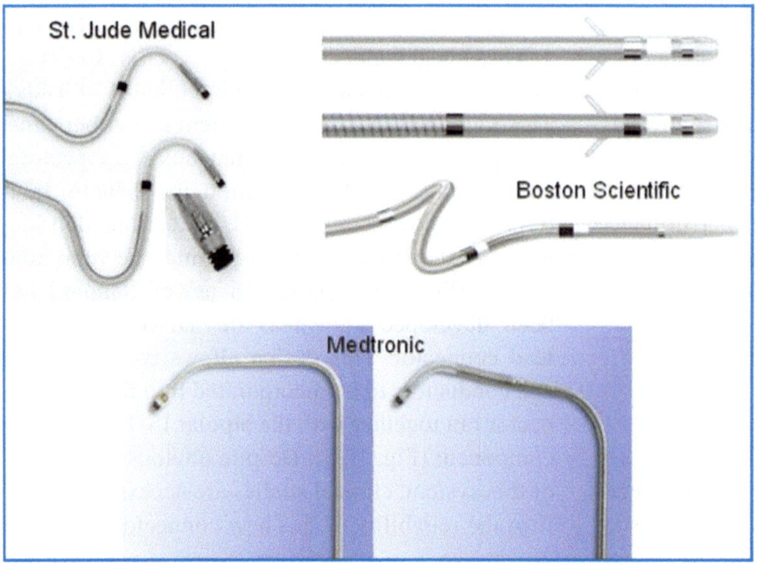

Fig. 1.27 Several types of left ventricular leads with different shapes (courtesy of St. Jude Medical, Boston Scientific, and Medtronic)

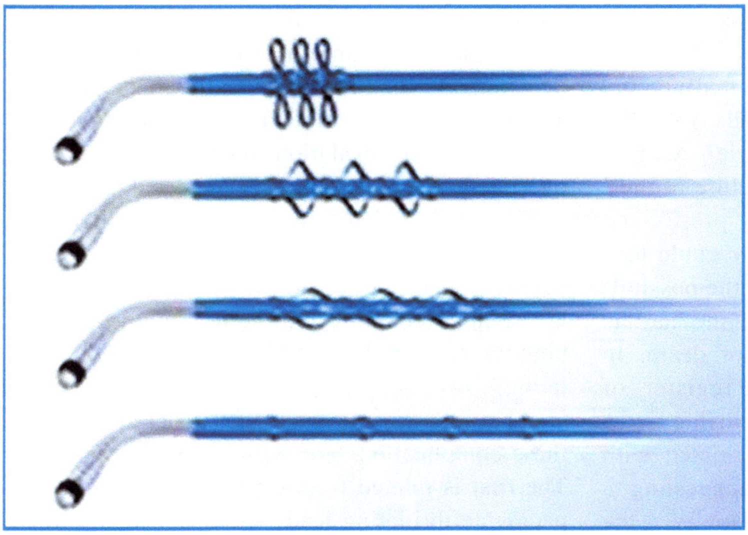

Fig. 1.28 Medtronic Attain StarFix® left ventricular lead. This lead is really nonisodiametric, offers great stability, but with the great cost of tissue ingrowth (courtesy of Medtronic)

1.1.5 Lead-related Problems and Extraction

We emphasize that cardiac stimulation system malfunction is often related to lead malfunction, the weakest part of the system. In this context, leads with a more complex design, such as defibrillation leads, have been subjected to recall by the manufacturers for an increased incidence of failure, with clinical manifestations characterized by impaired pacing and sensing function, as well as delivery of inappropriate shocks and, in rare cases, loss of therapy. Medtronic's Transvene coaxial defibrillation leads have a high incidence of malfunction caused by fracture of the high-voltage conductor or by insulation defect in general of the P80A middle layer (rarely the outer layer) [20]. Although the incidence of malfunction reported by the manufacturer is particularly high (average possibility 40% after 8 years from implant), the number of leads implanted is not so high, and number of those still in use is very low, making it an irrelevant clinical problem. On the contrary, the Medtronic's Sprint Fidelis, a small defibrillation lead implanted in large numbers represents a significant clinical problem. In 2008, a published review of 6,181 leads implanted in Canada revealed a significant incidence of failure of 1.29% after 21 months of implantation [21]. The clinical manifestation of the failure was mainly related to the delivery of inappropriate shocks for ventricular oversensing caused, in most cases, by a fracture of the conductor. The two critical areas involved in the fracture were predominantly the distal region near the anode and the proximal region at the anchoring sleeve. The presence of alternating sections of high rigidity and reduced stiffness to reduce the possibility of perforation of the RV is likely to be the pathophysiological mechanism of fracture of the conductor. The construction features of the Sprint Fidelis, and particularly the reduction in the size of the lead body obtained by eliminating the compression lumens, has been identified as a possible mechanism to explain the high number of malfunctions, estimated in a percentage of 6.3% after 42 months of implantation, probably increasing with time. Many patients with this kind of lead were referred during 2009 to electrophysiological centers for an extraction procedure.

In 2007, an alert was published about an increased incidence of perforation at the apex of the RV in patients with St. Jude Riata defibrillation lead. The complication was probably linked to increased rigidity of the catheter, caused by the reduced body size. A further large independent review in 4,273 Riata implants showed an incidence of perforation of 0.33% [22]. This was interpreted as not being associated with the lead Riata itself but to the use of a very small defibrillation catheter (7-F) in a high-risk perforation area such as that of the apex of the RV.

Complications related to electrode malfunction are not exclusive to defibrillation leads. In 1994, Telectronics issued a recall on atrial Accufix leads, reporting the possibility of fracture of the J retention wire in the body of this pre-formed active fixation atrial lead. The fracture could lead to protrusion of the same J wire, with the possibility of embolization or perforation of the cardiac chambers, indicating potential risk of death. In 1999, results of an international register of Accufix implants were published, reporting a low risk of morbidity and mortality associated with wire fracture (0.0048%/year) and suggesting a conservative management approach. However, the high number of leads implanted associated with the presence of the same identified characteristics (J wire material, electrode position on cine fluoroscopic X-ray, magnitude of movement of the lead in the heart chambers) identified a significant group of patients with increased risk of morbidity and in whom the indication for extraction procedure was reasonable [23].

1.1.6 What Do Lead Extractors Want to See Improved in Future Cardiac Lead Design and Materials?

Due to evolving indications, the number of ICD implanted has consistently increased in recent years and is expected to increase further. Implantation in younger patients and prolonged life expectancy will require multiple interventions during the follow-up periods and, as a consequence, we expect an increased and widespread use of lead extraction procedures. The purely practical reasons for this are linked to both infective and noninfective complications. The latter are conductors and/or insulation fractures, macro- and microdislodgments, and sensing and/or pacing and/or defibrillating failures. These conditions can be lead-related, patient-related, or implant-related, but many studies have shown that lead malfunction is the most common long-term complication for both pacing (atrial, RV and LV leads) and defibrillating leads [24–26].

The instruments necessary for overcoming these complications are prevention and treatment. The first is related to durability and reliability of pacing/defibrillating leads and the second to their extractability profile. Both issues apply to each component of a pacing/defibrillating lead.

1.1.6.1 Connectors

The connector's tail could be a fragile region in ICD leads. Sometime during the housing manoeuvre of the device, the tail is submitted to torsion and stretching forces, and in case of chronic stress, conductor or insulation could fracture, as shown respectively in Figures 1.29 and 1.30. Moreover, the more material present inside a PM/ICD pocket, the greater the risk of an important fibrous reaction, as well as related infection in case of a lengthy implant procedure or device replacement. In this situation, tail debridement could be challenging during lead extraction. To solve this problem, some companies have designed defibrillation leads with linear pins (Fig. 1.31).

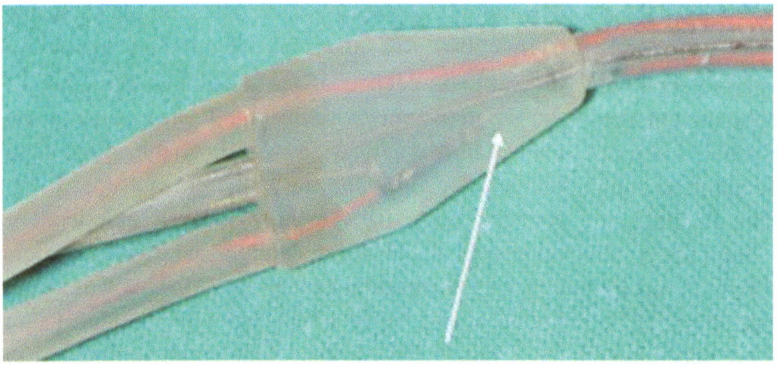

Fig. 1.29 Coil fracture in the Y region of an implantable cardioverter–defibrillator lead

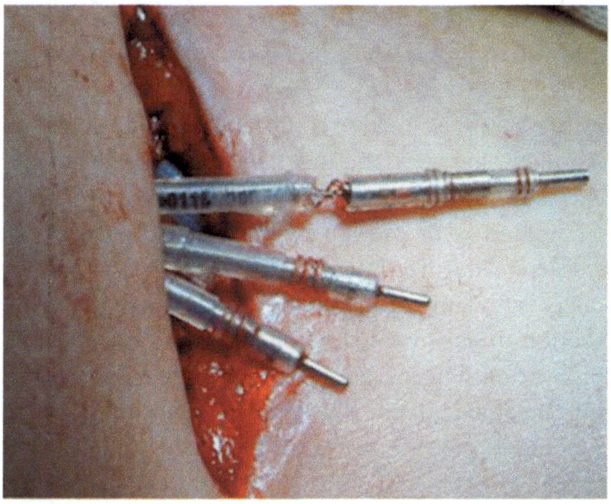

Fig 1.30 Insulation fracture of the pacing and sensing connector of an implantable cardioverter–defibrillator lead

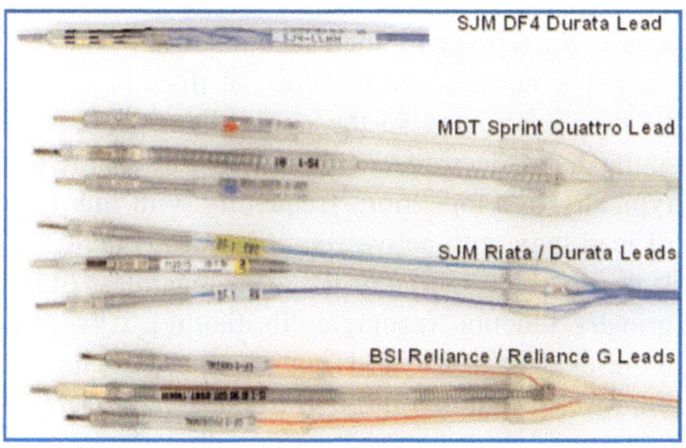

Fig. 1.31 Comparison of a new implantable cardioverter–defibrillator (ICD) lead (*top*) with linear pins to previous ICD leads from the same and other companies (courtesy of St. Jude Medical, Boston Scientific and Medtronic)

1.1.6.2 Conductors

As previously described, there are different designs for the conductor component of pacing and defibrillating leads. Each design has advantages and disadvantages, both for lead durability and reliability and in the lead extraction procedure. For the latter, the primary focus of this chapter, we emphasize the following aspects. Cables have been designed to create a stiffer lead with a high tensile strength and that does not need locking stylet insertion during a lead extraction procedure. However, when using mechanical dilation, this design is not optimum because of the impossibility to stretch the lead in order to reduce its cross-section dimensions, thus facilitating advancement of the mechanical sheath dilator. This is possible, however, with leads with a coaxial or co-radial design on condition that the locking stylet not be used. Use of this kind of stylet would cause enlargement of the cross-section lead dimensions, thus obstructing advancement of the mechanical sheath.

1.1.6.3 Insulating Materials

As described previously, many attempts have been made over the years to improve the durability and reliability of insulating materials (Fig. 1.32). Recently, good results have been achieved with the copolymer. This is a silicone rubber-polyurethane chemical mesh specifically created for cardiac

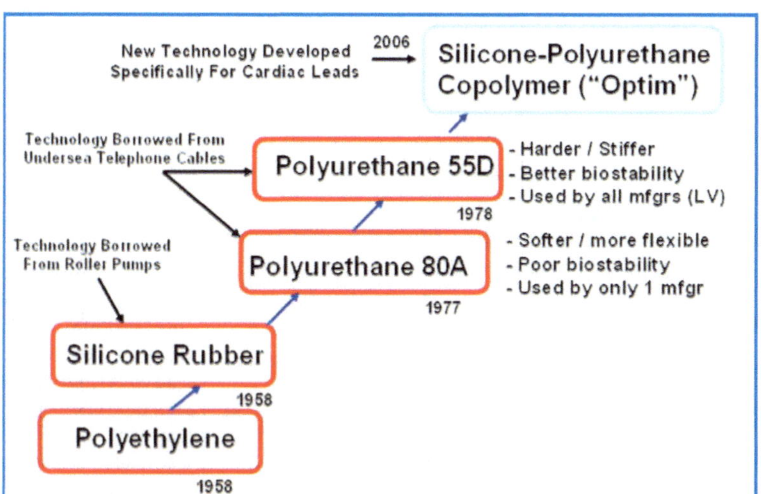

Fig. 1.32 Insulating material evolution – from silicone rubber developed in 1958 to the latest copolymer used for the first time in 2006

leads, after five decades of borrowed insulation technology, in order to combine the flexibility and biostability of silicone rubbers with the strength/tear resistance, abrasion resistance, and lubricity of P55D. What we expect from this innovation is a decreasing of the number of revisions and lead extraction procedures performed due to loss of insulation along the pacing/defibrillating lead.

1.1.6.4 Coils

At the level where the coil wires are in contact with the endocardium or the endothelial tissue, fibrous tissue proliferation occurs in the interstices between helical turns of the coiled wire anchoring the lead to the venous system, the endocardial wall, or the tricuspid valve. This fibrous reaction could make any attempt at lead extraction quite difficult and potentially dangerous (Fig. 1.33). Some studies indeed have shown that extraction could be easier and safer if fibrotic tissue is not allowed to grow between and underneath the shock coils [16–18]. As described earlier, a great deal of effort has been made to this purpose (Fig. 1.34). Another characteristic that can influence ICD lead extractability is coil electrode connection type. Compared with proximal connection, where lead extension during the extraction manoeuvre (obviously not using a locking stylet) allows lead cross-section dimension reduction, in distal connection, this action will increase the coil dimensions, making mechanical sheath advancement more challenging during the extraction procedure.

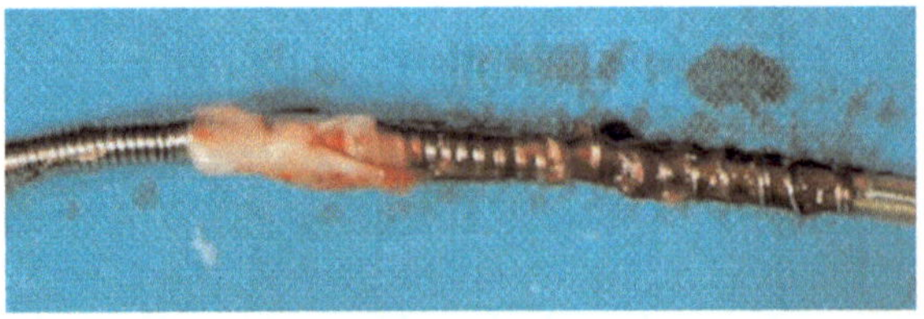

Fig. 1.33 Tenacious adhesion of superior vena cava along the proximal coil of an implantable cardioverter–defibrillator lead with a free-floating filar coil design. Note coil despiralization in the proximal end as a consequence of lead extraction

1.1.6.5 Fixation Mechanisms and Dimensions

The type of fixation mechanisms could influence lead extractability by their isodiametric or nonisodiametric design. The presence of tines in passive fixation leads, and so the nonisodiametric design at the distal electrode, is the reason why scar tissue typically develops more frequently with this type of lead than with active fixation leads (Fig. 1.35). If this is true for atrial or RV leads regardless of the primary function (pacing/defibrillating), it is even more evident in LV leads, in which the attempt to improve tip fixation through extendable/retractable tines could provoke serious difficulties during lead extraction. In addition to using conventional sheaths, this would require modified coronary sinus lead delivery in order to release the tip from the adherences present in the vein [27] (Fig. 1.36).

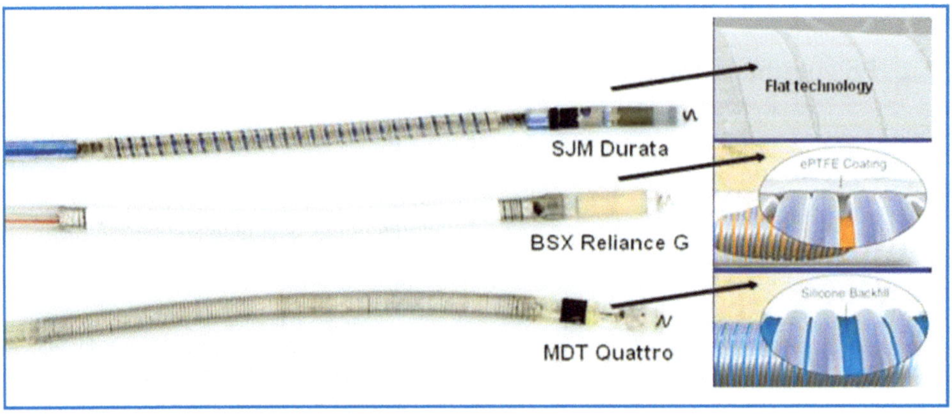

Fig. 1.34 Different methods of covering implantable cardioverter–defibrillator lead coils from different companies (courtesy of St. Jude Medical, Boston Scientific, and Medtronic)

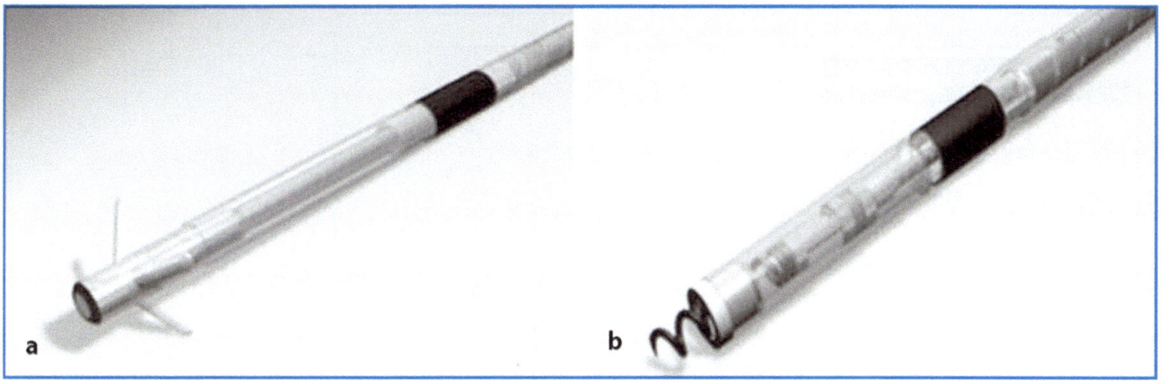

Fig. 1.35 Passive tined fixation lead (a). Active fixation extendable/retractable screw-in lead (b)

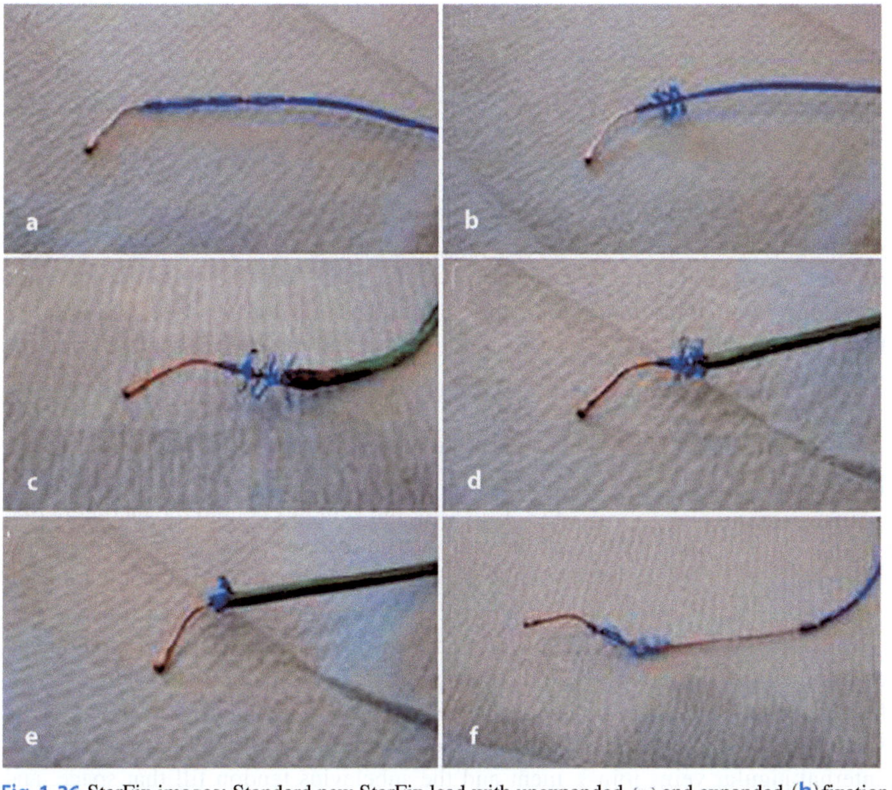

Fig. 1.36 StarFix images: Standard new StarFix lead with unexpanded (a) and expanded (b) fixation lobes. Ineffective mechanical dilatation using the complete lead delivery (c). Effective mechanical dilatation using the cutted lead delivery (without soft tip) (d) and sheath over lobe advancement (e). Lead appearance after removal (f). Note the push-tubing fracture around the lead body, the result of ineffective attempts to withdraw the deployed lobes

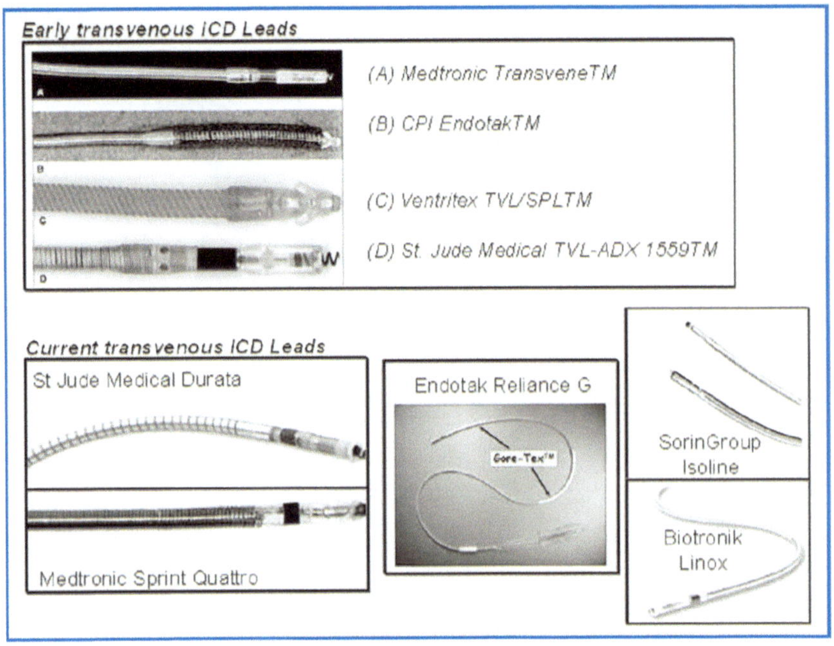

Fig. 1.37 Old and new generations of implantable cardioverter–defibrillator leads in terms of dimensions and isodiametric design (courtesy of St. Jude Medical, Boston Scientific, Medtronic, SorinGroup, and Biotronik)

As we know, adherences on a pacing/ defibrillating lead are present not only at the tip but frequently along its entire course. For this reason, the isodiametric or nonisodiametric design is an important issue, not only in regard to the tip region, but to the entire lead (Fig. 1.37).

1.2 Patient Anatomy

1.2.1 Vein Anatomy

1.2.1.1 Subclavian Vein

Each subclavian vein is a continuation of the axillary vein and runs from the outer rim of the first rib to the medial rim of the anterior scalene muscle. Here the subclavian and internal jugular veins join inside the anterior edge of the superior thoracic opening and create right and left innominate veins behind the sternal manubrium. The vein usually has a pair of valves about 2 cm from its end. The heads of clavicles extend posteriorly into the superior thoracic opening, displacing the veins posteriorly from the sternum. Because of the anteroposterior slope of the superior aperture, the arteries are more cephalad and more posterior than the veins (Fig. 1.38) [28].

The pleuras cupola and the lung apex project into the aperture behind the vessels. The anterior scalene muscles attach to the first ribs between the subclavian veins and arteries. The subclavian vein crosses the first rib at its anterior ending and lies between the anterior scalene muscle and the posterior bulge of the clavicle's head. As shown in Fig. 1.39 [29], the vein lies behind the medial region of the clavicle, not between the last and first rib, as usually believed. Two structures connect the medial region of the clavicle to the costal cartilage of the first rib: the costoclavicular (Halsted's) ligament and the tendon of the subclavius muscle. As described earlier, the subclavian vein does not lie between the rib and clavicle. Only Halsted's ligament and the subclavius tendon fill that space, and the first marks the transition from axillary to subclavian vein at the lateral limit of the first rib. During subclavian vein puncture, whereas the brachial plexus nerves are relatively protected by their posterior position, the thoracic duct, near the junction of the left internal jugular and subclavian veins, and the phrenic nerves, which enter the chest at the medial rim of the first ribs, are subject to injury.

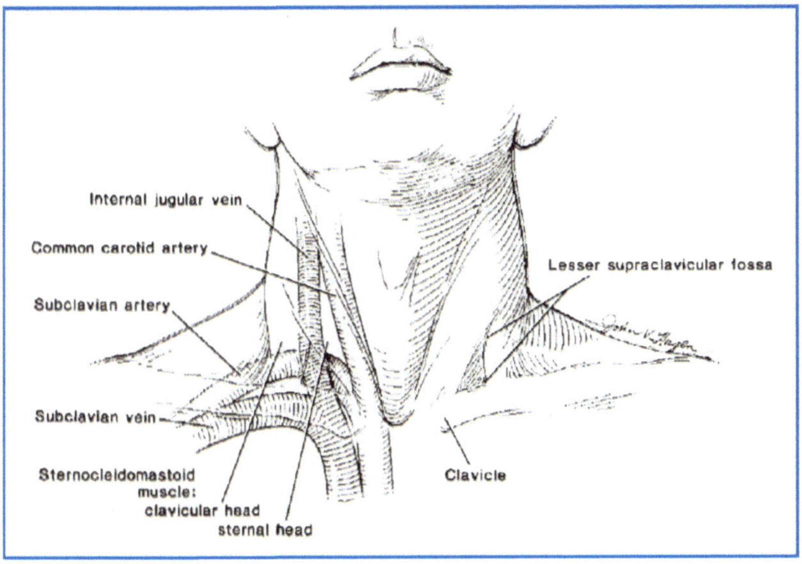

Fig. 1.38 Subclavian vein course and its relationships with adjacent anatomical structures (from [28], by permission of Mayo Foundation for Medical Education and Research. All rights reserved)

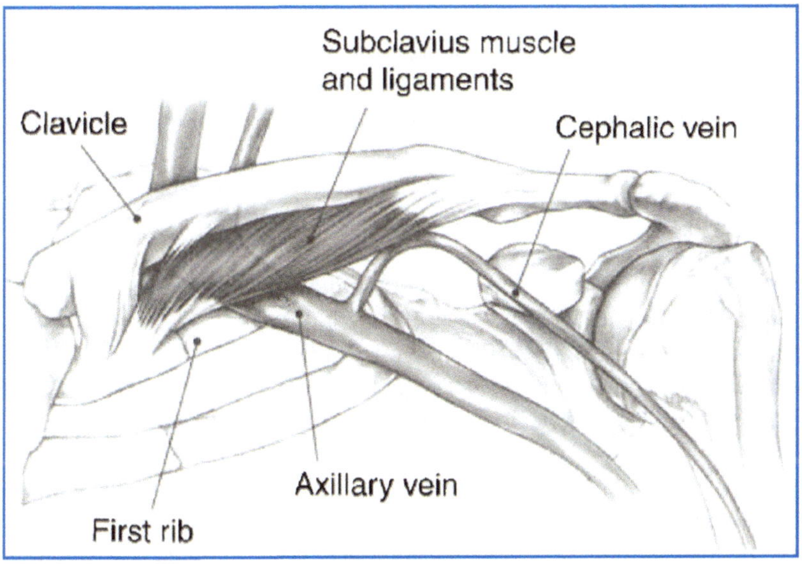

Fig. 1.39 Subclavian venous system and skeletal landmarks relevant to percutaneous access. Subclavius muscle and costoclavicular ligament complex are shown between the clavicle and the first rib (from [29], Chap. 5, p. 212, by permission of Mayo Foundation for Medical Education and Research. All rights reserved)

1.2.1.2 Femoral Vein

The femoral vein lies within the femoral triangle (of Scarpa), an anatomical region of the upper, inner human thigh (Fig. 1.40). The superior rim of the triangle is formed by the inguinal ligament, the medial rim by the adductor longus muscle, and the lateral rim by the sartorius muscle. The apex of the triangle is formed by the sartorius crossing the adductor longus muscle. The roof of the triangle is composed of the skin, subcutaneous tissue, the cribriform fascia, and the fascia lata. The concave floor is formed of underlying adductor longus, adductor brevis, pectineus, and iliopsoas muscles.

Within the triangle in a medial-to-lateral position is the neurovascular bundle represented by the femoral sheath, which has three components: the lateral one contains the femoral artery, the intermediate one the femoral vein, and the medial, and smallest, compartment is called the femoral canal. The neurovascular bundle encases efferent lymphatic vessels and a lymph node embedded in a

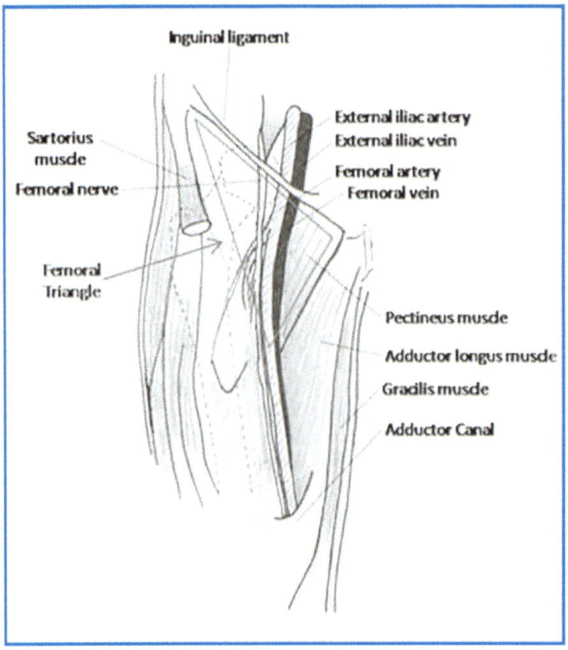

Fig. 1.40 Femoral vein course and anatomical Scarpa triangle

small amount of areolar tissue. It is conical and approximately 2-cm long.

Beginning at the adductor opening – as the continuation of the popliteal vein – the femoral vein runs down next to its artery, ending posterior to the inguinal ligament as the external iliac vein. During its course, the relation of the femoral vein to the femoral artery changes. In the distal region of the adductor canal, it runs posterolaterally to the femoral artery; more proximally in the canal and in the apex of the distal femoral triangle, it runs posterior to the artery, whereas at the superior region of the triangle (the base), it runs medial and slightly posterior to the femoral artery. In this region, both the vein and the artery are somewhat superficial. There are commonly five valves in the femoral vein: one of these is consistently found near the inguinal ligament.

1.2.1.3 Internal Jugular Vein

The internal jugular vein is located in the anterior neck. It channels blood from the skull, brain, superficial regions of the face, and much of the neck. The more cephalad portions of the vein are located somewhat deep within the neck, whereas the caudal portions are more superficial. It runs down to the carotid sheath and joins with the subclavian vein, creating the brachiocephalic vein posterior to the sternal rim of the clavicle. Near its terminal, the vein dilates into the inferior bulb. From above, the anterior and middle scalenus muscles, the cervical plexus, the phrenic nerve, the thyrocervical trunk, the vertebral vein, and the first part of the subclavian artery all lie posterior to the vein. Laterally, the internal jugular vein crosses anterior to the thoracic duct. Medially to the vein are the internal and common carotid arteries and the vagus nerve: the latter lies between vein and arteries but posteriorly. The anatomical position of the vein is best understood in relation to the sternocleidomastoid muscle (Fig. 1.38). For much of its run, the vein runs directly beneath the muscle. However, the more cephalad section lies just medial to the sternal head of the muscle. Its medial portion runs through a triangle formed by the sternal and clavicular heads of the sternocleidomastoid muscle. As the vein moves caudally, it runs medial to the clavicular head of the muscle.

1.2.2 Venous Approaches

For permanent cardiac pacing, physicians have always used the right chambers. In order to access to these anatomical regions, many different veins can be used, including the cephalic, axillary, subclavian, external or internal jugular, and the ileofemoral.

Classically, the venous approach establishes where the device will be implanted. Historically, the venous approach used for lead implantation was the ileofemoral vein. Once a small incision immediately below the inguinal ligament was performed, the operator had to carry the dissection down to the fascia above the vein. At this point, the iliac vein was entered with a standard puncture technique, and after lead implantation, it was tunneled to the abdominal pocket. For this venous approach, the device was actually housed in the abdominal region. The pocket was created lateral to the umbilicus and superficial to the rectus sheath [30, 31]. This is not the standard method for PM implantation used today, but it is important to know this approach in the event that more commonly used venous routes are not accessible or in case of a lead extraction procedure. In the latter, problems could arise particularly for ventricular leads. During dilation, the adhesions present on the lead along its course into the inferior vena cava can make advancing the sheath into the RV next the tricuspid region challenging for the short angle forming in the area between the sheath and the lead. This is a situation in which the "Pisa approach" [32] could be successful.

Another venous lead implantation approach of historical interest is the jugular vein. The first method to acces the vein was nonpercutaneous, in which two incisions are required. The first skin incision, performed above the clavicle between the posterior rim of the sternocleidomastoid muscle and the anterior rim of the trapezius muscle, is necessary to reach the external jugular vein or, extended forward, the carotid sheath wherein internal jugular vein is present. A second infraclavicular incision is then necessary to fashion the pocket over the pectoral muscle. Only the latter is required for the percutaneous approach, but regardless of the method used, in both cases, the lead must be tunneled to the pocket (usually over the clavicle). These techniques have been abandoned due to frequent complications related to lead failure. Outside the vein, the lead must run at an acute angle to reach the pocket, which is the reason for the recurrent lead fracture related to this venous approach. However, this is probably the better approach in case of lead extraction.

Currently, the cephalic, axillary, and subclavian veins are the most common venous approaches for lead implantation, with the generator housed subcutaneously in the adjacent infraclavicular region. Despite all the advantages of these approaches, one anatomically critical region remains a challenge to be overcome during lead extraction, especially when intrathoracic subclavian puncture is used. This is the costoclavicular region, which is discussed the following section.

1.2.3 Critical Anatomical Regions for Lead Extraction

Two anatomical points, in particular, can be critical during lead extraction: the costoclavicular region, and the junction between the innominate vein and SVC. The first region can impede the procedure *per se*, making the sheath advancement across the medial part of the costoclavicular region impossible, where Halsted's ligament and the tendon of the subclavius muscle are present. In the second region, there is a high risk of vein tearing because of the sharp angle between the sheath and the SVC during the dilation maneuver, especially when the sheath is entering from the right side or a powered sheath is used.

1.2.3.1 Costoclavicular Region

The type of technique and the venous access used for lead implantation play an important role with respect to lead performance and extraction. Historically, before 1979, the most frequently used venous approach was the cephalic vein through a cutdown in the deltopectoral groove, and when it was not exploitable, the ipsilateral external or internal jugular vein was used. Subclavian or axillary vein cutdowns were performed rarely because of the common lack of cardiologist skill in deep-vein dissection. For this reason, percutaneous use of the subclavian vein for endocardial pacing developed over the following years [33–39]. Because subclavian vein cannulation has demonstrated success more than 95% of the time, the percutaneous technique has rapidly become the most common approach for PM lead implantation [40, 41]. Initially, subclavian puncture was intrathoracic and was the preferred venous route at one time. In order to avoid possible complication with this type of puncture, such as pneumohemothorax or lung laceration, many surgeons have converted to an extrathoracic subclavian or axillary vein approach. This proved to be a safer technique not only during implantation but also for lead survival over the time.

Historically, surgeons believed that the subclavian vein could be entered at the junction of the middle and the inner thirds of the clavicle, creating a very medial approach to the vein. There is now evidence, however, that this traditional percutaneous subclavian approach predisposes the lead to crush injury between the clavicle and the first rib. At this point, the lead may become entrapped between the subclavian muscle and the costoclavicular ligament [42, 43]. Forces exerted on leads in this position may predispose them to insulation failure, especially for some polyurethane leads (P80A) and under conditions of chronic mechanical stress on the lead, such as higher activity in young patients, restricted anatomic circumstances in female patients, or if multiple leads are present in the vein [44, 45]. When a medial approach to the subclavian vein is used, the periosteum can be penetrated during needle advancement to access the vein, and this often results in a band of calcification around the lead. Under these circumstances, especially many years after the implant procedure, lead extraction can be challenging due to the great deal of friction and pressure exerted on the extraction sheath during the dilating maneuver.

One solution is to use a telescopic technique with progressively larger sizes to enlarge the costoclavicular route. Therefore, because the subclavian vein is compressed between the clavicle and anterior scalene muscle when the shoulder is displaced posteriorly and downward, it is advantageous to have the shoulder in neutral position with no roll during sheath advancement to keep the vein wide open. When sheath advancement is not possible or unsuccessful despite using the telescopic technique, and if the lead is free from adhesions, the Pisa approach [32] may be helpful.

1.2.3.2 Superior Vena Cava

The SVC is a critical region because of the short angle between this vein and the right or left innominate vein. Particularly in cases in which tenacious adhesions are present in this region, advancing the dilating sheaths, especially if powered, exposes the patient to the risk of vein tearing. During this maneuver, the anatomical landmarks on fluoroscopy are helpful: the second rib joining the sternal angle marks the midpoint of the SVC and the third marks the caval right-atrial junction. As described later, one solution to this challenging situation is moving to the Pisa approach [32], which uses access through the internal jugular vein to reduce the short angle between the sheath and the SVC during the dilating maneuver.

1.3 Patient–Lead Interaction

1.3.1 Fibrous Response to Intravascular Foreign Bodies

To approach an extraction procedure with more consciousness, it is important to be aware of the complications related to human body response after implantation of a pacing or defibrillating lead [46]. When a transvenous permanent lead is implanted, it stays in close contact with some points of the venous endothelium and endocardium. At these points, the lead may be responsible of chronic traumatism on the endothelium/endocardium, causing an inflammatory response of the vessel or endocardial wall, with thrombus formation and subsequent scarring [47–49].

Endothelial damage, in fact, is one of the factors included in Virchow's triad about thrombosis pathogenesis. In this case, the thrombus that develops in the sites of contact between the lead and the venous/cardiac wall is the initial response to placement of a lead, which represents an intravascular foreign body. Within 2 weeks after implantation, there is a proliferative response of fibroblasts and granulation tissue, which frequently results in endothelialization along the lead. Therefore, the thrombus eventually develops fibrosis, and fibrosis can then propagate along the lead, even beyond the areas of contact with the endothelium/endocardium. In this way, the lead becomes increasingly dense with time.

In their study, Esposito et al. [50] made morphologic and immunohistochemical observation of tissue surrounding retrieved leads. Immunohistochemical analysis revealed a tissue generally devoid of inflammatory and immune cells. The fibrous capsule surrounding the lead resulted in partially or completely being covered with a monolayer of CD34-expressing endothelial cells. Endothelialization of the fibrous encapsulation indicates a functionalization of blood-contacting surfaces around PM materials, thus providing a mechanism for long-term persistence of foreign materials in the blood.

The fibrous response is related not only to actually pacing leads, but also to nonfunctional leads, indicating that it is the simple presence of the lead – with its traumatic action on the endothelium/ endocardium regardless of its electrical properties and function – that elicits the fibrous response. In case of defibrillating leads, however, the endocardial injury due to eventual electrical discharges is an important pathogenetic step contributing to the fibrous response of the myocardium. In their study, Epstein et al. [51] examined eight hearts, five taken after transplantation and three after patient death. The electrode–myocardial interfaces were characterized by intense endocardial fibrosis and were remarkably consistent. Each lead was encased by a ring of fibroelastic tissue, and there was fibrosis of the RV myocardium adjacent to the leads (Fig. 1.41). Microscopically, interstitial fibrosis was adjacent to each lead in the current path of ICD shocks. Acute cell injury was present only in hearts that had received recent shocks. The authors concluded that the fibrosis associated with endocardial ICD leads and the cumulative acute damage produced by defibrillation discharges may explain changes in the defibrillation and pacing thresholds and the difficulty of lead extraction that can be encountered with transvenous ICD systems.

The sites most likely to develop severe fibrosis are the venous entry site, the junction between the anonymous vein and the SVC, and the region of the lead that runs from the anode ring to the tip. In these sites, calcium often incorporates into the fibrous matrix, especially in young patients and very old leads, cases in which a robust fibrous tissue usually develops [46]. Compared with atrial leads, ventricular leads contact more tissue because of their longer length, sometimes making extraction more difficult. The larger ICD coils (especially when not coated) often present aggressive fibrosis, and this is particularly problematic for the coil in the SVC, which stimulates aggressive fibrosis at an area of high risk for vascular tear [51]. Fibrosis not only binds leads to the vessel wall, but also infiltrates between leads, binding them together. The tissue reaction and fibrous encapsulation may in part be protective against thrombus formation. However, if an overwhelming tissue reaction ensues, the fibrosis itself may produce a significant obstruction or create an environment of impaired venous flow, which may in turn promote thrombus formation. It is clear that freeing the lead from all binding sites safely is the main goal of extraction tools and techniques that have been developed [46, 52, 53].

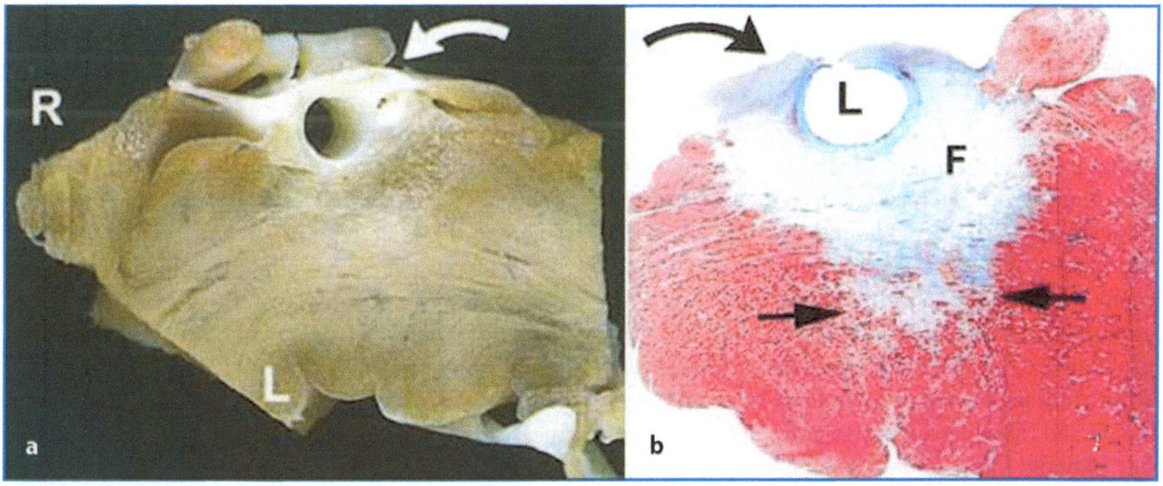

Fig. 1.41 Section of interventricular septum from a patient who underwent cardiac transplantation 676 days after implantable cardioverter–defibrillator lead implantation and 7 days after last defibrillator shock (**a**). Right ventricular surface of interventricular septum (*R*) is at the top and left ventricular surface (*L*) at bottom. Characteristic fibroelastic tissue encircles the lead (*curved arrow*). Trichrome-stained section of tissue (**b**): band of fibroelastic tissue (*curved arrow*) encircles lead (*L*), and beneath, in myocardium, lies fibrous connective tissue (*F*). Area of confluent fibrous connective tissue immediately adjacent to lead also extends into surrounding myocardium, forming radial pattern of interstitial fibrosis (*arrows*), suggesting that shocks have caused lines of electrical injury (courtesy [51])

1.3.2 Vascular Complications Related to Fibrous Response

Numerous reports of thrombotic venous complications following a PM/ICD system implantation, such as stenosis, occlusion, and SVC syndrome (SVCS), have been published, and their number is increasing. All these manifestations share the same pathogenetic root: thrombus formation, as described above, is the initial step of these processes, but it is still not well known why in some patients it does not limit itself to creating fibrosis around the lead or which are the risk factors for such venous complications [54–56].

1.3.2.1 Superior Vena Cava Syndrome

SVCS can be caused by an intrinsic or extrinsic obstruction of the SVC. Neoplastic, traumatic, or infectious processes in the mediastinum are common causes of extrinsic obstruction. Symptomatic stenosis and SVC occlusion due to vessel thrombosis or fibrosis secondary to an indwelling catheter or transvenous permanent PM/ICD leads – although very rare (<0.1% of patients) – are also well-recognized entities. Different studies report different incidence rates: many patients with this condition often remain largely asymptomatic, and so the variation in the assessed incidences may result from varying degrees of sensitivity in making the diagnosis [57, 58]. Symptomatic patients usually present with dyspnea and progressive arm, neck, and head swelling, which facilitates the clinical diagnosis. Other common symptoms are the inability to bend over without developing flush and headache, and exercise-induced flush. Patients often describe these symptoms as constant, with almost no significant variation over time: they are often able to successfully adapt their lifestyle and daily routines to reduce symptoms to a minimum. Acute and rapidly progressive cases are infrequent, but patients can rapidly develop cerebral edema and intracranial thrombosis, which can lead to coma and even death. SVC obstruction, as said, is often asymptomatic, when a slow onset allows the development of a sufficient collateral circulation. Collateral vessels, such as azygos, hemiazygos, and thoracoabdominal subcutaneous veins, can compensate the flow in obstructed SVC, and clinical symptoms of SVCS can develop gradually over several years (Fig. 1.42). SVCS, in fact, may develop at any time after a PM/ICD implantation but usually occurs after several years. Early obstruction usually results from thrombosis, whereas the later type of obstruction may be the result of subsequent fibrotic inflammatory process, probably sustained by a chronic reaction to the insulator materials of the lead body. For diagnosis, spiral computed tomography (CT) venography with bilateral upper-extremity contrast injection is the gold standard [58].

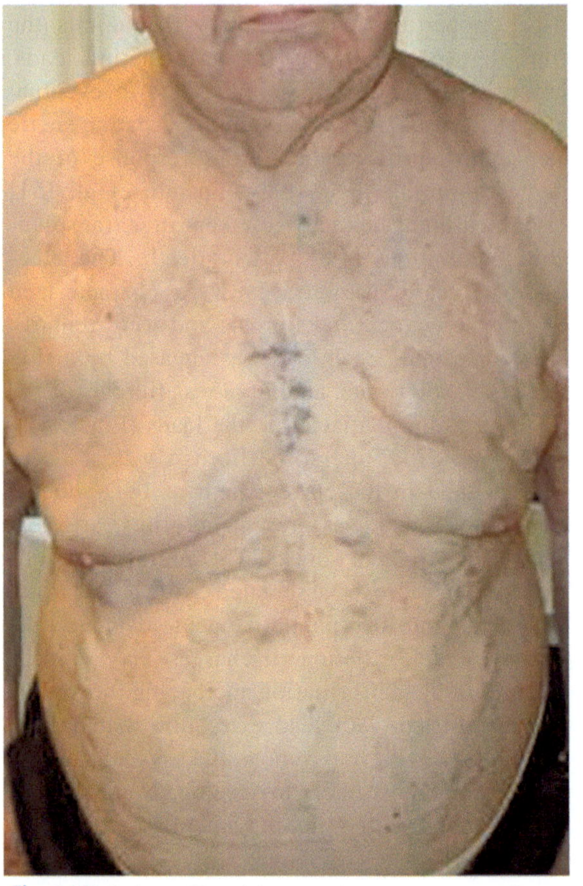

Fig. 1.42 Patient affected by superior vena cava syndrome. Note well-developed collateral vessels

1.3.2.2 Venous Stenosis/Thrombosis

Various degrees of upper-extremity deep-venous thrombosis, in most cases asymptomatic, are relatively frequent following permanent PM or ICD implantation, occurring in nearly one fourth of patients who are candidate for generator change, lead revision, or device upgrade. These follow-up procedures may be difficult or impossible due to obstruction in the access vein [59, 60].

In their study, Lickfett et al. [55] enrolled 105 consecutive patients admitted for their first elective ICD generator replacement. All patients underwent bilateral contrast venography. Venous obstruction of various degrees was found in 25% of patients. Complete occlusion was found in 9%, severe stenosis (>75% diameter reduction) in 6%, and moderate stenosis (>50–75% diameter reduction) in 10%. The incidence of venous obstruction was increased in patients with a PM prior to initial ICD system implantation (67%). No difference was found in patients with a single defibrillator lead compared with patients who had an additional SVC shocking coil. However, the presence of a second shocking coil in the SVC incorporated in a single ICD lead was associated with an increased incidence of venous obstruction. No difference was found between silicone- and polyurethane-insulated leads. The authors concluded that venous obstruction occurs relatively frequently after ICD implantation and that contrast venography should always be obtained if malfunction of a preexistent lead is suspected or if a system upgrade is considered.

Clinical features of venous occlusive disease of the upper extremity veins should routinely be considered in follow-up of all patients with transvenous endocardial leads. Symptoms depend on the site and extent of thrombus/stenosis. Patients frequently complain of vague shoulder or neck discomfort. Axillary/subclavian/innominate venous occlusion may result in edema of the ipsilateral upper extremity, with cyanosis, development of dilated collateral cutaneous circulation around the shoulder and across the chest, and jugular vein dilatation. This may be transient and mild or permanent and severe; the latter case is more likely when thrombosis is more peripheral, where collateral drainage is limited. Pulmonary embolism in these patients is not uncommon (16–36%). All these symptoms, however, are not specific and may occur in patients with lymphoedema, muscle injury, or superficial thrombophlebitis; for this reason, it is important to assess the diagnosis with objective testing. Spontaneous recanalization of the vessel or dilation of collateral vessels to drain the affected limb usually leads to resolution of the clinical manifestations. To confirm the clinical diagnosis, different imaging modalities are available and used: ultrasonography, contrast venography [55], spiral CT venography, and magnetic resonance angiography (MRA) after PM/ICD system removal (Fig. 1.43).

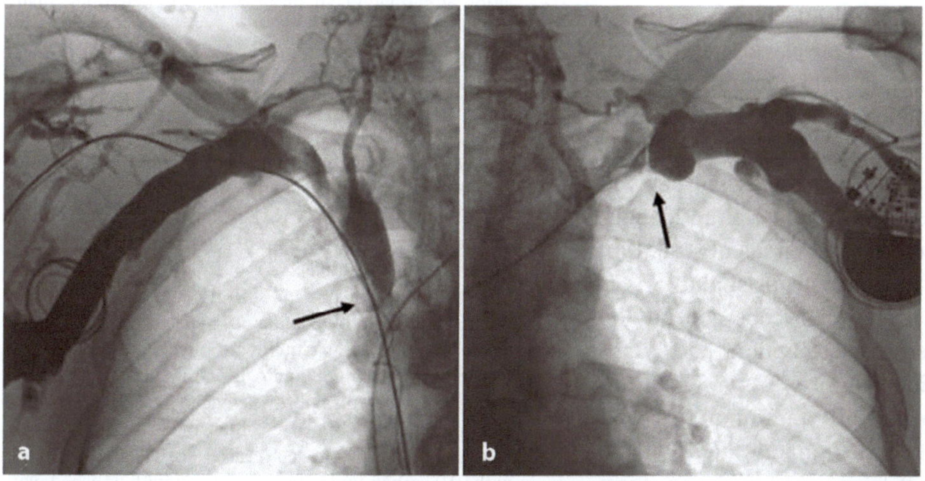

Fig. 1.43 Contrast venography of both subclavian veins in a patient with superior vena cava syndrome. He carried a monocatheter pacing system on the left (implanted 4 years earlier) and had two abandoned leads on the right (the pacemaker, implanted 21 years earlier, had been removed from the right pocket due to local infection). Subocclusive obstruction between the right subclavian and innominate veins (**a**). Total obstruction is visible in the first tract of the superior vena cava (*arrow*). Occlusive obstruction visible in the middle tract of the left subclavian vein (**b**) (*arrow*)

Although no clear risk factors have been identified, several predictors of venous occlusion in PM/ICD carriers have been reported [55, 56, 59, 61]. These include a history of device upgrades, the presence of temporary endocardial PM wires before implantation of a permanent device, the presence of multiple endocardial leads, retention of severed leads, lead infection, use of dual-coil leads, female hormone therapy, history of venous thrombosis, and gene-based predisposing factors for thrombophilia. In contrast, long-term anticoagulation therapy seems to offer a protective effect.

In a study by Haghjoo et al. [56], contrast venography was performed in 100 consecutive patients who were candidates for generator change, lead revision, or device upgrade to determine the predictors of venous obstruction after transvenous device implantation and to assess the effects of antiplatelet/anticoagulant drugs in preventing venous thrombosis. The incidence of venous obstruction was 26%, with 9% of patients having total obstruction and 17% exhibiting partial obstruction (considered as >70% diameter reduction). No statistically significant differences between obstructed and nonobstructed patients were seen for age, sex, indication for device implantation, atrial fibrillation, cardiothoracic ratio, insulation material, operative technique (in particular, access site: subclavian puncture vs. cephalic cut down), device type, and manufacturer. In a univariate analysis, multiple leads and presence of dilated cardiomyopathy were associated with higher risk of venous obstruction, whereas anticoagulant/antiplatelet therapy significantly reduced incidence of venous obstruction. Multivariate logistic regression analysis showed that only lead number and antiplatelet/anticoagulant therapy were predictors of venous obstruction.

The treatment of venous stenosis and SVCS caused by intravenously inserted leads depends on the site of venous obstruction, duration, and symptoms. Acute presentation with severe symptoms suggests prompt treatment with thrombolytics and maybe percutaneous transluminal angioplasty, which improves short-term results. Long term results show that anticoagulation with heparin and warfarin leads to similar clinical outcomes, and there is some debate as to whether to give prophylactic anticoagulation therapy in high-risk patients or not.

In the literature, there are several case reports of venous obstruction and even SVCS in patients with a PM/ICD system who were treated by balloon venoplasty [62] and vein stenting [63, 64]. In 2008, Worley [65] published his experience in dealing with venous obstructions during implant procedures in approximately 15% of patients with prior leads. The author described the safety and high success rate of 130 subclavian and 250 coronary venoplasty procedures and their substantial lack of acute or chronic clinical consequence to the patient. An extraction procedure, with the newly developed interventional technologies and the appropriate use of venoplasty, allow opportunities to create a conduit through the occluded vein by using the existing lead. In this way, is possible to avoid having to use the opposite or more medial site in cases of necessary reimplantation or upgrade procedures [66]. Given the efficacy and safety of modern lead extraction procedures, since 2000, Korley et al. [67] proposed ICD systems upgrading as an indication for transvenous lead removal, considering the significant morbidity and cost burden of potential complications that may arise with abandoned leads.

References

1. Cuvillier E (2009) Handbook of leads for pacing, defibrillation & cardiac resynchronization. Eric Cuvillier, Juana Dìaz
2. Barold SS, Stroobant RX, Sinnaewe AF (2004) Cardiac pacemaker step by step – an illustrated guide. Blackwell, Malden
3. Amundson DC, McArthur W, Mosharrafa M (1979) The porous endocardial electrode. Pacing Clin Electrophysiol 2(1):40–50
4. MacCarter DJ, Lundberg KM, Corstjens JP (1983) Porous electrodes: concept technology and results. Pacing Clin Electrophysiol 6(2 Pt 2): 427–435
5. Skalsky M, Maddison D (1985) Evaluation of a new low polarisation high impedence Pt/Ir coated porous 6 mm 2 dish electrode. Pacing Clin Electrophysiol 8:788 [abstract]
6. Garberoglio B, Inguaggiato B, Chinaglia B, Cerise O (1983) Initial results with an activated pyrolytic carbon tip electrode. Pacing Clin Electrophysiol 6(2 Pt 2): 440–448
7. Mugica J, Henry L, Attuel P et al (1986) Clinical experience with 910 carbon tip leads: comparison with polished platinum leads. Pacing Clin Electrophysiol 9(2 Pt 2):1230–1238
8. Thuesen L, Jensen PJ, Vejby-Christensen H et al (1989) Lower chronic stimulation threshold in the carbon-tip than in the platinum-tip endocardial electrode: a randomized study. Pacing Clin Electrophysiol 12(10):1592–1595

9. Mond H, Hunt D (1990) A second generation steroid eluting electrode Cardiostim 90. RBM Seventh International Congress Nice 12:62
10. Danilovic D, Breivik K, Hoff PI, Ohm OJ (1997) Clinical performance of steroid-eluting pacing leads with 12–mm2 electrodes. Pacing Clin Electrophysiol 20(11):2799–2809
11. Hua W, Mond HG, Strathmore N (1997) Chronic steroid-eluting lead performance: a comparison of atrial and ventricular pacing. Pacing Clin Electrophysiol 20(1 Pt 1):17–24
12. Jenney C, Tan J, Karicherla A et al (2005) A new insulation material for cardiac leads with potential for improved performance. Heart Rhythm 2:S318–S319
13. Calfee RV, Saulson SH (1986) A voluntary standard for 32 mm unipolar and bipolar pacemaker leads and connectors. Pacing Clin Electrophysiol 9(6 Pt 2):1181–1185
14. Mirowski M, Reid PR, Mower MM et al (1980) Termination of malignant ventricular arrhythmias with an implanted automatic defibrillator in human beings. N Engl J Med 303(6):322–324
15. Haqqani HM, Mond HG (2009) The implantable cardioverter-defibrillator lead: principles, progress, and promises. Pacing Clin Electrophysiol 32:1336–1353
16. Wilkoff BL, Belott PH, Love CJ et al (2005) Improved extraction of ePTFE and medical adhesive modified defibrillation leads from the coronary sinus and great cardiac vein. Pacing Clin Electrophysiol 28(3):205–211
17 Kouht AR, Grammes J (2009) The ePTFE coated ICD leads are easier to remove than standard ICD leads up to 50 months implant duration. Hearth Rhythm 6 (5):S132 [abstract]
18. Di Cori A, Bongiorni MG, Zucchelli G et al (2010) Transvenous extraction performance of expanded polytetrafluoroethylene-covered ICD leads in comparison to traditional ICD leads in humans. Pacing Clin Electrophysiol [Epub ahead of print]
19. Helland J, St Jude Medical Personal communication
20. Hauser RG, Cannom D, Hayes DL et al (2002) Long-term structural failure of coaxial polyurethane implantable cardioverter defibrillator leads, Pacing Clin Electrophysiol 25(6):879–882
21. Krahn AD, Champagne J, Healey JS et al (2008) Outcome of the Fidelis implantable cardioverter-defibrillator lead advisory: a report from the Canadian Heart Rhythm Society Device Advisory Committee. Heart Rhythm 5(5):639–642
22. Epstein AE, Baker JH 2nd, Beau SL et al (2009) Performance of the St Jude Medical Riata leads. Heart Rhythm 2009 6(2):204–209
23. Kay GN, Brinker JA, Kawanishi DT et al (1999) Risks of spontaneous injury and extraction of an active fixation pacemaker lead: report of the Accufix Multicenter Clinical Study and Worldwide Registry. Circulation 100(23):2344–2352
24. Fortescue EB, Berul CI, Cecchin F et al (2004) Patient procedural and hardware factors associated with pacemaker lead failures in pediatrics and congenital heart disease. Heart Rhythm 1(2):150–159
25. Ellenbogen KA, Wood MA, Shepard RK et al (2003) Detection and management of an implantable cardioverter defibrillator lead failure: incidence and clinical implications. J Am Coll Cardiol 41(1):73–80
26. Knight BP, Desai A, Coman J et al (2004) Long-term retention of cardiac resynchronization therapy. J Am Coll Cardiol 44(1):72–77
27. Bongiorni MG, DI Cori A, Zucchelli G et al (2010) A modified transvenous single mechanical dilatation technique to remove a chronically implanted active-fixation coronary sinus pacing lead. Pacing Clin Electrophysiol [Epub ahead of print]
28. Holmes DR Jr (1986) Permanent pacemaker implantation. In: Furman S, Hayes DL, Holmes DR Jr (eds) A practice of cardiac pacing. Futura, Mount Kisco, pp 97–127
29. Ellenbogen KA, Wood MA (2005) Cardiac pacing and ICDs 4th edn, Blackwell
30. Ellestad MH, French J (1989) Iliac vein approach to permanent pacemaker implantation. Pacing Clin Electrophysiol 12(7 Pt 1):1030–1033
31. García Guerrero JJ, De La Concha Castañeda JF, Fernández Mora G et al (2005) Permanent transfemoral pacemaker: a single-center series performed with an easier and safer surgical technique. Pacing Clin Electrophysiol 28(7):675–679
32. Kennergren C (2008) European perspective on lead extraction: part II. Heart Rhythm 5(2):320–323
33. Vellani CW, Tildesley G, Davies LG (1969) Endocardial pacing: a percutaneous method using the subclavian vein. Br Heart J 31(1):106–111
34. Mobin-Uddin K, Smith PE, Lombardo C, Jude J (1967) Percutaneous intracardiac pacing through the subclavian vein. J Thorac Cardiovasc Surg 54(4):545–548
35. Jachuck SJ, Gill BS, Petty AH. (1974) Permanent cardiac pacing through the subclavian vein. Br J Surg 61(5):373–376
36. Littleford PO, Spector SD (1979) Device for the rapid insertion of a permanent endocardial pacing electrode through the subclavian vein: preliminary report. Ann Thorac Surg 27(3):265–269
37. Friesen A, Klein GJ, Kostuk WJ, Ahuja SP (1977) Percutaneous insertion of a permanent transvenous pacemaker electrode through the subclavian vein. Can J Surg 20(2):131–135
38. Kessinger JM, Holter AR, Geha AS (1982) Implantation of permanent transvenous pacemaker via subclavian vein. Arch Surg 117(8):1105–1107
39. Vander Salm TJ, Haffajee CI, Okike ON (1981) Transvenous insertion of double sets of permanent electrodes through a single introducer: clinical application. Ann Thorac Surg 32(3):307–310
40. Bernstein AD, Parsonnet V (1992) Survey of cardiac pacing in the United States in 1989. Am J Cardiol 69(4):331–338
41. Goldman BS, Fraser JD, Morgan CD (1991) Survey of cardiac pacing in Canada. Can J Cardiol 7(9):391–398
42. Jacobs DM, Fink AS, Miller RP et al (1993) Anatomical and morphological evaluation of pacemaker lead compression. Pacing Clin Electrophysiol 16(3 Pt 1):434–444
43. Magney JE, Flynn DM, Parsons JA et al (1993) Anatomical mechanisms explaining damage to pacemaker leads defibrillator leads and failure of central venous catheters adjacent to the sternoclavicular joint. Pacing Clin Electrophysiol 16(3 Pt 1):445–457

44. Kleemann T, Becker T, Doenges K et al (2007) Annual rate of transvenous defibrillation lead defects in implantable cardioverter-defibrillators over a period of >10 years. Circulation 115(19):2474–2480
45. Takahashi T, Bhandari AK, Watanuki M et al (2002) High incidence of device-related and lead-related complications in the dual-chamber implantable cardioverter defibrillator compared with the single-chamber version. Circ J 66(8):746–750
46. Smith MC, Love CJ (2008) Extraction of transvenous pacing and ICD leads. Pacing Clin Electrophysiol 31(6):736–752
47. Rozmus G, Daubert JP, Huang DT et al (2005) Venous thrombosis and stenosis after implantation of pacemakers and defibrillators. J Interv Card Electrophysiol 13(1):9–19
48. Contini C, Papi L, Pesola A et al (1973) Tissue reaction to intracavitary electrodes: effect on duration and efficiency of unipolar pacing in patients with A-V block. J Cardiovasc Surg (Torino) 14(3):282–290
49. Pauletti M, Pingitore R, Contini C (1979) Superior vena cava stenosis at site of intersection of two pacing electrodes. Br Heart J 42(4):487–489
50. Esposito M, Kennergren C, Holmström N et al (2002) Morphologic and immunohistochemical observations of tissues surrounding retrieved transvenous pacemaker leads. J Biomed Mater Res 63(5):548–558
51. Epstein AE, Kay GN, Plumb VJ et al (1998) Gross and microscopic pathological changes associated with nonthoracotomy implantable defibrillator leads. Circulation 98(15):1517–1524
52. Byrd CL, Schwartz SJ, Hedin N (1991) Intravascular techniques for extraction of permanent pacemaker leads. J Thorac Cardiovasc Surg 101(6):989–997
53. Bongiorni MG, Soldati E, Zucchelli G et al (2008) Transvenous removal of pacing and implantable cardiac defibrillating leads using single sheath mechanical dilatation and multiple venous approaches: high success rate and safety in more than 2000 leads. Eur Heart J 29(23):2886–2893
54. Korkeila P, Nyman K, Ylitalo A et al (2007) Venous obstruction after pacemaker implantation. Pacing Clin Electrophysiol 30(2):199–206
55. Lickfett L, Bitzen A, Arepally A et al (2004) Incidence of venous obstruction following insertion of an implantable cardioverter defibrillator. A study of systematic contrast venography on patients presenting for their first elective ICD generator replacement. Europace 6(1):25–31
56. Haghjoo M, Nikoo MH, Fazelifar AF et al (2007) Predictors of venous obstruction following pacemaker or implantable cardioverter-defibrillator implantation: a contrast venographic study on 100 patients admitted for generator change lead revision or device upgrade. Europace 9(5):328–332
57. Aryana A, Sobota KD, Esterbrooks DJ, Gelbman AI (2007) Superior vena cava syndrome induced by endocardial defibrillator and pacemaker leads. Am J Cardiol 99(12):1765–1767
58. Melzer C, Lembcke A, Ziemer S et al (2006) Pacemaker-induced superior vena cava syndrome: clinical evaluation of long-term follow-up. Pacing Clin Electrophysiol 29(12):1346–1351
59. van Rooden CJ, Molhoek SG, Rosendaal FR et al (2004) Incidence and risk factors of early venous thrombosis associated with permanent pacemaker leads. J Cardiovasc Electrophysiol 15(11):1258–1262
60. Sticherling C, Chough SP, Baker RL et al (2001) Prevalence of central venous occlusion in patients with chronic defibrillator leads. Am Heart J 141(5):813–816
61. Bracke F, Meijer A, Van Gelder B (2003) Venous occlusion of the access vein in patients referred for lead extraction: influence of patient and lead characteristics. Pacing Clin Electrophysiol 26(8):1649–1652
62. Worley SJ, Gohn DC, Pulliam RW (2008) Over the wire lead extraction and focused force venoplasty to regain venous access in a totally occluded subclavian vein. J Interv Card Electrophysiol 23(2):135–137
63. Bakir I, La Meir M, Degrieck I et al (2005) Contralateral replacement of pacemaker and leads following laser sheath extraction and concomitant stenting for superior vena cava syndrome. Pacing Clin Electrophysiol 28(10):1131–1134
64. Gilard M, Pérennes A, Mansourati J et al (2002) Stent implantation for the treatment of superior vena cava syndrome related to pacemaker leads. Europace 4(2):155–158
65. Worley SJ (2008) Implant venoplasty: dilation of subclavian and coronary veins to facilitate device implantation: indications frequency methods and complications. J Cardiovasc Electrophysiol 19(9):1004–1007
66. Borek PP, Wilkoff BL (2008) Pacemaker and ICD leads: strategies for long-term management. J Interv Card Electrophysiol 23(1):59–72
67. Korley VJ, Hallet N, Daoust M, Epstein LM (2000) A novel indication for transvenous lead extraction: upgrading implantable cardioverter defibrillator systems. J Interv Card Electrophysiol 4(3):523–528

2 From Guidelines: Definitions, Indications, Facilities, and Outcomes of Transvenous Lead Extraction

Roberto Verlato, Maria Stella Baccillieri and Pietro Turrini

2.1 Introduction

Lead removal is removal of a pacing or defibrillator lead using any technique. It includes two completely different procedures: lead explant and lead extraction. Lead explant is the removal of a lead using simple traction techniques, which is usually possible for leads implanted for less than 1 year. Lead extraction is removal of a lead implanted for more than 1 year or that requires the assistance of specialized equipment in order to be removed. Lead extraction is by far the more complex procedure. As it carries some risks for the patient, clear indications, expertly trained personnel, adequate tools, and appropriate environment and facilities are mandatory for its safe removal [1, 2].

When considering indications for lead extraction, whatever they be, it is important to first evaluate the strength of the indication and the risks of the intervention on an individualized patient basis. Thereafter, the risk/benefit ratio of each patient should be balanced with the level of experience of the operator. Age, sex, body mass index, lead implant duration, number of leads, even small calcifications of fibrosis along the lead, venous thrombosis, systemic infection, presence of large vegetations, pacemaker dependency, and physical characteristics of the lead (intrinsic fragility and tensile robustness) are all factors associated with increased procedural risk [2]. Infections, lead malfunction, actual or potential lead failure, interference between multiple leads, lead-induced life-threatening arrhythmias, lead interference with malignancy treatment, chronic pain, and subclavian vein/superior vena cava (SVC) thrombosis are clinical situations most commonly requiring lead removal/extraction in order to be completely alleviated.

Indications for transvenous lead removal, first published in 2000 as a North American Society of Pacing and Electrophysiology (NASPE) Policy Statement [1], have been recently revised and reported in the format established for the American College of Cardiology/American Heart Association's methodology for practice guidelines (Class I, Class II, and Class III, Level of Evidencea, b, and C) [3] in a Heart Rhythm Society Expert Consensus on Training, Facilities and Indications for Management of Patients requiring lead extraction [2]. These indications are summarized in Tables 2.1–2.5.

2.2 Indications for Lead Removal: Infections

Cardiovascular implantable electronic device (CIED)-associated infections are the strongest indication for complete removal of the device and leads [4–20]. Initially described in the early 1970s [21, 22], CIED infection has been subsequently reported to occur in 1–7% of patients [23–27]. Cabell et al. recently reported the CIED infection rate among Medicare beneficiaries from 1994 to 1999 [28] . During this period CIED implantation rates substantially increased by 42%, from 2.37 to 3.16 procedures/1,000 beneficiaries, respectively, from 1994 to 1999. During this same period, rates of device infections increased by 124%, from 0.94 to 2.11 cases/1,000 beneficiaries. The rates of hospitalization for CIED infection continued to

R. Verlato (✉)
Interventional Electrophysiology Unit, Cardiovascular Department, P. Cosma Hospital, Camposampiero (PD), Italy

M. G. Bongiorni (Ed.), *Transvenous Lead Extraction*.

Table 2.1 Indications for transvenous lead extraction: infection

Recommendations	Level of evidence
Class I	
1. Complete device and lead removal is recommended in all patients with definite CIED system infection, as evidenced by valvular endocarditis, lead endocarditis, or sepsis	A
2. Complete device and lead removal is recommended in all patients with CIED pocket infection as evidenced by pocket abscess, device erosion, skin adherence, or chronic draining sinus without clinically evident involvement of the transvenous portion of the lead system	B
3. Complete device and lead removal is recommended in all patients with valvular endocarditis without definite involvement of the lead(s) and/or device	B
4. Complete device and lead removal is recommended in patients with occult gram-positive bacteremia (not contaminant)	B
Class IIa	
1. Complete device and lead removal is reasonable in patients with persistent occult gram-negative bacteremia	B
Class III	
1. CIED removal is not indicated for a superficial or incisional infection without involvement of the device and/or leads	C
2. CIED removal is not indicated to treat chronic bacteremia due to a source other than the CIED, when long-term suppressive antibiotics are required	C

CIED, cardiovascular implantable electronic device

Table 2.2 Indications for transvenous lead extraction: chronic pain

Recommendations	Level of evidence
Class IIa	
1. Device and/or lead removal is reasonable in patients with severe chronic pain, at the device or lead insertion site, that causes significant discomfort for the patient, is not manageable by medical or surgical techniques, and for which there is no acceptable alternative	C

Table 2.3 Indications for transvenous lead extraction: thrombosis or venous stenosis

Recommendations	Level of evidence
Class I	
1. Lead removal is recommended in patients with clinically significant thromboembolic events associated with thrombus on a lead or a lead fragment	C
2. Lead removal is recommended in patients with bilateral subclavian vein or SVC occlusion precluding implantation of a needed transvenous lead	C
3. Lead removal is recommended in patients with planned stent deployment in a vein already containing a transvenous lead, to avoid lead entrapment	C
4. Lead removal is recommended in patients with SVC stenosis or occlusion with limiting symptoms	C
5. Lead removal is recommended in patients with ipsilateral venous occlusion preventing access to the venous circulation for required placement of an additional lead when there is a contraindication for using the contralateral side (e.g., contralateral AV fistula, shunt or vascular access port, mastectomy)	C
Class IIa	
1. Lead removal is reasonable in patients with ipsilateral venous occlusion preventing access to the venous circulation for required placement of an additional lead, when there is no contraindication for using the contralateral side	C

SVC, superior vena cava; *AV*, atrioventricular

Table 2.4 Indications for transvenous lead extraction: functional leads without infection

Recommendations	Level of evidence
Class I	
1. Lead removal is recommended in patients with life-threatening arrhythmias secondary to retained leads	B
2. Lead removal is recommended in patients with leads that, due to their design or their failure, may pose an immediate threat if left in place (e.g., Telectronics ACCUFIX J-wire fracture with protrusion)	C
3. Lead removal is recommended in patients with leads that interfere with the operation of implanted cardiac devices	B
4. Lead removal is recommended in patients with leads that interfere with the treatment of a malignancy (radiation/reconstructive surgery)	C
Class IIa	
1. Lead removal is reasonable in patients who require specific imaging techniques (e.g., MRI) that cannot be imaged due to the presence of the CIED system for which there is no other available imaging alternative for diagnosis	C
Class IIb	
1. Lead removal may be considered in patients with an abandoned functional lead that poses a risk of interference with the operation of the active CIED system	C
2. Lead removal may be considered in patients with functioning leads that, due to their design or their failure, pose a potential future threat if left in place (e.g., Telectronics ACCUFIX without protrusion)	C
3. Lead removal may be considered in patients with leads that are functional but not being used (i.e., RV pacing lead after upgrade to ICD)	C
4. Lead removal may be considered to permit implantation of an MRI-conditional CIED system	C
Class III	
1. Lead removal is not indicated in patients with functional but redundant leads if patients have a life expectancy <1 year	C
2. Lead removal is not indicated in patients with known anomalous placement of leads through structures other than normal venous and cardiac structures (e.g., subclavian artery, aorta, pleura, atrial or ventricular wall or mediastinum) or through a systemic venous atrium or systemic ventricle. Additional techniques including surgical backup may be used if the clinical scenario is compelling	C

MRI, magnetic resonance imaging; *RV*, right ventricle; *ICD*, implantable cardioverter–defibrillator; *CIED*, cardiovascular implantable electronic device

increase faster than rates of device implantations and at an accelerate rate from 1996 to 2003, with a dramatic increase after 2000 [29]. Pacemaker infection increased in this period 2.8-fold and implantable cardioverter–defibrillator (ICD) infection sixfold. The exact reasons of such an increase are not clear. However, the shift toward ICD use for primary prevention of sudden death and for cardiac resynchronization therapy (CRT) alone, but mostly with a defibrillation backup, to treat patients with advanced refractory heart failure [25–27], may play a role primarily due to the disadvantaged health status of such cohorts of patients. Longer interventions and more leads are other factors that might explain the increased risk of postimplant infection. On the other hand, the improved survival rates in patients bearing cardiac devices probably leads to an increase in the number of "at risk" days for an infective complication to appear [29]. A population-based study of all adult patients with cardiac devices and who resided in Olmsted County, Minnesota, USA, from 1975 to 2004 reported an incidence of definite device infection of 1.9/1,000 device-years. The

Table 2.5 Indications for transvenous lead extraction: nonfunctional leads without infection

Recommendations	Level of evidence
Class I	
1. Lead removal is recommended in patients with life-threatening arrhythmias secondary to retained leads or lead fragments	B
2. Lead removal is recommended in patients with leads that, due to design or failure, may pose an immediate threat if left in place (e.g., Telectronics ACCUFIX J-wire fracture with protrusion)	C
3. Lead removal is recommended in patients with leads that interfere with the operation of implanted cardiac devices	B
4. Lead removal is recommended in patients with leads that interfere with the treatment of a malignancy (radiation/reconstructive surgery)	C
5. Lead removal is recommended for patients who require specific imaging techniques (e.g., MRI), for which there is no other available imaging alternative for diagnosis, and cannot be imaged due to the presence of the CIED system	C
Class IIa	
1. Lead removal is reasonable in patients with leads that, due to design or failure, pose a threat that is not immediate or imminent if left in place (e.g., Telectronics ACCUFIX without protrusion)	C
2. Lead removal is reasonable in patients if a CIED implantation would require more than four leads on one side or five through the SVC	C
3. Lead removal is recommended in order to permit implantation of an MRI-conditional CIED system	C
Class IIb	
1. Lead removal may be considered in patients with nonfunctional leads if contraindications are absent	C
Class III	
1. Lead removal is not indicated in patients with nonfunctional leads if patient's life expectancy is <1 year	C
2. Lead removal is not indicated in patients with known anomalous placement of leads through structures other than normal venous and cardiac structures (e.g., subclavian artery, aorta, pleura, atrial or ventricular wall, or mediastinum) or through a systemic venous atrium or systemic ventricle. Additional techniques including surgical backup may be used if the clinical scenario is compelling	C

SVC, superior vena cava; *MRI,* magnetic resonance imaging; *CIED,* cardiovascular implantable electronic device

Legends of Tables 2.1–2.5 Classification of recommendations and level of evidence according to the American College of Cardiology/American Heart Association [3]

Classification of recommendations

Class I: Conditions for which there is evidence and/or general agreement that a given procedure or treatment is useful and effective.

Class II: Conditions for which there is conflicting evidence and/or a divergence of opinion about the usefulness/efficacy of a procedure or treatment.
- IIa: Weight of evidence/opinion is in favor of usefulness/efficacy
- IIb: Usefulness/efficacy is less well established by evidence/opinion

Class III: Conditions for which there is evidence and/or general agreement that the procedure/treatment is not useful or effective and in some cases may be harmful

Level of evidence

A Data derived from multiple randomized clinical trials or meta-analyses

B Data derived from a single randomized trial, or non-randomized studies

C Consensus opinion of experts, case studies, or standard of care

Note: Assigning a Level of Evidence B or C should not be construed as implying that the recommendation is weak. Many important clinical questions addressed in this document either do not lend themselves to experimentation or have not yet been addressed by high-quality investigations; the authors of this document feel it was important to include all recommendations.

incidence of pocket infection without systemic infection was 1.37/1,000 device-years, and the incidence of pocket infection with systemic infection or lead endocarditis was 1.14/1,000 device-years [4]. The cumulative probability of device infection was higher among patients with ICD compared with those with pacemaker. By applying these infection-rate incidences to the 3.25 million patients with a functioning CIED worldwide [11], we can extrapolate that at least 7,500 new CIED infections will occur yearly.

Several host- and procedure-related risk factors have been reported to increase the probability of permanent CIED infection. In a retrospective analysis, Sohail et al. [5] identified previous CIED infection, malignancy, long-term corticosteroid use, multiple device revisions, a permanent central venous catheter, the presence of more than two leads, and a lack of antibiotic prophylaxis at the time of CIED implant or replacement as risk factors for subsequent pacing system infection. The large multicenter Prospective Evaluation of Pacemaker Lead Endocarditis (PEOPLE) study reported by Klug et al. in 2007 [6] found that fever within 24 h before the implantation procedure, use of temporary pacing before implantation procedure, and early reinterventions were positively correlated with infection occurrence. Implantation of a new system and antibiotic prophylaxis were negatively correlated with risk of infection in this study. The usefulness of antibiotic prophylaxis before the implantation procedure to reduce infection risk was also found in a meta-analysis of all published studies [30]. Re-opening the CIED pocket for any reason and CIED replacement both increase the infection rate. Harcombe et al. [31] studied 2,861 patients who underwent transvenous pacemaker implantation or replacement. The global infection rate during follow-up was 1.48%. However, patients who underwent pacemaker replacement had significantly higher infection rates (6.48% vs 1.4%, $P < 0.001$) compared with patients who underwent their first implant. Wilkoff [10] observed that generator changes or device upgrades are associated with increased risk of infection compared with primary implants – 3% vs 0.5%, respectively. Another recent experience suggests that even apparently simple reinterventions such as ICD replacement carry a high risk of complications [32]. In this study, ICD generator replacement in patients with advisory devices was associated with a substantial rate of complications, including infections and death. Among 2,915 patients with recalled ICDs at 17 Canadian centers, 533 (18.3%) had their device replaced. Among them, complications occurred in 43 patients (8.1%). In particular, infection occurred in 1.9%, pocket hematoma requiring reintervention in 2.3%, and lead malfunction requiring further reoperation in 1.5% of patients. All the above-mentioned studies suggest that opening the pocket of an implanted CIED is a risky maneuver that should be performed only if strictly necessary.

More than two thirds of CIED infections will occur in the pacemaker generator pocket; lead endocarditis and systemic infection account for the remaining cases [11, 12]. The absolute rates of septicemia and endocarditis in published studies are actually in the range of 0.5–2% [10, 12, 16, 20, 24, 25]. Staphylococci genes account for the vast majority of device-related infections [33]. Either coagulase-negative staphylococci or *S. aureus* are the most common pathogens identified according to the case series reported [9–16]. Other types of skin flora produce infection less frequently. Gram-negative organisms are rarely involved in CIED infection, even in the presence of Gram-negative bacteremia [7]. Other Gram-positive cocci and fungi, particularly *Candida* species, cause a minority of device-related infections. Multidrug resistance is common and reflects the nosocomial origin of many of these infections. A major mechanism contributing to either pacemaker- or lead-related intravascular infection is biofilm formation capability [18,34–36] by most of *S. epidermidis* strains obtained from patients with CIED infection. Biofilm, consisting of infecting microorganisms and extracellular matrix, forms on the surface of an indwelling medical device and serves as a protected environment for microorganisms. It is believed that mature biofilm formation is predominantly responsible for the inability of the host immune response and antimicrobial therapy to clear device-related infections [34–36]. Because of this protected environment, device removal to achieve infection cure is usually required.

Current indications for lead extraction to cure CIED infections are summarized in Table 2.1. There are four Class I indications for transvenous lead extraction. The first is the presence of a definite CIED system infection, as evidenced by valvular endocarditis, lead endocarditis, or sepsis. The modified Duke Criteria for Infective Endocarditis should be used to make this diagnosis [37]. A diagnosis of infective endocarditis is based on the presence of either major or minor criteria. Major criteria in the Duke strategy include pathological and clinical findings. Microorganisms demonstrated by culture or histological examination of a vegetation, an embolized vegetation, an intracardiac abscess specimen, and vegetation or intracardiac abscess confirmed by histological examination showing active endocarditis are the major pathological criteria for definitive diagnosis. The two major clinical criteria are more than one positive blood culture and positive echocardiogram defined as follows: oscillating intracardiac mass on valves or on supporting structures in the path of regurgitant jets or on implanted material in the absence of an alternative anatomic explanation, abscess, new partial dehiscence of prosthetic valve, or new valvular regurgitation. To make the correct echocardiographic diagnosis of lead-related endocarditis, transesophageal echocardiogram is mandatory. The sensitivity of transthoracic echo for detecting endocarditis is indeed very low, at around 30%. The addition of transesophageal echo increases sensitivity to 100% [38] (Fig. 2.1). The reason is that in pacemaker/ICD infective endocarditis, vegetation formation is not limited to the tricuspid valve but can be found anywhere along the course of the electrode; transesophageal imaging is therefore necessary to visualize masses, especially at the SVC level. Minor criteria for infective endocarditis are represented by fever, vascular phenomena, major arterial emboli, septic pulmonary infarcts, mycotic aneurysm, intracranial hemorrhage, conjunctival hemorrhages, Janeway lesions, immunologic phenomena (glomerulonephritis, Osler's nodes, Roth's spots, and rheumatoid factor), one positive blood culture, or serological evidence of active infection with organism consistent with infective endocarditis. A definite CIED-related endocarditis should be diagnosed in the presence of two major criteria, one major criterion and three minor criteria, or five minor criteria.

Several sources for infection of CIED pocket and leads have been postulated. One possible source is contamination at the time of device implantation. Pocket infection can also complicate cutaneous erosion of the generator or defibrillator. Microorganisms from the pacemaker/ICD pocket can spread along the electrode to the endocardium and the electrode tip. Additional possible sources of CIEDs include hematogenous seeding of the endovascular electrode during transient bacteremia related to a pocket infection or to an unrelated infection site [33].

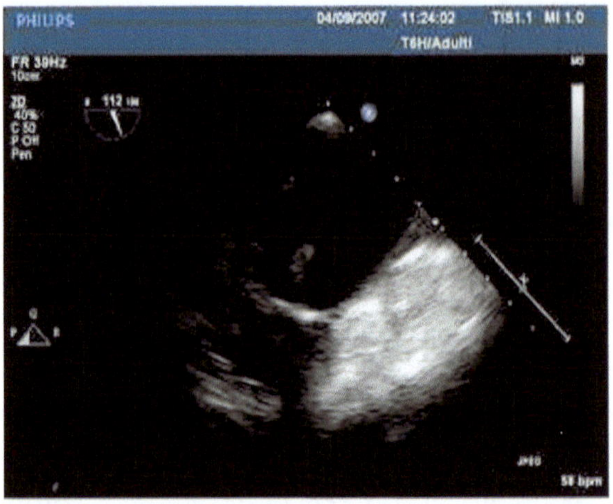

Fig. 2.1 Transesophageal echocardiographic view of the right atrium and the right ventricle. There is an oblong mobile vegetation adherent to the pacing lead as it crosses the tricuspid valve attached to its ventricular portion. Patient had positive blood cultures for *Staphylococcus lugdunensis*. Both these findings are major criteria for the diagnosis of lead endocarditis

There are no prospective studies that compare cure rates for antibiotic treatment alone vs antibiotic therapy combined with CIED system removal. However, the high rate of uncontrolled or relapsing bacteremia, even after prolonged medical therapy, makes removal of the entire CIED system optimal. In one recent retrospective case analysis [11] that included patients with an infected pacemaker or ICD, infection relapse was strongly associated with failure to completely remove all hardware. This case series included 123 patients, 119 (97%) of whom had transvenous implanted leads. Only one (0.86%) of 117 patients who underwent removal of their entire system had infection relapse. In contrast, three of six (50%, $P = 0.003$) without complete hardware removal suffered relapse. The only patient who had hardware removal and still had infection relapse had a new generator implanted in an old pocket site. All other patients had new devices placed at different sites at a later date. The mortality rate in patients with pacemaker/ICD endocarditis treated with antibiotics alone ranges from 31% to 66% [15, 39, 40]. In contrast, the mortality rate in patients who had combined antibiotics and electrode removal was only 18% (range 13–33%) in one literature review [41]. Another series also reported failure to remove an infected indwelling intravascular device to be associated with increased all-cause mortality [42]. Patients whose infected pacemaker or ICD was not removed had an almost threefold (47.6% vs 16.7%) increased risk of dying.

New embolization without clinical sequelae has been reported during intravascular extraction in 30% of 33 patients with vegetations >10 mm [15]. Surgical extraction is favored by some for patients with larger vegetations; however, two deaths from septic complications occurred in ten patients after surgical lead extraction [15]. Others have found no evidence that endovascular removal of larger vegetations is deleterious [12, 42, 43]. In a recent experience [12], 189 patients with CIED infection, 23% of them with device-related endocarditis, underwent complete device and lead removal. The diameter of vegetations ranged from 0.3 to 7 cm in the longest dimension. None of the patients developed clinical manifestations of pulmonary embolism as a complication of percutaneous lead extraction. Ninety-six percent of patients were completely cured of infection with complete system removal and antibiotic administration. Based on all the above-mentioned studies, lead extraction performed without delay is necessary to cure and improve clinical outcome of patients with CIED-related systemic infection.

CIED pocket infection as evidenced by pocket abscess, device erosion, skin adherence, or chronic draining sinus (Figs. 2.2–2.4), without clinically evident involvement of the transvenous portion of the lead system have become the second Class I indication for lead extraction in the new guidelines [2]. In the 2000 NASPE Policy Statement on Lead Extraction [1], these CIED infections were considered a Class II indication, (conditions for which leads were often removed, but there was some divergence of opinion with respect to the benefit vs risk of removal) when the lead could be cut through a clean incision totally separated from the infected area. This criterion is not mentioned in current guidelines. Indeed the experience with local treatment of CIED devices has been disappointing through the years [10–12, 44–47]. There is now enough evidence that complete removal of all device hardware is critical to consistently and effectively treat any infected device systems [10–12]. As there is usually a long time period

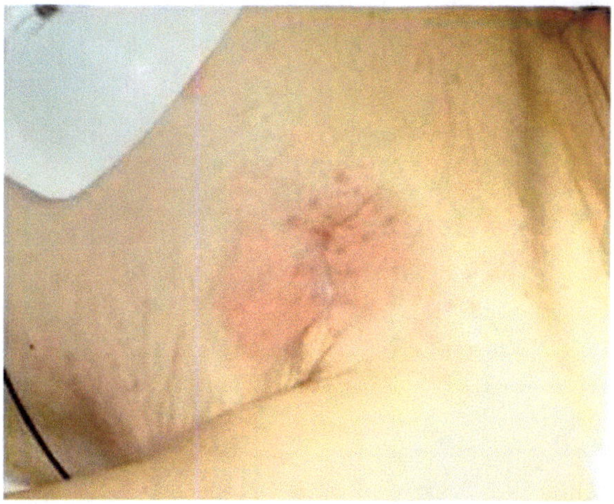

Fig. 2.2 Superficial cellulitis, local adhesion, and modest remodeling of the anterior chest wall tissues caused by fat necrosis due to a pacemaker pocket infection. There is a small amount of bruising in the middle of the erythema. This represents an infection recurrence after three attempts of local debridement to cure pocket infection without lead extraction

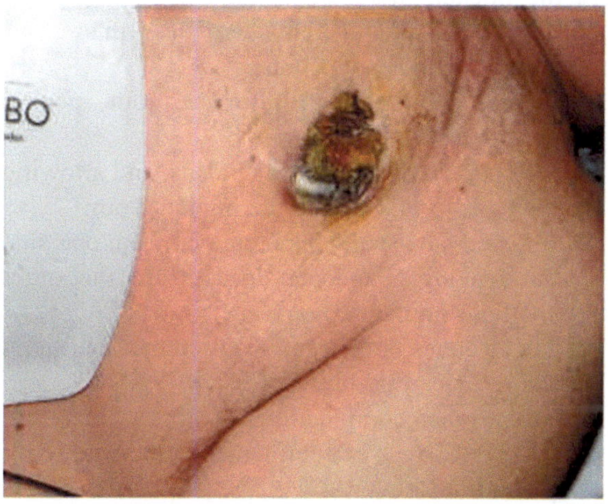

Fig. 2.3 Implantable cardioverter–defibrillator (ICD)-pocket erosion. Part of the ICD header and can are visible. There is evidence of drainage of purulent material and blood from the ulceration without cellulitis. There is a slight bluish discoloring of tissues immediately caudal to the exposed portion of the ICD. Also note multiple scars (five) due to previous attempts to cure pocket infection without extraction of all the hardware, ICD, and leads

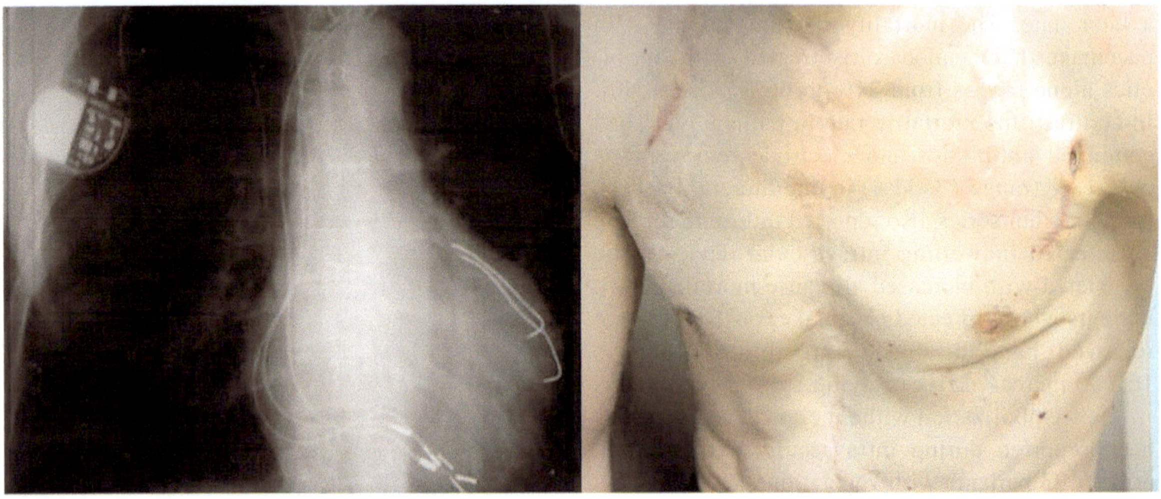

Fig. 2.4 *Left panel*: Multiple endocardial and epicardial leads are visible. A functional lead is connected with a right-sided pacemaker. *Right panel*: Lead erosion. Part of the lead body is exposed. No cellulitis is visible. Infection and lead erosion recurred despite multiple local interventions on the left side without lead removal

between local treatment and infection recurrence in the pocket, there are a number of reports of apparently successful cures with less than complete removal. These include:

1. Device removal with or without pocket debridement;
2. Device removal, cutting the leads, and allowing the ends to retract into the implant vein;
3. Infected device and lead removal from one side but leaving abandoned leads from the other shoulder implanted;
4. Transvenous device and lead removal but leaving in epicardial leads;
5. Many other combinations of approaches with various degrees of debridement and acute reimplantation.

All of these approaches will work but will not ultimately prove to be consistently effective, particularly when the duration of follow-up is extended (Figs. 2.3–2.5). Effectiveness is also dependent on the virulence of the infecting pathogen. Several patients will finally undergo lead extraction after seven or eight prior revisions, often with years in between recurrent manifest infections. To avoid open surgical extractions and multiple disfiguring scars and chest remodeling (Fig. 2.4), it is best to perform at the beginning complete extraction of all hardware, complete debridement of the infected scar tissue, no reimplantation at the primary extraction procedure, sustained antibiotic therapy (minimum 2 weeks), and reimplantation of a new CIED at a remote anatomic location [2, 10]. Another reason to perform lead extraction at the beginning is the high prevalence of involvement of the intravascular segment of the lead in patients with only local symptoms of pocket infection. Klug et al. [18] studied 105 patients with local inflammatory findings, impending or frank pocket or lead exteriorization, but without signs of systemic infection. After lead extraction was performed, both intravascular and extravascular lead segments were collected and blood and lead-segment cultures were performed. Swab cultures from the CIED pocket were performed as well. Regardless of the initial presentation, the intravascular part of the leads gave positive cultures in 79.3% of patients. Additionally, 91.6% of the extravascular lead segments were positive, in contrast to only 38.1% positivity for wound swab cultures. After extraction, infection recurred in 4/8 patients (50%) without complete lead body extraction and in only 1/97 (1%) whose leads had been completely extracted. These data suggest that a definite risk of progression from local to systemic infection exists and this should prompt the extraction of the leads even in the absence of other infectious manifestations [18].

Complete device and lead removal is recommended also in all patients with valvular endocarditis without definite involvement lead and/or

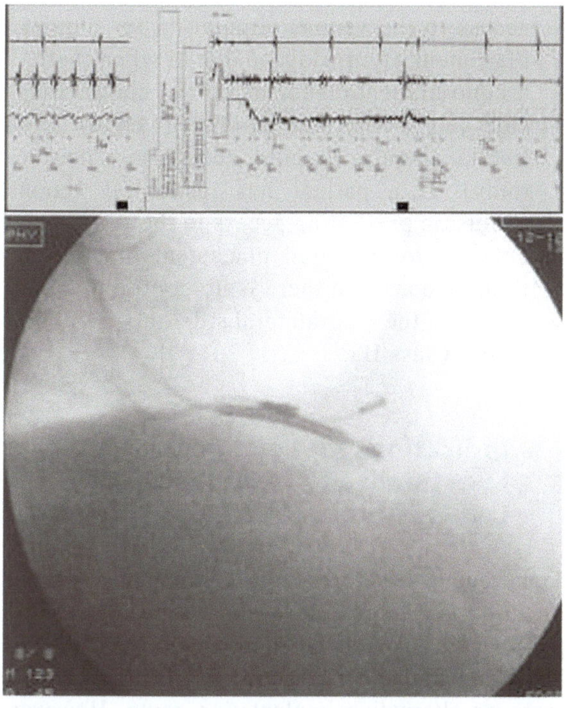

Fig. 2.5 *Upper panel*: Stored intracardiac electrogram of a ventricular tachycardia (VT) episode from a cardiac defibrillator in a patient with two right ventricular leads. A true VT with atrioventricular dissociation is present, and an implantable cardioverter–defibrillator 11-joules shock is appropriately delivered. Postshock noise oversensing is clearly visible, causing inhibition of pacing and ventricular fibrillation oversensing. The noise is due to interference between an abandoned single-pass atrioventricular pacing–sensing lead and a functioning defibrillation lead. *Lower panel*: Close-up of chest X-ray demonstrating the close proximity between a bipolar ventricular lead, which had been abandoned, and the proximal coil of a functional defibrillation lead

device involvement. It is impossible in such cases to exclude CIED system involvement as the source of bacteremia. On the other hand, the immunological depression induced by endocarditis and the persistent endocarditis-related bacteremia are heavy risk factors for a secondary seeding of the intravascular lead portion, finally resulting in a lead endocarditis.

Complete device and lead removal is also recommended in patients with occult Gram-positive bacteremia (not contaminant) [11, 13, 15, 21–37], in particular, if *S. aureus* is isolated [41]. Gram-negative bacteremia is not usually indicative of CIED-related infection [7]. However, in case of persistent occult Gram-negative bacteremia, complete device and lead extraction is reasonable. This is the only Class II indication for CIED infection mentioned in the recent Heart Rhythm Society (HRS) Expert Consensus [2]. In the presence of a superficial or incisional infection without involvement of the device and/or leads as well as of chronic bacteremia due to a source other than the CIED, when long-term suppressive antibiotics are required, lead extraction is never indicated and should not be performed.

2.3 Indications for Lead Removal: Chronic Pain

Device and/or lead removal is reasonable in patients with severe chronic pain at the device or lead insertion site that causes significant discomfort, is not manageable by medical or surgical techniques, and for which there is no acceptable alternative. This is a Class IIa indication for lead extraction with a level of evidence C based on the personal experience and opinion of HRS Expert Consensus members.

2.4 Indications for Lead Removal: Venous Stenosis or Occlusion

Whereas symptomatic subclavian vein occlusion with pacemaker/ICD leads is rare, occurring in the range of 0.35–3.5% [48, 49], some degree of asymptomatic obstruction may be seen in up to 50% of patients [50]. The results of numerous randomized trials demonstrating the efficacy of cardiac defibrillators in preventing sudden cardiac death and of cardiac resynchronization therapy to treat patients with advanced congestive heart failure [25–27] have led to an ever-expanding population of candidates for such device therapy. A significant proportion of patients with congestive heart failure have existing transvenous right atrial (RA) and right ventricular (RV) leads, which may further impair systolic and diastolic left ventricular (LV) function by inducing wall-motion abnormalities [51, 52]. Such patients may therefore have the most to gain from an upgrade of their existing pacemaker or ICD to biventricular systems, along with potential upgrade of existing pacemaker to prophylactic ICD therapy. The existence of central venous stenosis or occlusion, even if asymptomatic, is an obstacle to device upgrade that can be managed by a variety of options: the existing system can be abandoned, with placement of an entirely new system on the contralateral side; a contralateral LV lead can be transvenously placed and tunneled across the chest to the existing system; an epicardial LV lead can be placed via thoracotomy. However, an alternative and feasible approach is an ipsilateral upgrade after extraction of the existing leads facilitated by the use of sheaths [53]. The vein is recanalized by the sheath, and venous access is gained through the same sheath after lead extraction. Subclavian vein angioplasty may be required to regain complete venous access in some patients [54]. The use of laser sheaths has been reported to be most effective for subclavian vein recanalization [53, 55]. In a minority of permanently paced patients, SVC obstruction develops due the presence of pacing leads, which is a serious complication often requiring thoracotomy and surgical treatment [56, 57], carrying a significant morbidity rate. During the past decade, several reports have been published demonstrating that SVC obstruction and the associated clinical syndrome can be effectively and safely treated by "one-step" percutaneous intervention [58–63]. The intervention consists of percutaneous retrieval of all the pacing leads, followed by venous revascularization with angioplasty and stenting, and finally installation of a new device. It would be inappropriate to stent open a vein, which would trap the pacing leads against the vein wall and prevent future safe lead extraction. Current recommendations for lead extraction in the presence of venous stenosis or occlusions are illustrated in Table 2.3. They include:

1. Significant thromboembolic events associated with thrombus on a lead or a lead fragment;
2. Bilateral subclavian vein or SVC occlusion precluding implantation of a needed transvenous lead;
3. Planned stent deployment in a vein already containing a transvenous lead to avoid lead entrapment;
4. SVC stenosis or occlusion with limiting symptoms;
5. Ipsilateral venous occlusion preventing access to the venous circulation for required placement of an additional lead when there is a contraindication for using the contralateral side [e.g., contralateral arteriovenous (AV) fistula, shunt or vascular access port, mastectomy]. If a patient has ipsilateral venous occlusion preventing access to the venous circulation for required placement of an additional lead, when there is no contraindication for using the contralateral side, this is considered a Class IIa.

2.5 Indications for Lead Removal: Functional and Nonfunctional Leads Without Infection

Transvenous lead extraction for patients without infection is a more controversial topic. It is often possible to abandon failed or no longer required leads and implant the needed lead(s) through the same or alternative implantation route. However, there are several important considerations that favor earlier lead extraction instead of abandonment. First of all, abandoned leads will be more difficult to remove with prolonged implant duration, with an increased risk of major complications [44, 64, 65]. The risk during extraction increases as interlead fibrosis thickens and covers more of the surface of the lead, especially if there are multiple leads [66, 67]. Lead fragility increases as implant duration lengthens due to chemical and mechanical stresses and calcifications [44, 64–68]. In particular, in young people with more than one implanted lead, implanting a new lead(s) without extracting the old ones is usually inadvisable. Whether it is really safe to abandon a nonfunctioning pacing or defibrillating lead remains controversial. Bohm et al. followed 60 patients with noninfected retained leads [69]. Complications were observed during follow-up in 12 patients (20%), including lead migration, skin erosion, venous thrombosis, and muscle stimulation. Suga et al. studied 433 patients with 531 abandoned leads [70]. Complications were observed during follow-up in 24 patients (5.5%), infection in eight, and other difficulties in 16. Young age at implant, the presence of three or more abandoned leads or four or more total leads, and two or more previous procedures were predictive factors of future complications. On the other hand, two recent studies suggested that abandoning a nonfunctioning lead does not pose a clinically significant additional risk of future complications during short/midterm follow-up [71, 72]. However, two of 18 children (>10%) with an abandoned lead developed lead endocarditis after 5 and 10 years, respectively, as reported by Silvetti and Drago [71]. Even if it has been suggested that a nonfunctioning defibrillation lead can be abandoned without risk of future complications [72], noise oversensing caused by interaction between the abandoned and functional endocardial ventricular leads has been definitely demonstrated [73, 74], and it is a frequent cause of inappropriate shocks in daily clinical practice (Fig. 2.5). Therefore, removal of an abandoned lead that could otherwise interfere with normal detection of arrhythmias by an ICD should always be considered. Another particular situation prompting lead extraction is represented by leads such as the Telectronics Accufix, which could fracture, leaving the J retention wire protruding outside the lead body, representing a life-threatening situation due to the risk of perforation of the heart and/or of the great vessels [75–78]. Indications for removal of functional or nonfunctional leads without infection are summarized in Tables 2.4 and 2.5. They include:

1. Life-threatening arrhythmias secondary to retained leads or lead fragments;
2. Leads that, due to their design or their failure, may pose an immediate threat to patients if left in place;
3. Leads that interfere with the operation of implanted cardiac devices;
4. Leads that interfere with treatment of a malignancy (radiation/reconstructive surgery);
5. Removal of the complete system, CIED and leads, is finally recommended for patients who require specific imaging techniques [e.g., magnetic resonance imaging (MRI)] and cannot be imaged due to the presence of the CIED system and for which there is no other available imaging alternative to reach a diagnosis.

Less certain indications are represented by:

1. Leads that due to their design or failure pose a threat to the patient and that is not immediate or imminent if left in place;
2. Patients in whom a CIED implantation would require more than four leads on one side or five leads through the SVC.

Removal of noninfected leads is not indicated (Class III) if patients have a life expectancy of less than 1 year and in patients with known anomalous placement of leads through structures other than normal venous and cardiac structures (e.g., subclavian artery, aorta, pleura, atrial or ventricular wall, or mediastinum) or through a systemic venous atrium or systemic ventricle. Additional techniques including surgical backup may be used if the clinical scenario is compelling.

References

1. Love CJ, Wilkoff BL, Byrd CL et al (2000) Recommendations for extraction of chronically implanted transvenous pacing and defibrillator leads: indications, facilities, training. Pacing Clin Electrophysiol 23(4):544–551
2. Wilkoff BL, Love CJ, Byrd CL et al (2009) Transvenous lead extraction: Heart Rhythm Society expert consensus on facilities, training indications and patient management. Heart Rhythm 6:1086-1104
3. ACC/AHA Task Force on Practice Guidelines (2006) Methodology manual for ACC/AHA Guideline Writing Committees. http://www.acc.org/qualityandscience/quality/quality.htm
4. Uslan DZ, Sohail MR, St Sauver JL et al (2007) Permanent pacemaker and implantable cardioverter defibrillator infection: a population-based study. Arch Intern Med 167:669–675
5. Sohail MR, Uslan DZ, Khan AH et al (2007) Risk factor analysis of permanent pacemaker infection. Clin Infect Dis 45:166–173
6. Klug D, Balde M, Pavin D et al (2007) Risk factors related to infections of implanted pacemakers and cardioverter-defibrillators: results of a large prospective study. Circulation 116:1349–1355
7. Urslan DZ, Sohail MR, Friedman PA et al (2006) Frequency of permanent pacemaker or implantable cardioverter-defibrillator infection in patients with gram-negative bacteremia. Clin Infect Dis 43:731–736
8. Bailey SM, Wilkoff BL (2006) Complications of pacemakers and defibrillators in the elderly. Am J Geriatr Cardiol 15:102–107
9. Klug D, Wallet F, Kacet S et al (2005) Detailed bacteriologic tests to identify the origin of transvenous pacing system infections indicate a high prevalence of multiple organisms. Am Heart J 149:322–328
10. Wilkoff BL (2007) How to treat and identify device infections. Heart Rhythm 4:1467–1470
11. Chua DY, Wilkoff BL, Lee I et al (2000) Diagnosis and management of infections involving implantable electrophysiologic cardiac devices. Ann Intern Med 133(8):604–608
12. Sohail MR, Uslan DZ, Khan AH et al (2007) Management and outcome of permanent pacemaker and implantable cardioverter-defibrillator infections. J Am Coll Cardiol 49:1851–1859

13. Road I (1998) Intravascular catheter-related infections. Lancet 351:893–898
14. Dy Chua J, Abdul-Karim A, Mawhorter S et al (2005) The role of swab and tissue culture in the diagnosis of implantable cardiac device infection. Pacing Clin Electrophysiol 28:1276–1281
15. Klug D, Lacroix D, Savoye C et al (1997) Systemic infection related to endocarditis on pacemaker leads: clinical presentation and management. Circulation 95:2098–2107
16. Mansur AJ, Grinberg M, Costa R et al (1984) Dura mater valve endocarditis related to retained fragment of postoperative temporary epicardial pacemaker lead. Am Heart J 108:1049–1052
17. Klug D, Wallet F, Kacet S et al (2003) Involvement of adherence and adhesion *Staphylococcus epidermidis* genes in pacemaker lead-associated infections. J Clin Microbiol 41:3348–3350
18. Klug D, Wallet F, Lacroix D et al (2004) Local symptoms at the site of pacemaker implantation indicate latent systemic infection. Heart 90:882–886
19. Rubio-Alvarez J, Duran-Munoz D, Sierra-Quiroga J et al (1989) Right heart endocarditis and endocardial pacemakers. Ann Thorac Surg 48:147–151
20. Schwartz IS, Pervez N (1971) Bacterial endocarditis associated with a permanent transvenous cardiac pacemaker. JAMA 218:736–737
21. Coman LC, Levison ME (1975) Sustained bacteremia and transvenous cardiac pacemakers. JAMA 233:264–266
22. Bluhm G (1985) Pacemaker infections. Acta Medica Scand Suppl 699:1–62
23. Arber N, Prass E, Copperman Y et al (1994) Pacemaker endocarditis: report of 44 cases and review of the literature. Medicine 73:299–305
24. Del Rio A, Anguera I, Miro JM et al (2003) Surgical treatment of pacemaker and defibrillator lead endocarditis. Impact of electrode lead extraction on outcome. Chest 124:1451–1459
25. Cleland JG, Daubert JC, Erdmann E et al, for the Cardiac Heart Failure (care-HF) Study Investigators (2005) The effect of cardiac resynchronization on morbidity and mortality. N Engl J Med 352:1539–1549
26. Young JB, Abraham WT, Smith AL et al, for the Multicenter Insynch ICD Randomized Clinical Evaluation (MIRACLE ICD) Trial Investigators (2003) Combined cardiac resynchronization and implantable cardioversion defibrillation in advanced chronic heart failure: The MIRACLE ICD Trial. JAMA 289:2719–2721
27. Moss AJ, Zareba W, Hall WJ et al (2002) Prophylactic implantation of a defibrillator in patients with myocardial infarction and reduced ejection fraction. N Engl J Med 346:877–883
28. Cabell CH, Heidenreich PA, Chu VH et al (2004) Increasing rates of cardiac device infections among Medicare beneficiaries: 1990–1999. Am Heart J 147:582–586
29. Voigt A, Shalaby A, Saba S (2006) Rising rates of cardiac rhythm management device infections in the United States: 1996 through 2003. J Am Coll Cardiol 48:590–592
30. Da Costa A, Kirkorian G, Cucherat M et al (1998) Antibiotic prophylaxis for permanent pacemaker implantation: a meta-analysis. Circulation 97:1796–1801
31. Harcombe AA, Newell SA, Ludman PF et al (1998) Late complications following pacemaker implantation or elective unit replacement. Heart 80:240–244
32. Gould PA, Krahn AD, for The Canadian Heart Rhythm Society Working Group on Device Advisories (2006) Complications associated with implantable cardioverter-defibrillator replacement in response to device advisory. JAMA 295:1907–1911
33. Baddour LM, Bettmann MA, Bolger AF et al (2003) Nonvalvular cardiovascular device-related infections. AHA scientific statement. Circulation 108: 2015–2031
34. Donlan RM (2001) Biofilm formation: a clinically relevant microbiological process. Clin Infect Dis 33:1387–1392
35. Bell M (2001) Biofilms: a clinical perspective. Curr Infect Dis Rep. 3:483–486
36. O'Gara JP, Humphreys H (2001) *Staphylococcus epidermidis* biofilms: importance and implications. J Med Microbiol 50:582–587
37. Baddour LM, Wilson RW, Bayer AS et al (2005) Infective endocarditis: diagnosis, antimicrobial therapy, and management of complications. A statement for healthcare professionals from the Committee on Rheumatic Fever, Endocarditis and Kawasaki Disease. Circulation 111:e394–e434
38. Fowler VG, Li J, Corey GR et al (1997) Role of echocardiography in evaluation of patients with *Staphylococcus aureus* bacteremia: experience in 103 patients. J Am Coll Cardiol 30:1072–1078
39. Bracke FA, Meijer A, van Gelder LM (2001) Pacemaker lead complications: when is extraction appropriate and what can we learn from published data? Heart 85:254–259
40. Cacoub P, Leprince P, Nataf P et al (1998) Pacemaker infective endocarditis. Am J Cardiol 82:480–484
41. Chamis AL, Peterson GE, Cabell CH et al (2001) *Staphylococcus aureus* bacteremia in patients with permanent pacemakers or implantable cardioverter-defibrillator. Circulation 104:1029–1033
42. Victor F, De Place C, Camus C et al (1999) Pacemaker lead infection: echocardiographic features, management and outcome. Heart 81:82–87
43. Ruttmann E, Hangler HB, Kilo J et al (2006) Transvenous pacemaker lead removal is safe and effective even in large vegetations: an analysis of 53 cases of pacemaker lead endocarditis. Pacing Clin Electrophysiol 29:231–236
44. Byrd CL (2007) Managing device-related complications and transvenous lead extractions. In Ellenbogen KA, Kay GN, Wilkoff BL, Lau CP (eds.) Clinical cardiac pacing, defibrillation and resynchronization therapy (3rd edn) Saunders, Philadelphia, pp 855–930
45. Lakkireddy DR, Verma A, Wilkoff BL (2005) Current concepts in intravascular pacemaker and defibrillator lead extraction. In: Wang, Paul J (ed) New arrhythmia technologies. Gerald V. Naccarelli, Michael R, Rosen NA, Mark Estes III, David L. Hayes, David E. Haines (co-eds). Blackwell-Futura Publishing, Malden pp 124–133
46. Borek PP, Wilkoff BL (2008) Pacemaker and ICD leads: strategies for long-term management. J Interv Card Electrophysiol 23:59–72
47. Jones SO, Eckart RE, Albert CM et al (2008) Large, single-center, single-operator experience with transvenous lead extraction: outcomes and changing indications. Heart Rhythm 5:520–525

48. Kar AK, Ghosh S, Majundar A et al (2000) Venous obstruction after permanent pacing. Indian Heart J 52:431–433
49. Barakat K, Robinson NM, Spurrell RA (2000) Transvenous pacing lead-induced thrombosis: a series of cases with review of the literature. Cardiology 93:142–148
50. Sticherling C, Chough SP, Baker RL et al (2001) Prevalence of central venous occlusion in patients with chronic defibrillators leads. Am Heart J 141:813–816
51. Tse HF, Lau CP (1997) Long-term effects of right ventricular pacing on myocardial perfusion and function. J Am Coll Cardiol 29:744–749
52. Pastore G, Noventa F, Piovesana PG et al (2008) Left ventricular dyssynchrony resulting from right ventricular apical pacing. Relevance of baseline assessment. Pacing Clin Electrophysiol 31:1456–1462
53. Gula LJ, Ames A, Woodburne A et al (2005) Central venous occlusions not an obstacle to device upgrade with the assistance of laser extraction. Pacing Clin Electrophysiol 28:661–666
54. Worley SJ, Gohn DC, Pulliam RW (2008) Over the wire lead extraction and focused force venoplasty to regain venous access in a totally occluded subclavian vein. J Interv Electrophysiol 23:135–137
55. Henrikson CA, Alexander D, Ringel RE et al (2006) Laser recanalization of the subclavian vein. Pacing Clin Electrophysiol 29:436:437
56. Jarvinen A, Harjiula A, Verkkala K (1986) Intrathoracic surgery for retained endocardial leads. Thorac Cardiovasc Surg 34:94–97
57. Dubernet J, Irarrazaval MJ, Lema G et al (1985) Surgical removal of entrapped endocardial leads without using extracorporeal circulation. Pacing Clin Electrophysiol 8:175–180
58. Chan AW, Bhatt DL, Wilkoff BL et al (2002) Percutaneous treatment for pacemaker-associated superior vena cava syndrome. Pacing Clin Electrophysiol 25:1628–1633
59. Crowe MT, Davies CH, Gaines PA (1995) Percutaneous management of superior vena cava occlusions. Cardiovasc Intervent Radiol 18:367–372
60. Shah R, Sabanathan S, Lowe RA et al (1996) Stenting in malignant obstruction of superior vena cava. J Thorac Cardiovasc Surg 112:335–340
61. Gross CM, Kramer J, Waigand J et al (1997) Stent implantation in patients with superior vena cava syndrome. AJR Am J Roentgenol 169:429–432
62. Schindler N, Vogelzang RL (1999) Superior vena cava syndrome. Experience with endovascular stents and surgical therapy. Surg Clin North Am 79:683–694
63. Oderich GS, Treiman GS, Schneider P et al (2000) Stent placement for treatment of central and peripheral venous obstruction: A long-term multi-institutional experience. J Vasc Surg 32:760–769
64. Byrd CL, Wilkoff BL, Love CJ et al (1999) Intravascular extraction of problematic or infected permanent pacemaker leads: 1994–1996. U.S. Extraction Database, MED Institute. Pacing Clin Electrophysiol 22:1348–1357
65. Wazni O, Epstein LM, RG Carrillo et al (2010) Lead extraction in the contemporary setting: The LExICon Study: An observational retrospective study of consecutive laser lead extractions. J Am Coll Cardiol 55:579–586
66. Anderson JM (1988) Inflammatory response to implants. ASAIO Trans 11:101–107
67. Schoen FJ, Harasaki H, Kim KM et al (1988) Biomaterial-associated calcification: pathology, mechanisms, and strategies for prevention. J Biomed Mater Res 22:11–36
68. Woscoboinik JR, Maloney JD, Helguera ME et al (1992) Pacing lead survival: performance of different models. Pacing Clin Electrophysiol 15:1991–1995
69. Bohm A, Pinter A, Duray G et al (2001) Complications due to abandoned noninfected leads. Pacing Clin Electrophysiol 24:1721–1724
70. Suga C, Hayes DL, Hyberger LK et al (2000) Is there an adverse outcome from abandoned pacing leads? J Interv Card Electrophysiol 4: 493–499
71. Silvetti MS, Drago F (2008) Outcome of young patients with abandoned, nonfunctional endocardial leads. Pacing Clin Electrophysiol 31:473–479
72. Glikson M, Suleiman M, Luria DM et al (2009) Do abandoned leads pose risk to implantable cardioverter-defibrillator patients? Heart Rhythm 6:65–68
73. Pfitzner P, Trappe HJ (1998) Oversensing in a cardiac defibrillator system caused by interaction between two endocardial defibrillation leads in the right ventricle. Pacing Clin Electrophysiol 21:764–768
74. Lickfett L, Wolpert C, Jung W et al (1999) Inappropriate implantable defibrillator discharge caused by a retained pacemaker lead fragment. J Interv Card Electrophysiol 3:163–167
75. Lloyd MA, Hayes DL, Holmes DR Jr et al (1996) Extraction of the Telectronics Accufix 330-801 atrial lead: the Mayo Clinic experience. Mayo Clin Proc 71:230–234
76. Daoud EG, Kou W, Davidson T et al (1996) Evaluation and extraction of the Accufix atrial J lead. Am Heart J 131:266–269
77. Kawanishi DT, Brinker JA, Reeves R et al (1998) Kaplan-Meier analysis of freedom from extraction or death in patients with an Accufix J retention wire atrial permanent pacemaker lead: a potential management tool. Pacing Clin Electrophysiol 21:2318–2321
78. Kawanishi DT, Brinker JA, Reeves R et al (1998) Spontaneous versus extraction related injuries associated with Accufix J-wire atrial pacemaker lead: tracking changes in patient management. Pacing Clin Electrophysiol 21:2314–2317

3 Perioperative Management of Transvenous Lead Extraction

Gianluca Solarino, Andrea Di Cori and Giulio Zucchelli

3.1 Introduction

Since the early 1990s, the development and use of the procedure for removing chronically implanted transvenous lead systems has progressed and involves an ever-growing number of physicians and centers. Due to the possibility of vascular catastrophe and life-threatening events during this procedure, perioperative management, including thorough patient evaluation and preparation, remain key points for a safe and effective procedure. This chapter focuses on appropriate patient management before, during, and after lead extraction.

3.2 Preoperative Evaluation

3.2.1 History and Physical Examination

The extraction process begins with a full patient evaluation, including a review of medical history and current therapy, followed by a complete physical examination. Patient history assessment should include a review of the previous indication for device implantation, the indication for extraction procedure, and control of systemic signs of infection. In case of local or systemic infection, it is very important to verify when symptoms or signs appeared. Physical examination should focus on the pocket device. The pocket should be examined to detect pocket device location (prepectoral or subpectoral position) and signs of local infection (inflammation, erythema, wound dehiscence, skin erosion, purulent drainage, generator exposure). Similarly, ipsilateral arm enlargement with edema, with or without chest-wall collateral veins distension, can suggest venous entry site thrombosis. All these factors may affect procedural duration and procedural-related pain, conditioning the anesthesiological strategy. Several clinical (patient-related) and technical [cardiovascular implantable electronic device (CIED)-related] factors may, indeed, affect not only procedural risk but also interventional strategy:

1. Implant duration: This represents the most important factor affecting difficulty, complexity, and outcome of the removal procedure, being directly related to the development of intravascular fibrosis. Usually, leads implanted 6 months earlier may be removed with manual traction alone [1], whereas procedure complexity and major complication risks increase progressively with implantation time [2]. In addition, the younger the patient at the time of implantation, the more challenging the extraction due to the development of thick, fibrous lead-binding sites.
2. Lead number: As shown in the Lead Extraction Registry [2] the risk of complications and procedural complexity is proportional to the number of leads present because of the possibility of lead–lead binding sites.
3. Lead location: Usually, ventricular leads are more resistant to removal than atrial leads because of their tendency to develop adhesions to the tricuspidal valve and ventricular wall [3]. Moreover, atrial tip detachment from the right appendage may be very challenging for the lead

G. Solarino (✉)
2nd Cardiovascular Department AOUP, Santa Chiara University Hospital, Pisa, Italy

M. G. Bongiorni (Ed.), *Transvenous Lead Extraction*.

course and wall thickness. Coronary sinus (CS) leads are easy to extract by simple traction in the majority of cases due to their low tendency to develop adhesions inside the CS and the relative short period of reimplantation. Sometimes, adhesions are present along the entire course of the lead body – and about 10% of leads inside the CS – and may require mechanical dilatation from the venous entry [4].

4. Lead type: Usually, implantable cardioverter–defibrillator (ICD) leads are considered more difficult to remove than are pacing leads [3]. Indeed, the presence of a large, exposed defibrillating coil can develop large and tenacious adhesions at the superior vena cava (SVC) and tricuspid valve level. However, in our experience, even if ICD lead removal is challenging, the success rate seems to be higher than the pacing lead success rate, with rare failure, fractures, or partial removal. Moreover, the latest generation of ICD leads, including Gore-Tex insulation and isodiametric structure, seems to be related with a lower rate of fibrosis development along the coil [5].
5. Fixation mechanism: Active fixation leads seem to have advantages and disadvantages. On the one hand, once the screw is retracted, the tip can be easily detached from the endocardium, and the lead, being isodiametric, can be removed more easily than the others [6, 7]. On the other hand, an unscrewed lead is more difficult than a tined one. Fixation mechanisms that cannot be unscrewed, such as the Vitatron Helifix, make the procedure more complex, increasing the risks of myocardial perforation and cardiac tamponade.
6. Lead damaged by previous unsuccessful removal attempts: After an unsuccessful transvenous lead extraction (TLE), leads could be seriously damaged. Coil or insulation fracture irreversibly modifies the lead body structure, reducing the procedural success and increasing procedure complexity and complications.
7. Intravascular leads: When no part of the lead can be approached outside the vascular system, a crossover to the transfemoral or transjugular approach is mandatory.
8. J-retention-wire fracture: The design of Telectronics Accufix and Encor leads included insertion and permanent retention of a J wire inside the lead. In some patients, the fractured J wire damaged the outer insulation, lacerating the heart, with fatal tamponade or mediastinal structure damage. If multiple fractures occur, wire fragments can migrate in the blood flow, reaching the pulmonary vein and pulmonary parenchymas (Fig. 3.1)

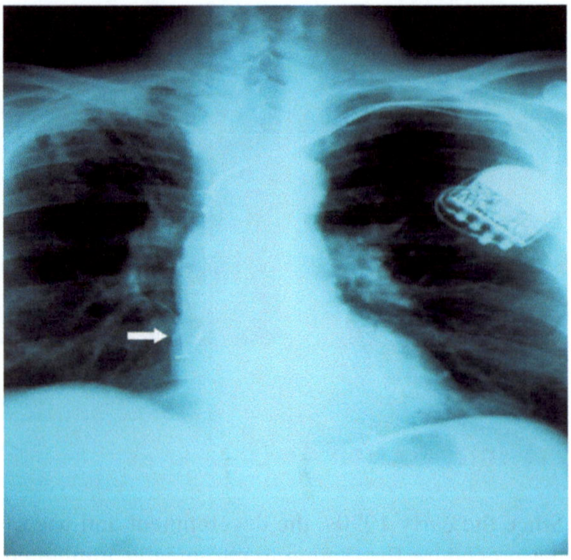

Fig. 3.1 Posteroanterior chest X-ray showing an Encor lead fracture with J-wire protrusion (*arrow*)

3.2.1.1 Medical Therapy

Current medications should be evaluated, with special attention to antibiotics and oral anticoagulants. Their peri-extraction management is related to their indication for anticoagulation. We suggest transitioning patients on oral anticoagulation therapy to subcutaneously administered low molecular weight heparin (LMWH), which may be given up to 12 h before planned procedure. Resumption of warfarin at its maintenance dose after postimplantation procedure with simultaneous LMWH for 3–5 days allows for outpatient transition back to orally administered anticoagulation.

Antibiotic prophylaxis is mandatory in case of local or systemic infection. Usually, coagulase-negative staphylococci (41 – 68%) represent the most frequent pathogens isolated in blood culture or in lead-tip cultures, followed by *S. aureus* (23-34 %) [8–10]. We routinely suggest beginning antibiotic therapy at least 2 weeks before admission, based on cultures (if available) or, alternatively, using a broad-spectrum antibiotic, including for methicillin-resistant strains [8], and continuing therapy for several days after implantation. In our experience, effective antibiotic therapy before lead removal allows fast reimplantation without risks of relapse. A strict collaboration with the infectious disease service is suggested for appropriate antibiotic selection, treatment duration, and patient follow-up.

3.2.1.2 Cardiac Rhythm

It is essential to determine whether the patient is pacemaker dependent and will require temporary pacing support during the procedure. As patients who are not pacemaker dependent prior to the procedure may become so during the procedure. In our daily practice, all patients receive a temporary pacing lead through the left femoral vein before original extraction.

3.2.2 Transvenous Lead Extraction Consensus

The explanting physician should discuss with the patient all aspects of the TLE procedure, from beginning to end, including potential risks and benefits. Moreover, the patient needs to be well informed about the risks related to disease progression and possible pacemaker (PM)/ICD malfunctions. Then, the patient must provide written informed consent.

Every patient situation is different, and interventional risks must be carefully tailored to every single case, considering several factors: patient age; lead implantation time; number of leads; comorbidities. Team experience is essential in predicting outcomes, and every patient should be informed about success rates, number of procedures and complication rates of the center and operator. Several studies demonstrate that centers with a high number of procedures per year have higher success rates and lower major complication rates [11, 12].

3.2.3 Laboratory Tests

Baseline laboratory values should be reviewed, including blood and platelet count, hemoglobin, creatinine, blood urea nitrogen, and International Normalized Ratio (INR). The patient should be typed and screened for blood products. According to guidelines, at least 4 U of blood should be available, and in case of a complicated procedure, it should be kept directly in the operating room [13].

3.2.4 Chest X-Ray

Posterolateral and anterolateral chest radiography should be performed in order to examine heart, lungs, and lead features (Fig. 3.2). When the explanting lead is very old, thick calcifications can

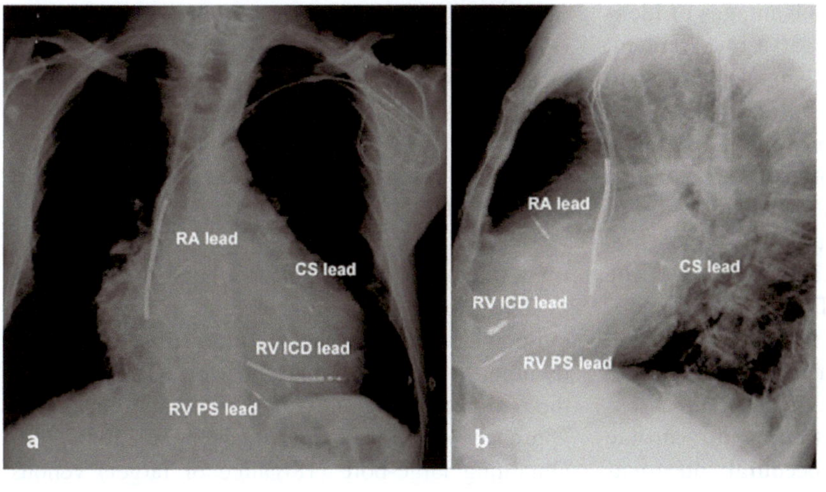

Fig. 3.2 Posteroanterior (a) and lateral (b) chest X-ray showing a patient with four screw in leads, including a coronary sinus (*CS*) active fixation lead (Medtronic Starfix). *RA*, right atrium, *RV*, right ventricle, *ICD*, implantable cardioverter–defibrillator, *PS*, pericardial space

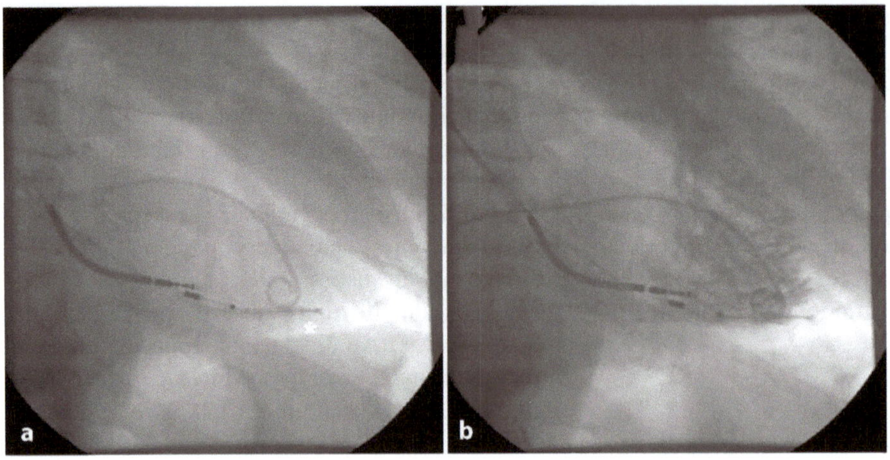

Fig. 3.3 Posteroanterior fluoroscopy: before right heart angiography (**a**); during iodine contrast injection (**b**). The angiography shows that the nonfunctioning implantable cardioverter–defibrillator lead tip (*) is lodged in the myocardial wall of the right ventricle, resulting in a high risk removal procedure.

be seen along its course, suggesting resistant binding sites that physician must consider carefully. Moreover, X-ray should exclude left-side lead implantation or extravascular course. When the lead course is suspect (subclavian arteriovenous fistula, left-side placement through a patent foramen ovale or atrial/ventricular septal defect, tip advancement into the pericardium), echocardiography, computed tomography (CT), or right-side cardiac angiography confirmation [14–16] may be necessary to characterize lead course and plan procedural strategy (Fig 3.3).

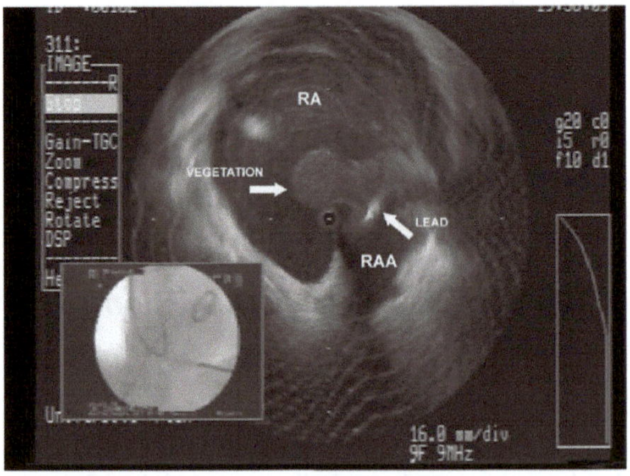

Fig. 3.4 Intracardiac echocardiography interrogation at the atrial plane showing a large, lead-related vegetation (>2 cm). *RA*, right atrium, *RAA*, right atrial appendage

3.2.5 Echocardiography

Echocardiography (transthoracic, transesophageal) is mandatory before lead removal, particularly in case of sepsis. It combines the advantages of identifying vegetations, prosthetics valve involvement, and severity of valve damage. It is also useful to predict prognosis and embolic risk [17]. Transthoracic echocardiography (TTE) is performed to assess cardiac performance. It can also detect presence, location, size, and relationship of vegetations with cardiac structure involvement. As TTE sensitivity is limited in comparison with the transesophageal approach (TEE) in cases of endocarditis (20–75% vs 55–90%, respectively) [8, 9, 18], a TEE should be performed in every patient with suspected CIED-related infection to assess vegetation and sizing. Sometimes, intracardiac echocardiography (ICE) preprocedural interrogation may be used as an additional imaging tool (Fig. 3.4). The information size is relevant in order to decide whether the patient can undergo TLE or requires a surgical approach (Table 3.1).

3.2.6 Patient Preparation

First, the thorax must be cleaned, and shaved if necessary. Considering the potential risk of cardiac tamponade or hemothorax requiring emergency treatment, the thorax must be well scrubbed from the epigastric region (for the pericardiocentesis approach) to the neck and from right side to the left. Obtaining large-bore (18-gauge or larger) venous

Table 3.1 Transvenous lead extraction check list 1: preoperative management

Transvenous lead extraction check list 1	
Preoperative management	
Patient admission	❒
12 ECG	❒
Chest X-ray	❒
TTE	❒
TEE	❒
CIED and lead features	❒
CIED interrogation	❒
Peripheral venous access	❒
Blood exams, typing, and screening for blood products	❒
Anesthesiological evaluation	❒
Cardiac surgeon warning	❒
Venography	❒
Fill TLE database	❒

ECG, electrocardiogram; *TTE*, transthoracic echocardiography; *TEE*, transesophageal echocardiography; *CIED*, cardiovascular implantable electronic device; *TLE*, transvenous lead extraction

access is suggested for fast emergency fluid and/or blood administration. Defibrillator pads, electrocardiogram (ECG), oxygen saturation, and invasive blood pressure (radial artery) monitoring are essential to control vital signs. Useful information about the venous system can be achieved by venography. In fact, in cases of uninfected lead extraction, it is extremely worthwhile to check venous system patency and the possibility of using the same venous access at reimplantation (usually performed during the same procedure). This is because silent thrombosis is not uncommon. Experience has shown a relative high incidence of stenosis (11%) and total occlusion (12%) in asymptomatic patients [19, 20]. Another possible indication for performing venography is suspicion of SVC syndrome (SVCS), when other reimplantation approaches or venoplasty then need to be planned, or when contralateral implantation is not possible for technical or clinical reasons (Table 3.2).

Table 3.2 Transvenous lead extraction check list 2: intraoperative management

Transvenous lead extraction check list 2		
Intraoperative management		
- Patient	ECG monitoring	❒
	O_2% monitoring	❒
	External defibrillation pad	❒
	ICD therapy/rate responsive mode switch off	❒
	Blood products availability check	❒
	Artery line access	❒
	Temporary pacemaker positioning	❒
- Room and facilities	Stylets	❒
	Sheaths	❒
	High-quality fluoroscopy	❒
	Additional tools (lasso, catcher, steerable catheters...)	❒
	Femoral workstation	❒
	Temporary PM and lead	❒
	Defibrillator	❒
	Intravascular echocardiography	❒
	TTE available	❒
	Anesthesiological support	❒
	Pericardiocentesis tray	❒
	Thoracotomy tray	❒
	Surgical standby	❒
	Fill the TLE database	❒

ECG, electrocardiogram; O_2%, monitoring blood oxygen saturation; *ICD*, implantable cardiac defibrillator; *PM*, pacemaker; *TTE*, transthoracic echocardiography; *TLE*, transvenous lead extraction

3.2.7 Equipment

3.2.7.1 Fluoroscopy

Independent of procedure location [cardiac catheterization (CAT) lab, electrophysiology (EP) lab or operating room (OR)] a high-definition fluoroscopy is recommended. The ability to clearly visualize leads and their courses, stylets, and sheaths is critical in order to follow all extractions steps and determine procedural success. It also helps to monitor potential complications, such as lead fractures during traction, lead-fragment migration in the venous system, or pleural bleeding due to vein or cardiac-wall avulsion during dilatation.

3.2.7.2 Temporary pacemaker

In all patients, we prefer positioning a temporary pacemaker through the left femoral vein, leaving the right one available for ICE or transfemoral workstation, if required. The temporary PM should be placed far from the permanent lead tip, reducing the risk of displacement during dilatation.

3.2.7.3 Echocardiography

Echocardiography should be readily available in case of complications. Some centers use TEE monitoring during the procedure. We use ICE monitoring in patients with systemic infection, and TTE is available in the EP room in the other cases.

3.2.7.4 Extraction Tools

Several tools should be checked before the procedure, such as mechanical polypropylene sheaths, stylets, snares (catcher, lassos), and transfemoral workstation. Also, standard implantation equipment can be necessary (introducer sheaths, guide wires, stylets). Please refer to the dedicated chapter of this book for a more complete and exhaustive discussion about these items.

3.2.7.5 Pericardiocentesis and Thoracotomy Trays

These items should be immediately available in case complications are encountered.

3.2.8 Staff

According to recent guidelines, TLE requires an appropriate team approach.

3.2.8.1 Primary Operator

The primary operator needs to be appropriately and adequately trained on device removal. A consistent number of procedures should be performed to complete the learning curve, and permanent, ongoing training is mandatory. Moreover, this operator should be trained in managing potential life-threatening complications.

3.2.8.2 Second Physician/Assistant

This team member must be available during the entire lead extraction procedure as support for equipment and tools management.

3.2.8.3 Anaesthesia Support

An anesthesiologist is often required during lead removal to manage and control procedure-related pain. According to the practice of the individual center, TLE can be performed under general anesthesia, or under local anaesthesia with sedation. The former is less stressful and painful for the patient, allowing the use of TEE monitoring to control periprocedural complications (for example, cardiac tamponade). The sedation approach is generally performed when general anaesthesia is contraindicated or if the procedure is foreseen as being simple.

3.2.8.4 Specialized Nurses' Support

These team members are essential for monitoring vital signs during extraction. They must be confident with the procedure, materials, and potential complications in order to activate emergency protocols.

3.2.8.5 Fluoroscopy Technician

This team member offers assistance with fluoroscopy control during dilatation monitoring every single step.

3.2.9 Intervention Room

Before any procedure, tools and equipment should be verified and safety measures established in order to prevent complications and to allow well-timed interventions in case of emergency. Depending on the center's facilities, TLE can be performed in the EP laboratory, in the CAT laboratory, or in the OR. Regardless of surgery location, the room must have an adequate size to contain all necessary materials and allow emergency interventions if necessary.

3.2.10 Standby Surgery

When interventions are performed in the EP laboratory, it is good practise to plan standby cardiac surgery, especially for high-risk procedures. The OR is preferred for direct and quick emergency sternotomy and cardiopulmonary bypass in case of complications, such as cardiac tamponade or hemothorax, or in case of transvenous approach failure (i.e., crossing to thoracotomy approach [21]). We usually perform TLE in the EP laboratory, considering the advantages of high-quality fluoroscopy, equipment availability (sheaths, snare, catcher, catheters, etc.), and the short distance to the operating room. Only in case of pediatric or high-risk procedures is the cardiac-surgery room preferred.

3.3 Postoperative Management

The key point in postoperative management of patients undergoing TLE is proper monitoring, which includes admission to the intensive care unit immediately after the procedure. Good monitoring depends on several factors (Table 3.3).

Systemic pressure monitoring with a small catheter in the radial artery (18–20 gauge) is usually performed for at least 12 h after the procedure and, in particular cases, we assess central venous pressure if a venous introducer is available.

At the end of the procedure, we prefer to position a temporary PM from the ipsilateral subclavian vein before removing the femoral one, because this permits leg motion and reduces the profound venous thrombosis risk. This is particularly important in patients who need to wait some days before attending a new reimplantation procedure. We usually maintain the temporary pacemaker for at least 24 h, even if the patient's spontaneous rhythm is adequate. We prefer its removal at the end of the procedure only in case of single-day extraction/reimplantation procedures.

It is advisable to perform a transthoracic echocardiogram monitoring to exclude bleeding in the pericardium and pulmonary embolism. In case of suspicion of a pulmonary embolism, the bene-

Table 3.3 Transvenous lead extraction check list 3: postoperative management

Transvenous lead extraction check list 3	
Postoperative management	
Blood pressure monitoring	❐
ECG monitoring	❐
Temperature monitoring	❐
Blood exams	❐
Blood cultures	❐
TTE monitoring	❐
Medical treatment	❐
Fill the TLE database	❐

ECG electrocardiogram, *TTE* transthoracic echocardiography, *TLE* transvenous lead extraction fits of heparin infusion can prevail over the risk of significant pericardial effusion, but the diagnosis must be certain and, initially, cardiac tamponade must be absolutely excluded.

Immediately after the procedure, it is desirable to collect blood cultures even in case of local infection indication to TLE, because a negative blood culture after >48 h (72 h according to current guidelines) will allow device reimplantation in few days. Additional blood cultures are considered necessary only in cases of fever and/or shivers. Blood examinations are routinely performed the day after the procedure, evaluating at least the white blood cell count, hemoglobin, urea, creatinine, and electrolyte levels. We anticipate their assessment in case of general anesthesia or complex procedures. After 24 h, we generally remove vacuum drainage from the old pocket if there is no bleeding.

In our practice, we consider three different settings in postoperative management of TLE:

1. TLE without reimplantation: Temporary PM, vacuum drainage, and arterial line (if still present) are removed the day after the procedure and the patient is completely mobilized. Chest X-ray is planned to confirm radiological success of the procedure and identify possible occult complications (i.e., pleural effusion, pulmonary embolism, mild pneumothorax). Discharge is feasible after 48 h if infective problems or other complications do not emerge. Sometimes, it is necessary to remove a PM from one side while another pacing system is present contralaterally. In such cases, the temporary PM is usually removed at the end of the procedure and the maintained system is checked before discharge, especially in case of complex procedures, in order to exclude a post extraction malfunction.
2. TLE with reimplantation in the same procedure: These procedures are typically performed when correction of a malfunctioning system in necessary. It is crucial to minimize the risk of infection, which is considerable in time-consuming procedures. No drainage is left inside the pocket at the end of the procedure, and the temporary PM is removed before the patient leaves the operating room. After 24 h, the patient is mobilized, and an X-ray of the thorax is required. Discharge is considered safe after 48 h if the patient is clinically stable, apyretic, and the white blood cell count is normal. We usually do not collect blood cultures after removal in these setting, but we look at lead-tip cultures for possible treatment of a superinfection, keeping in mind the possibility of contamination.
3. TLE followed by reimplantation after >48 h: This situation is typical in case of infection of the old system. Particular attention in the postoperative period must be paid to PM-dependent patients to evaluate the correct functioning of the pacing system, because dislodgment of the temporary pacing lead could have dramatic consequences. For this reason, in very rare cases, when a lengthy time period is necessary before reimplantation, screw-in leads are used for temporary pacing. Otherwise, after temporary PM removal, light mobilization is desirable before reimplantation in order to reduce the risk of venous thromboembolism. Low weight molecular heparin should be used after 24 h from TLE, particularly if the patient is not able to stand, reimplantation is delayed, and/or temporary PM is not removed. In these cases, an echocardiographic re-evaluation of the pericardium is desirable. Reimplantation timing in such patients will depend on clinical condition (including body temperature), blood tests, blood and tip cultures drawn after TLE, and – above all – prior diagnosis of lead and/or valve vegetations.

3.3.1 Antibiotic Treatment

Antibiotic treatment is generally used as prophylactic therapy in case of extraction without reimplantation. However, we prefer to continue antibiotic administration for 1 week in cases in which the contralateral PM was implanted before TLE or extraction immediately followed by reimplantation. Although there is no clear evidence pertaining to this practice, we consider these situations high risk for infection.

Antibiotic therapy is one of the key points in treating infective complications of cardiovascular devices. Therefore, we usually treat the patient for at least 2 weeks in case of local infection and for 3–4 weeks or more in case of endocarditis or systemic bacteremia. Therapy after lead extraction is obviously based on the results of blood and tip cultures, and a local infective diseases specialist is available on call to determine the correct treatment. Usually, we use more then one antibiotic class in combination, and patients are discharged when intravenous administration can be replaced with oral administration.

When there is neither growth in blood/tip cultures nor previously documented infection, we administer an empiric combination of different antibiotical class against the most common pathogenic agents (e.g. Moxifloxacin and Rifampicin) based on the usual antibiotic sensitivity in positive tip cultures. Blood tests are repeated at 1, 2, and 4 weeks, including inflammatory response indicators. Follow-up is necessary to document recovery from the infection and particularly regression of endocarditis lesions.

References

1. Bracke F, Meijer A, Van Gelder B (2002) Extraction of pacemaker and implantable cardioverter defibrillator leads: patient and lead characteristics in relation to the requirement of extraction tools. Pacing and Clin Electrophysiol 25:1037–1040
2. Byrd CL, Wilkoff BL, Love CJ et al (1999) Intravascular extraction of problematic or infected permanent pacemaker leads: 1994–1996. U.S. Extraction Database, MED Institute. Pacing Clin Electrophysiol 22:1348–1357
3. Smith MC, Love CJ (2008) Extraction of transvenous pacing and ICD leads. Review. Pacing Clin Electrophysiol 31:736–752
4. Bongiorni MG, Zucchelli G, Soldati E et al (2007) Usefulness of mechanical transvenous dilation and location of areas of adherence in patients undergoing coronary sinus lead extraction. Europace 9:69–73
5. Wilkoff BL, Belott PH, Love CJ et al (2005) Improved extraction of ePTFE and medical adhesive modified defibrillation leads from the coronary sinus and great cardiac vein. Pacing Clin Electrophysiol 28:205–211
6. Smith HJ, Fearnot NE, Byrd CL et al (1994) Five years experience with intravascular lead extraction, Pacing Clin Electrophysiol 17:2016–2020
7. Field ME, Jones SO, Epstein LM (2007) How to select patients for lead extraction. Hands on. Heart Rhythm 4(7):978–985
8. Sohail MR, Uslan DZ, Khan AH et al (2008) Infective endocarditis complicating permanent pacemaker and implantable cardioverter-defibrillator infection. Mayo Clin Proc. 83(1):46–53
9. Sohail MR, Uslan DZ, Khan AH et al (2007) Management and outcome of permanent pacemaker and implantable cardioverter defibrillator infections. J Am Coll Cardiol 49:1851–1859
10. Borek PP, Wilkoff BL (2008) Pacemaker and ICD leads: strategies for long-term management. J Interv Card Electrophysiol 23(1):59–72
11. Bongiorni MG, Soldati E, Zucchelli G et al (2008) Transvenous removal of pacing and implantable cardiac defibrillating leads using single sheath mechanical dilatation and multiple venous approaches: high success rate and safety in more than 2000 leads. Eur Heart J 29:2886–2893
12. Kennergren C, Bjurman C, Wiklund R et al (2009) A single-centre experience of over one thousand lead extractions. Europace 11(5):612–617
13. Wilkoff BL, Love CJ, Byrd CL, Bongiorni MG et al (2009) Transvenous lead extraction: Heart Rhythm Society expert consensus on facilities, training, indications, and patient management: this document was endorsed by the American Heart Association (AHA). Heart Rhythm 6(7):1085–1104
14. Henrikson CA, Leng CT, Yuh DD, Brinker JA (2006) Computed tomography to assess possible cardiac lead perforation. Pacing Clin Electrophysiol 29:509–511
15. Kennergren CA (2008) European perspective on lead extractions: part II. Heart Rhythm 5(2):320–323
16. Yavari A, Khawaja ZO, Krishnamoorthy et al (2009) Perforation of right ventricular free wall by pacemaker lead detected by multidetector computed tomography. Europace 11(2):252–254
17. Thuny F, Di Salvo G, Belliard O et al (2005) Risk of embolism and death in infective endocarditis: prognostic value of echocardiography: a prospective multicenter study. Circulation 112:69–75
18. Dumont E, Camus C, Victor F et al (2003) Suspected pacemaker or defibrillator transvenous lead infection. Prospective assessment of a TEE-guided therapeutic strategy. Eur Heart J 24:1779–1787
19. Goto Y, Aabe T, Sekine S et al (1998) Long-term thrombosis after transvenous permanent pacemaker implantation. Pacing Clin Electrophysiol 21:1192– 1195
20. Zuber M, Huber P, Fricker U et al (1998) Assessment of the subclavian vein in patients with transvenous pacemaker leads. Pacing Clin Electrophysiol 21:2621–2630
21. Henrikson CA, Brinker JA (2008) How to prevent, recognize and manage complications of lead extraction. Part III: procedural factors. Heart Rhythm 5:1352–1354

4 Tools, Techniques, and Approaches

Luca Segreti, Ezio Soldati and Maria Grazia Bongiorni

4.1 Definitions

The following are defined in the dictionary available at www.wordreference.com [1]:

1. Tools: the means whereby some act is accomplished.
2. Technique: a practical method or art applied to some particular task.
3. Approach: ideas or actions intended to deal with a problem or situation.

According to the North American Society of Pacing and Electrophysiology (NASPE) Policy Statement [2] and the Heart Rhythm Society (HRS) Expert Consensus on Transvenous Lead Extraction [3], the following concepts are defined as:

1. Lead removal: removal of pacing and defibrillating lead using any technique.
2. Lead explant: manipulation of a pacing or defibrillator lead so that the lead exits the vasculature via the implant vein using tools typically supplied for lead implant, with the addition of manual traction for a lead that has been implanted for less than 1 year.
3. Lead extraction:
   a. Removal of a lead with the assistance of specialized equipment regardless of the implant duration. This may include, but is not limited to, the use of specialized stylets that are not included as part of the typical implant package, sheaths with or without additional cutting capability (e.g., Teflon, polypropylene, metal composition, laser, and radiofrequency current), snares, grasping devices, or other devices used to engage or entrap and remove the lead or lead fragments.
   b. Removal of a lead from a route other than via the implant vein.
   c. Removal of any lead that has been implanted for more than 1 year.

So, within the general category of lead removal, distinctions must be made between:

- Lead explant: simple procedures that can be performed via the implant vein without specialized tools; and
- Lead extraction: removal of leads involving more complex procedures and specialized tools.

Making this distinction is necessary when designing training programs, for classifying procedures in registries and databases, and for appropriate reimbursement levels for the different procedures.

4.1.1 Lead Extraction Basis

Leads are usually removed via the implant vein, which is the venous access by which the lead was inserted. However, sometimes, alternative venous access is required from a nonimplant vein. Examples of alternative approaches to subclavian vein include femoral and jugular veins. Relative contraindications for transvenous lead removal [2] are addressed in this chapter to emphasize that the unavailability of the necessary equipment represents a contraindication to transvenous lead removal:

L. Segreti (✉)
2nd Cardiovascular Department AOUP, Santa Chiara University Hospital, Pisa, Italy

M. G. Bongiorni (Ed.), *Transvenous Lead Extraction*.

1. Presence of calcification visible by X-ray involving the lead in the atrium or superior vena cava (SVC).
2. Unavailability of required equipment.
3. Patient is an unsuitable candidate for emergent thoracotomy.
4. Known anomalous placement of the lead through structures other than the normal venous and cardiac structures (e.g., subclavian artery, pericardial space).

Pacing and implantable cardioverter–defibrillator (ICD) leads are designed to be stable in their position and not to be easily removed. The major obstacle to lead removal is the body's response to an intravascular foreign body. Moreover, the tensile strength of fibrous lead encapsulation increases over time (Fig. 4.1). After a few months from implant, leads are fixed at binding sites along their course and at the tip, mainly by the growth of fibrous tissue that surrounds the lead itself [4]. Usually, leads implanted for 1 year or more are not likely to be removed by simple traction, particularly in the presence of ICD leads, where the defibrillating coils are usually responsible for significant growth of fibrous adhesions. The sites where binding is most likely to be present are at lead insertion into the subclavian vein, the junction between innominate vein and SVC and right atrium, the lead tip, and – in the case of ventricular leads – the tricuspid valve [4–6]. The key point in lead removal is to free the lead at these binding sites – from the venous entry point to the tip. Most available techniques combine traction with dissection of binding sites, and the most important difference between the techniques is the energy used to dissect the binding sites. No single technique for transvenous lead removal should be considered standard and applicable in all cases. Conversely, different tools and approaches must be tailored to each individual case [7]. Every patient and lead is unique. Clinical and technical factors play a remarkable role in degree of difficulty, results, and complications of lead removal [8, 9]. Independent of technique, transvenous lead removal is a procedure affected by a significant risk of serious complications, including death [10, 11]. The importance of the necessary equipment, specialist facilities, and operator skill are recommended in the guidelines [2, 3].

4.2 Extraction Tools

The following equipment is necessary for successful lead extraction [3]:

1. Implant tools: typically supplied for lead implant, allowing manipulation of the lead so that the lead exits the vasculature via the implant vein. These tools include such items as standard stylets (nonlocking) and fixation-screw retraction clips.
2. Traction devices: specialized locking stylets, snares, sutures, grasping, or other devices used to engage or entrap and remove the lead or lead fragments.
3. Mechanical sheaths: sheaths composed of metal, Teflon, polypropylene, or other materials; they require manual advancement over the lead and rely on the mechanical properties of the sheath to disrupt fibrotic adhesions.
4. Laser sheaths: sheaths that employ fiberoptics

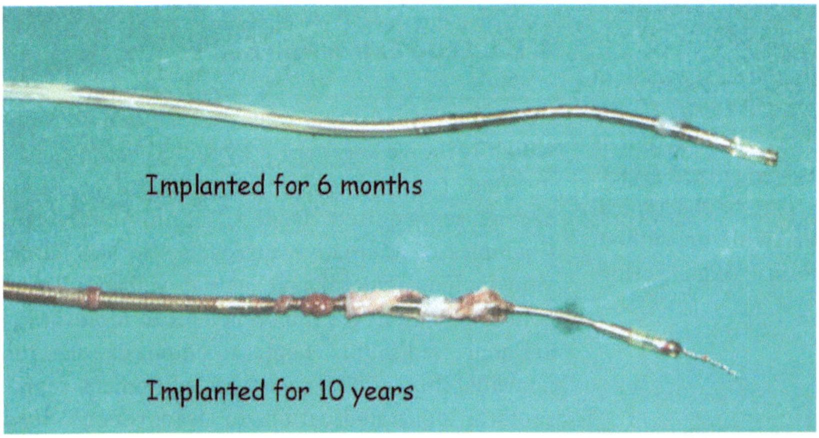

Fig. 4.1 Leads extracted. Binding sites develop, increase, and strengthen over time. No significant adhesions in the lead with 6 months' dwelling time; fibrotic adhesions in the lead with 10 years dwelling time

to transmit laser light to disrupt the fibrotic adhesions.
5. Electrosurgical sheaths: sheaths that use radiofrequency energy (such as that found in an electrosurgical unit) emitted between two electrodes at the sheath tip to disrupt the fibrotic adhesions.
6. Rotating threaded-tip sheath: sheaths equipped with a rotationally powered mechanism that bore through and disrupt fibrotic adhesions with a threaded screw mechanism at the sheath tip.
7. Other extraction devices: bulldog lead extender; soft-grip hemostat; coil expander; lead clippers; pin vise.
8. Femoral tools: tools developed for retrieving leads by the femoral approach. Many of these tools have come from other disciplines.

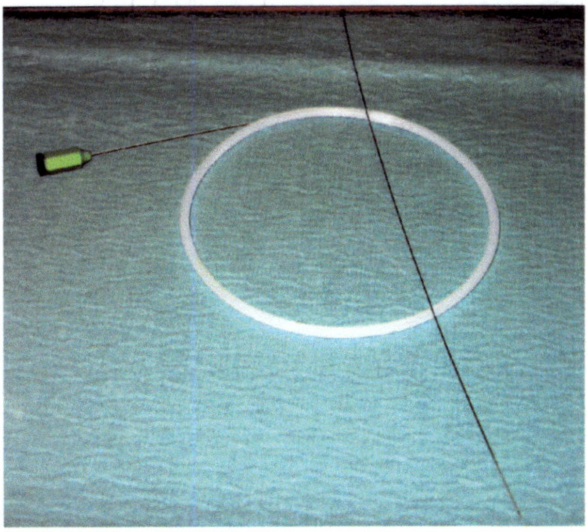

Fig. 4.2 Stylet wires

4.2.1 Implant Tools

These tools are typically supplied for lead implant and allow lead manipulation so that the lead exits the vasculature via the implant vein and include such items as standard stylets (nonlocking) and fixation-screw retraction clips. They sometimes permit lead removal using simple traction. All lead extractions require some degree of direct traction (pulling), and direct traction is the most basic technique. Simple traction means pulling on the lead with varying degrees of force to separate the lead from vascular and endocardial binding sites. Simple direct traction on the proximal portion of the lead can be sufficient to remove recently implanted leads. Some authors suggest adding five to ten lead rotations to increase the effectiveness of simultaneous gentle traction [12]. Lead explant is defined as manipulation of a pacing or defibrillator lead so that the lead exits the vasculature via the implant vein using tools typically supplied for lead implant, with the addition of manual traction, for a lead that has been implanted for less than 1 year [2, 3].

Stylet wires (Fig. 4.2) are used to stiffen leads for removal. Moreover, stylet wires can be used to débride foreign matter inside the lead body, confirm patency, and measure lead length. Stylet wires improve the effectiveness of lead removal when using either direct traction or mechanical sheaths. In fact, by stiffening the lead, stylet wires minimize the chance of lead breakage during traction and assist sheath advancement, which results in the extraction of a greater amount of intact lead. In other words, stylet wires, as do locking stylets, improve tensile strength of the leads and thus minimize the chance of lead breakage; however, they do not eliminate the other complications associated with traction.

4.2.2 Traction Devices

Specialized locking stylets are here reported. Other traction devices include snares, sutures, and grasping or other tools used to engage or entrap and remove the lead or lead fragments.

4.2.2.1 Locking Stylets

Locking stylets lock inside the inner lumen of the lead with different locking mechanisms, and recently introduced devices can be unlocked and repositioned if necessary. Even though different kinds of locking stylets have been used in the past, there are only a few types now in use:

1. Wilkoff locking stylet (Cook Vascular Inc., Leechburg, PA, USA) (Fig. 4.3): this stylet has a small flange at the tip that is locked into the conductor coil when a thin, preloaded cylinder

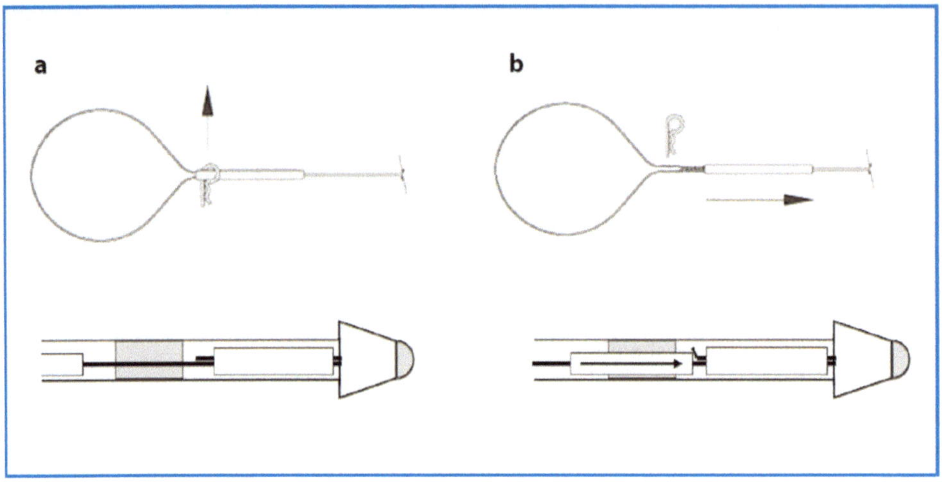

Fig. 4.3 Wilkoff Locking Stylet: after the stylet is advanced to the tip of the lead, unlatch the tubular handle of the locking mechanism by removing the pin (a) and lock the stylet in the lead by firmly advancing the tubular handle forward while holding the loop handle in place (b)

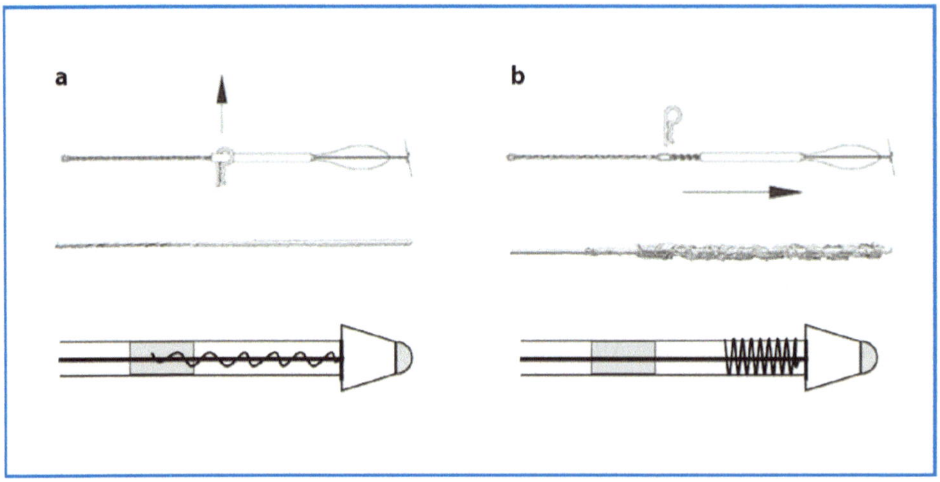

Fig. 4.4 Liberator Locking Stylet: after the stylet is advanced to the tip of the lead, unlatch the tubular handle of the locking mechanism by removing the pin (a) and lock the stylet in the lead by firmly advancing the tubular handle forward while holding the wire extender in place (b)

is advanced. This mechanism can be reversed and relocked by retracting or advancing the cylinder mechanism and does not tolerate the rotation that causes stylet retraction. This stylet cannot be used in active fixation leads and when conduction coil diameter is 0.016 inches or less.

2. Liberator (Cook Vascular) (Fig. 4.4): this stylet has a wound spring at the distal portion that is compressed and locked into the conductor coil when a thin, preloaded cylinder is advanced. Therefore, the mechanism is activated by advancement of the cylinder, which causes the wound spring portion to lock in place. This type of locking stylet is universal: one size fits all leads with lumen diameter of 0.016 to 0.032 inches.
3. VascoExtor viper stylet (Vascomed GmbH, Binzen, Germany) (Fig. 4.5): This stylet was introduced at the end of the 1990 [13–15]. It is inserted through the lead coil to the lead tip. By manipulation of the stylet handle, the fixation tip can be spread, and the stylet is fixed directly in the coil in the area of the lead tip, and the extraction force can be applied directly on the lead tip. There are two advantages of this stylet: first, the extraction stylet can be removed from the lead by unlocking (if the lead is not too damaged); second, it can be universally applied to most existing pacing and defibrillator lead designs. (The Wilkoff, Liberator, and VascoExtor viper stylets provide traction at the lead tip.)

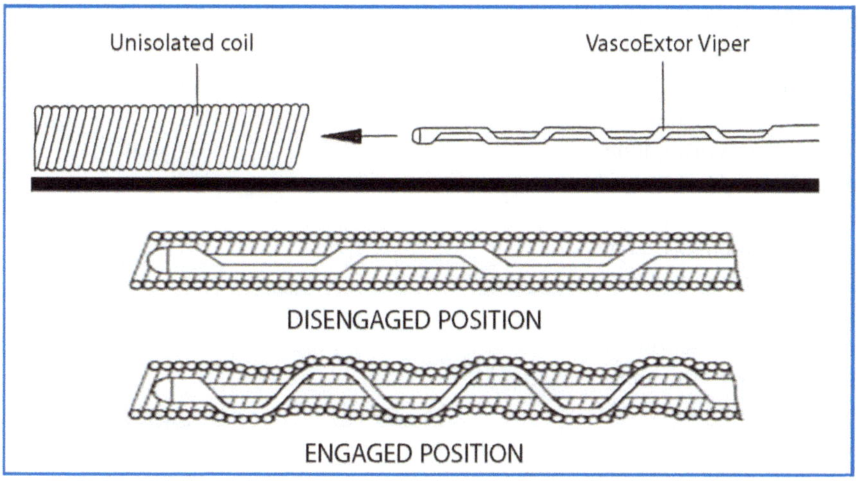

Fig. 4.5 VascoExtor Viper Stylet: disengaged and engaged positions

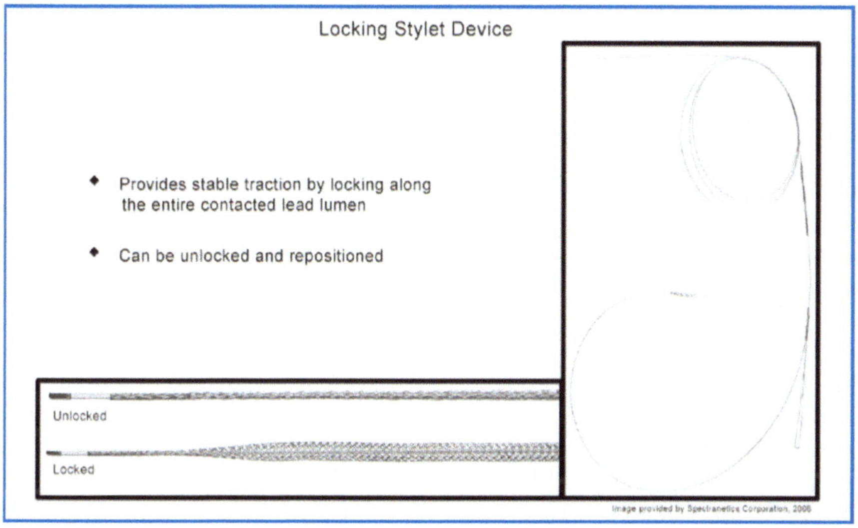

Fig. 4.6 Spectranetics Lead Locking Device: stylet in unlocked and locked positions. When the mesh is expanded (locked position), it binds the lead lumen at various points

4. Spectranetics Lead-Locking Device (Spectranetics, Colorado Springs, CO, USA) (Fig. 4.6): this device has an expandable mesh over the entire length of the stylet body [16]. When the mesh is retracted, the entire length of the stylet is isodiametric with the stylet tip for insertion. When the mesh is expanded, it binds the lumen of the lead at various points along its length: this allows this stylet to provide traction on multiple areas along the length of the lead. The proximal end of the entire mesh is connected to a proximal connector that is used to deploy and lock the stylet into the lead. This stylet has three sizes (Lead-Locking Device 1,2 and 3) to fit all leads.

4.2.3 Mechanical Sheaths

The first approach to freeing chronically implanted leads from binding sites was using mechanical force. Mechanical sheaths for lead extraction were introduced in clinical practice by Byrd in the late 1980s using tools developed by Cook Vascular [17, 18]. This system is provided with locking stylets and dilator sheaths and is the first choice when the proximal end of the lead is exposed (venous entry approach). The sheaths are designed for use to percutaneously dilate tissue surrounding cardiac leads, indwelling catheters, and foreign objects: they are used to advance over the lead and, by breaking binding sites, free it from fibrous adhesions. Sheaths consist of a pair of long and moderately flexible cannulae, one fitting coaxially inside the other and capable of moving freely. Many sheath systems are available for extraction. Sheaths vary in material (Teflon, polypropylene, and stainless), size (from 7 F to 16 F), and method of advancement (unpowered, powered by laser, cautery, or rotating-tip mechanism). The inner and outer telescoping sheaths provide flexibility and strength as they are passed over the lead to the endocardial surface. Balanced traction on the stylet or locking stylet allows first the inner and then the outer sheath to break through the scar tissue and down over the lead to the endocardium.

- Characteristics of Teflon and polypropylene sheaths: these sheaths are available in various lengths. Extra-long sheaths are designed for patients with lateral (especially left-side) venous entry sites, tall patients, and those with large thoracic anatomy. All sheaths are radiopaque. The leading edges of the sheats are beveled. Teflon sheaths are the most flexible, but cuts through tissue poorly. Polypropylene is stiffer than Teflon and so better overcomes adhesions (Figs. 4.7 and 4.8 and Table 4.1). Among the mechanical sheaths, polypropylene sheaths are the most frequently used due to their favorable profile of flexibility, stiffness, and cutting capacity (Table 4.2).
- Stainless sheaths: stainless sheaths are designed for use in percutaneous dilation of tissues surrounding pacemaker/defibrillator leads and other indwelling catheters with a central lumen in order to facilitate venous access. The material composition at the vein entry sites ranges from inflammatory tissue response to fibrous or fibrocalcified tissue to bone. These very stiff stainless sheaths allow obstacles along the vein to be overcome, but the sheaths must be advanced only a few centimeters into the vein and cannot be advanced beyond any curve in the vein. Therefore, they must be replaced by appropriately sized Teflon or polypropylene sheaths once venous access has been established (Fig. 4.9 and Table 4.3).

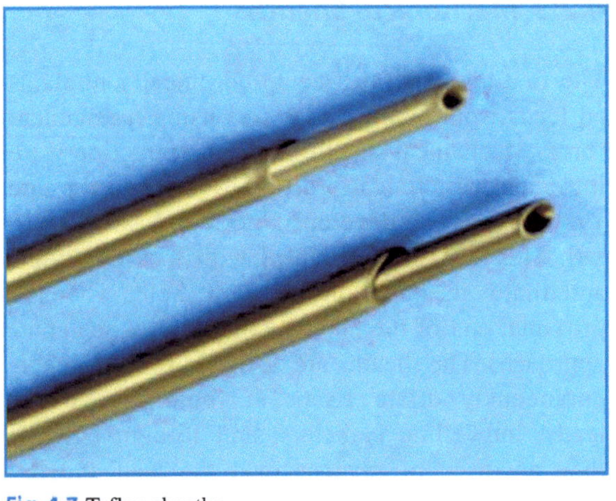

Fig. 4.7 Teflon sheaths

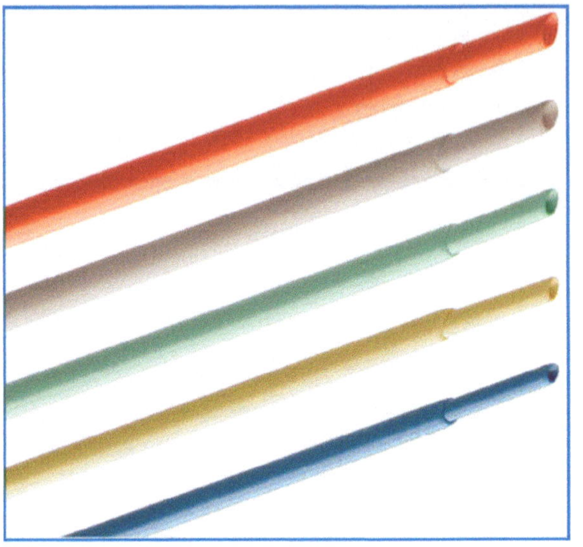

Fig. 4.8 Polypropylene sheaths

Table 4.1 Teflon and polypropylene sheath specifications: inner (ID) and outer (OD) diameter in French (Cook Vascular)

Color	Inner sheath ID/OD	Outer sheath ID/OD
	Teflon	
Black	8.5/12.0	12.8/16.0
Black	9.5/13.0	14.3/18.0
	Polypropylene	
Blue	7.0/9.3	10.0/12.3
Yellow	8.5/10.7	11.6/13.9
Green	10.0/12.1	13.1/15.2
White	11.5/13.6	14.1/16.3
Orange	13.0/15.3	16.0/18.1

Table 4.2 Teflon, polypropylene and stainless sheaths: features

	Flexibility	Stiffness capacity	Cutting capacity	Risk of vascular injury
Teflon	+++	+	+	+
Polypropylene	++	++	++	++
Stainless	+	+++	+++	+++

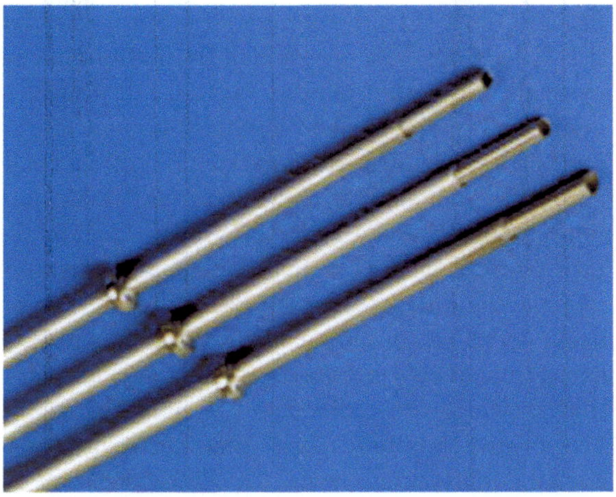

Fig. 4.9 Stainless sheaths

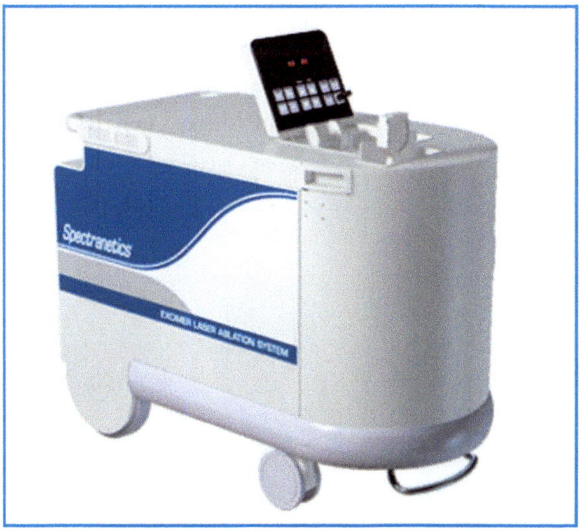

Fig. 4.10 Spectranetics CVX-300® Excimer laser system

Table 4.3 Stainless sheath specifications: inner (ID) and outer (OD) diameter in French (Cook Vascular)

Color	Inner sheath ID/OD	Outer sheath ID/OD
Metal	8.7/10.3	11.5/12.6
Metal	10.4/11.9	12.7/13.7
Metal	12.3/13.8	14.5/15.6

4.2.4 Laser Sheaths

To improve the effectiveness of lead extraction, powered sheaths equipped with an energy source that performs dissection were developed in the 1990s. The first technological advance consisted of light amplification by stimulated emission of radiation (laser)-assisted sheaths [19] that consist of a focused beam of light created by the excitation of atoms to a high energy level. The Spectranetics CVX-300® Excimer laser system (Fig. 4.10) generates 308 nm of laser energy by electrically charging two gases, xenon and chloride (XeCl). The laser energy is transmitted along flexible fiberoptic strands encased in catheters and sheaths, which are passed through the veins. There are three sizes of laser extraction sheaths: 12 F, 14 F, and 16 F (Fig. 4.11). The ultraviolet light energy is delivered from the sheath tip, where the fibers are arranged in a ring-shape and are focused on the tissue requiring treatment; the laser beam is effective for about 1 mm. Excimer laser ablation produces either solid photochemical destruction or liquid vaporization: this process is called photoablation, which frees cardiac pacemaker and ICD leads from binding scar tissue. Laser sheaths are supplemented with an outer Teflon sheath that provides counterpressure and countertraction. Thus, laser energy is delivered to the tissue at the edge of a dedicated sheath in the presence of fibrous binding sites. Once the lead is free, the sheath is advanced to the next adhesion. This laser process is stopped before the tip is reached due to the high risk of wall tears. The tip is then freed by a combination of traction from a locking stylet combined with sheath advancement. In an ideal situation, the sheath is passed over the lead, dissecting each binding site until the sheath reaches a point about 1 cm from the heart wall. An outer sheath is used as a workstation and for counterpressure and countertraction. The lead is then removed from the heart wall using countertraction.

The modified Spectranetics laser system (SLS) II sheath, which has improved mechanical properties enhancing advancement over the lead, has recently been developed as the second-generation laser sheath. In comparison with the previous model, the sheath is 10 cm longer, and its distal 10-cm segment is more flexible. Moreover, the 15° bevel tip makes it easier to pass the sheath over the acute vascular and lead angles, and the sheath composition provides either an inner lubricious coating or an increased body torsional strength.

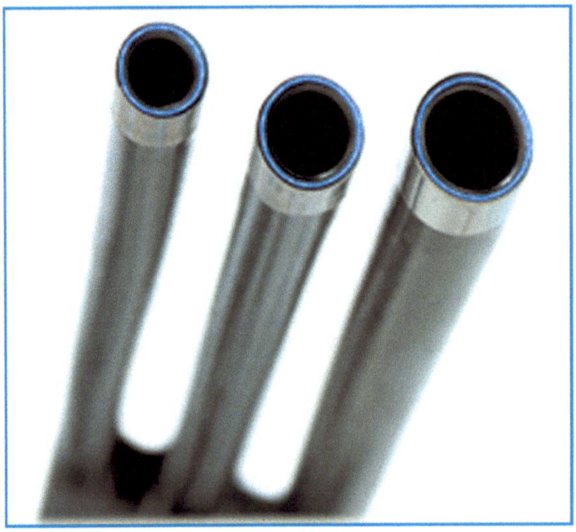

Fig. 4.11 Spectranetics laser sheaths

4.2.5 Electrosurgical Sheaths

PERFECTA® Electrosurgical dissection sheaths (EDS) by Cook Vascular, which use radiofrequency energy, represent another advance in transvenous lead removal. The dilating polytetrafluoroethylene sheath is connected to a radiofrequency generator (compatible generators are Valleylab Force FX®, Valleylab Force FX-8®) with an interface adapter; energy delivery induces a thermal effect at their distal end, therefore allowing fibrous tissue to be cut at the adhesions. Radiofrequency energy conducted between bipolar tungsten electrodes (which are radiopaque) is used to locally dissect the binding tissue that surrounds and anchors transvenous leads. The electrodes are at the leading edge of the bevel: EDS electrodes should be kept on the inner curve of the lead during advancement into the SVC to prevent its perforation. The tapered distal end of the electrosurgical dissection sheaths can also be used to mechanically disrupt these adhesions: significant rotational torque may need to be applied to the sheath. An outer sheath is used as a workstation and for counterpressure and countertraction (Fig. 4.12 and Table 4.4).

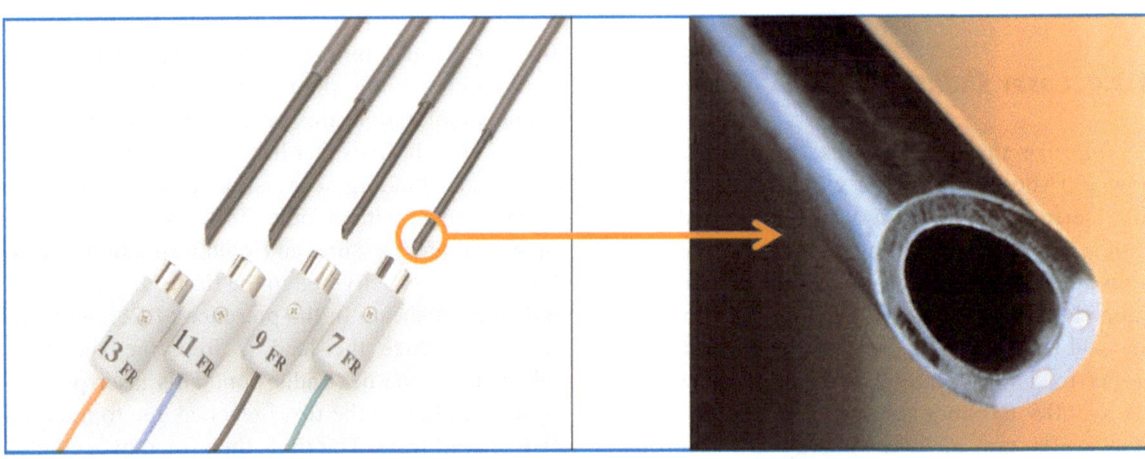

Fig. 4.12 PERFECTA® Electrosurgical sheaths

Table 4.4 Electrosurgical sheath specifications: inner (ID) and outer (OD) diameter in French

Color	Inner sheath ID/OD	Outer sheath ID/OD
Green	7.0/11.0	12.0/15.0
Black	9.0/13.0	14.0/17.0
Blue	11.0/15.0	16.0/19.0
Orange	13.0/17.0	18.0/21.0

4.2.6 Rotating Threaded-Tip Sheath

The EVOLUTION® mechanical dilator sheath set (Cook Vascular) is composed of an inner plastic sheath with a threaded metal tip and an outer telescoping polymer sheath. The inner sheath has a stainless steel tip at its distal end, and no electrical energy supply is required. This sheath is mounted on a pistol capable of mechanically rotating the sheath. Multiple sheath sizes are available: 7 F, 9 F, 11 F, and 13 F. A shortle version, with a shorter sheath length, is also available. Although this sheath has the capability of dissecting through all types of tissues, even calcified adhesions, there are only limited experiences reported in literature [20, 21], and some complications related to this tool are described [22] (Fig. 4.13).

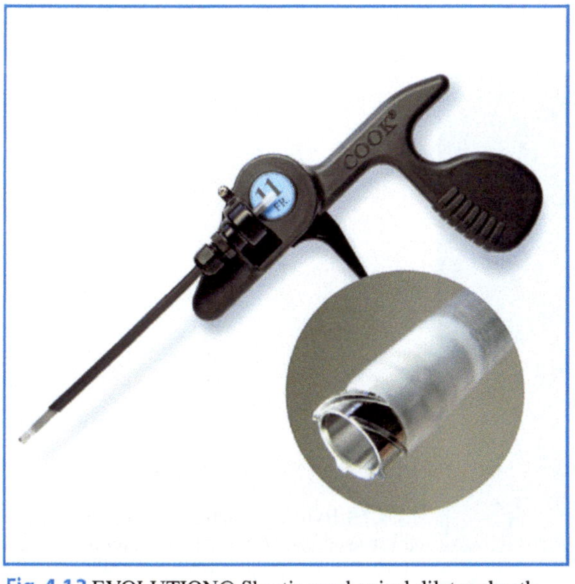

Fig. 4.13 EVOLUTION® Shortie mechanical dilator sheath

Reports in the literature suggest that powered sheaths are more effective than mechanical sheaths [10]; in some experiences, their use is associated with a higher incidence of major complications and is undoubtedly more expensive. In the near future, the cost/benefit ratio of both techniques will require careful evaluation; probably, most procedures could be performed by mechanical techniques, whereas powered sheath techniques should be reserved for select cases.

4.2.7 Other Extraction Devices

Images of the following extraction devices are shown in Fig. 4.14a–e):

1. BulldogTM lead extender: The bulldog lead extender (Cook Vascular) consists of a metal loop and a sleeve for closing the loop. It is used to extend the exposed portion of the lead to perform lead traction: the exposed end is placed into the loop and the sleeve is advanced down the loop, closing it over the lead. This mechanism allows extension and direct traction of lumenless cardiac leads (that incorporate a cable design instead a helical coil). In these cases, the end of the lead and conductors are placed into the metal loop, and the sleeve is advanced over the loop to close it, allowing a firm grasp of the lead components.
2. Soft-grip hemostat: these devices are used to hold the pacing or defibrillator lead firmly without damaging the inner coil of the lead. They are particularly useful in case of limited exposed end of the lead submitted to removal.
3. Coil expander: these are used in preparing the cut lead coil to allow proper sizing using gauge pins. Gauge-pin stylets allow the diameter of the lead lumen to be determined in order to select the appropriate locking stylet, the size of which corresponds to the largest gauge pin accepted by the lead.
4. Lead clippers: these are used to separate the connector from pacemaker or defibrillator lead wire. They cleanly cut the lead so that the inner coil is exposed.
5. Pin vise: using allows the plastic sheath to be grasped, making progression and the application of torsion forces easier.

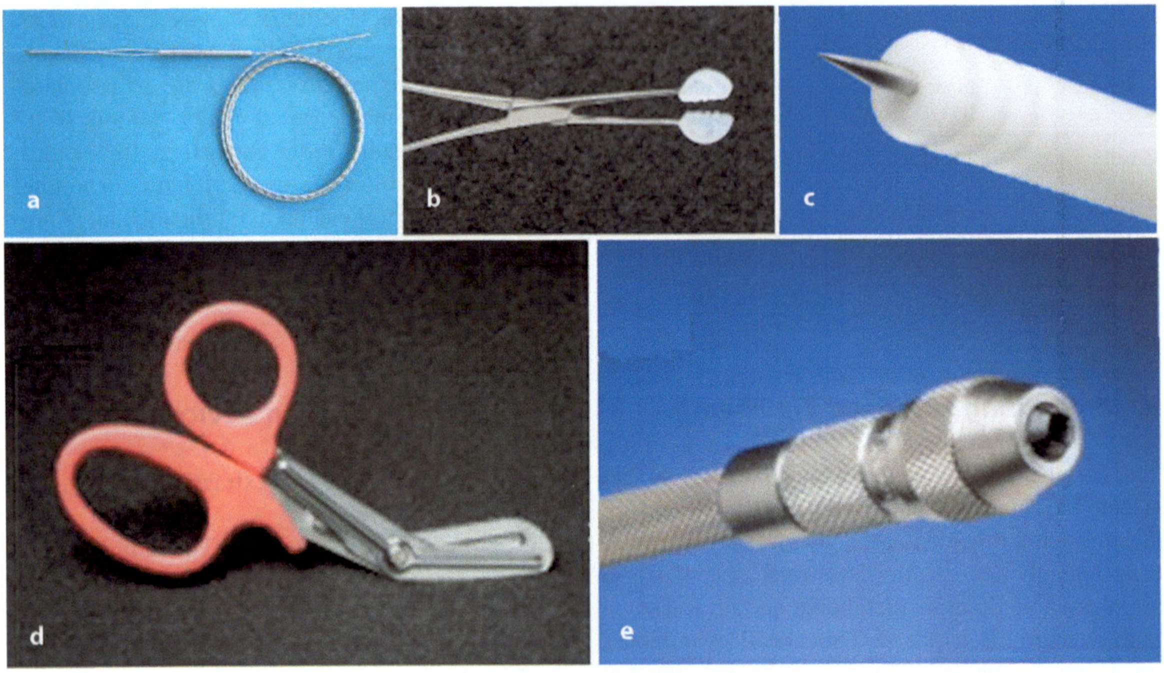

Fig. 4.14 Other traction devices: Bulldog™ lead extender (a); Soft-Grip hemostat (b); coil expander (c); lead clippers (d); pin vise (e)

4.2.8 Femoral Tools

Femoral tools were developed to retrieve leads via the femoral approach. Many of these tools come from other disciplines. The most common procedure for extracting leads using the femoral approach is employed using the Byrd Workstation™ femoral intravascular retrieval set. With this system, as described later under "Femoral Approach", leads are removed through a large sheath with the use of a combination of snares.

1. The Byrd Workstation helical loop basket and tip-deflecting wire guide (Fig. 4.15). Components included in the Byrd Workstation are: (a) 16-F workstation check-flow introducer sheath set; (b) 12-F straight inner femoral sheath; (c) helical

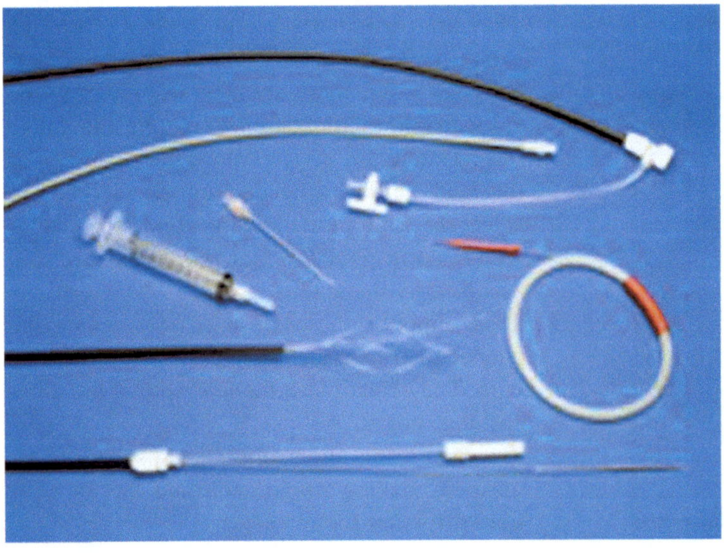

Fig. 4.15 Byrd Workstation femoral intravascular retrieval set: 16-F sheath containing a coaxial 12-F inner sheath preloaded with a Dotter helical loop basket and a tip-deflecting wire guide

loop basket and tip-deflecting wire guide. These devices are used to snare and extract transvenous cardiac leads via the femoral vein [17]. The Byrd Workstation is 16 F with an approximately 30-cm-long sheath equipped with a check-flow valve that serves to irrigate the sheath continuously to prevent clot formation. The 12-F inner sheath is a long, flexible cannula that carries the basic Dotter helical loop basket and tip-deflecting wire guide through the inferior vena cava (IVC) and into the right atrium. The transfemoral workstation works as a conduit inside which it is possible to use positioning and grasping tools to capture and remove the leads via the femoral approach. These tools, called snares, are inserted through the Byrd Workstation in order to grasp the lead and pull it down from the superior veins and then from the heart. The helical loop basket and tip-deflecting wire guide, and the Needle's Eye snare (Cook Vascular) are commonly used to capture and remove leads from the femoral route. The preloaded cannula (12-F inner sheath) passes through the outer cannula (16-F workstation) to carry these two instruments, via the femoral vein, into the right atrium. A 12-F curved femoral introducer sheath can be alternatively used to add directional control to the helical loop basket/tip-deflecting wire guide combination when the intra-atrial position of the lead is difficult to access with the straight inner femoral sheath.

2. The Needle's Eye® snare (Cook Vascular). This is another extraction tool (Fig. 4.16) that can be inserted through and used in conjunction with the Byrd Workstation [23]. As with the tip-deflecting wire guide and helical loop basket, it is a transfemoral grasping tool that forms a basket snare around the lead body. It is delivered to the vicinity of the lead through a long, flexible, 12-F cannula placed coaxially within a larger, outer, 16-F cannula that has a hemostasis valve at its proximal end. The flush port is continuous with the snare's innermost lumen. The Needle's Eye snare is designed to grasp straight or configured objects with or without free ends, providing quick-release capability by simply retracting the threader mechanism. It is compatible either with the straight or curved (for added position ability) inner femoral sheath.

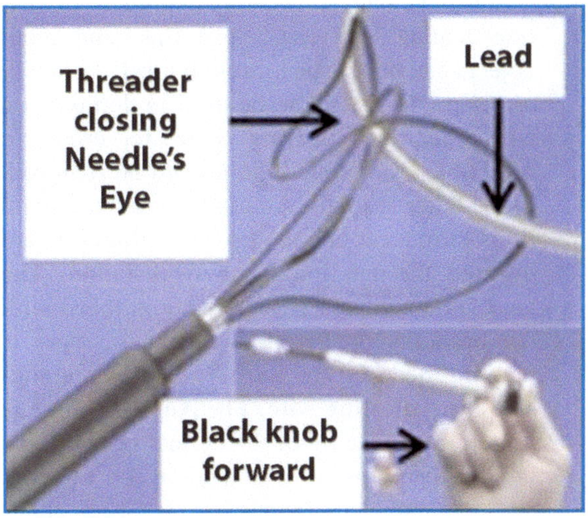

Fig. 4.16 Needle's Eye® snare

4.2.8.1 Other Femoral Tools

In addition to the previously described tools, there are other tools that can be used following the transfemoral approaches to lead extraction. They are classified depending on their use in catheters and snares. Usually, these tools can be used either in one- or two-step approaches (described later in under "Femoral Approach"). Briefly, when a lead's free proximal end is accessible, the one-step femoral approach is adopted. Otherwise, a two-step approach must be used, with the former step used to create a loop around the lead to pull the proximal end of the lead in the IVC.

1. Catheters: electrophysiology deflectable leads can be used to perform a reversible loop around the indwelling lead in the two-step approach; the pigtail catheter can be used in similar way, even if its grasp on the lead is sometimes not strong enough to extract the lead. These catheters are usually preferred to the tip-deflecting wire in the presence of despiralization of the lead that is to be removed in order to avoid possible irreversible entrapment between lead spirals and the tip-deflecting wire. Lassos and the Amplatz gooseneck snare are examples of snares used in lead extraction through the femoral vein. The lasso snare is generally used either to retrieve leads that have free ends or as a second step in the two-step approach.
2. Amplatz gooseneck 25-mm snare can be used

either in the one- or two-step approach. In fact, free-floating lead ends, lead tips, and other objects can be grasped through a 6-F introducer. Alternatively, it can be used in conjunction with the tip-deflecting wire to create a reversible loop around the lead to be removed. In the latter case, the Amplatz gooseneck snare in its introducer and the tip-deflecting wire are inserted through the Byrd Workstation. The lead to be removed is selectively grabbed with the tip-deflecting wire; the Amplatz snare is then inserted into the Byrd Workstation alongside the deflecting wire. The Amplatz snare is used to grasp the tip of the deflecting wire; the loop is then closed by advancing the catheter. At this point, a continuous loop has been created around the lead to be removed. This process of snaring is reversible; in fact, releasing the Amplatz snare liberates the tip-deflecting wire.

4.3 Techniques for Lead Extraction

Any technique used for extraction should have a good lead control. The finality of lead control is to allow traction-force application uniformly over the entire length of the lead. Lead control is important for improving success rate and reducing complications. First, lead control is obtained by securing the inner coil with a stylet. Second, a suture is used as an additional traction device. Finally, once the lead is prepared, lead control is obtained by constantly assessing the lead's tensile properties during traction. Changes in tensile response may be due to stylet detachment from the lead, freeing of the lead from binding sites, inner conductor's unravelling, or outer insulation's rupture. Lead traction, counterpressure and countertraction, progressive dissection and mechanical dislodgement are the techniques used for lead extraction [11, 18, 24–26].

4.3.1 Lead Traction

Simple traction is the most primitive method of lead removal. It was the only method of lead extraction during the early years of pacing, when leads to be removed had large and strong bodies, no effective fixation mechanisms, and low dwelling time [27] (Table 4.5). In the past, when manual traction was ineffective, weighted traction was used [28, 29]. Traction was performed either manually for minutes or using various weights or elastic bands for days [27]. The exposed lead was attached to the Buck's traction (Fig. 4.17) that provided continuous traction. This process was performed by progressive increase of weights until premature atrial or ventricular contraction occurred or the sound of the weights hitting the floor confirmed successful removal.

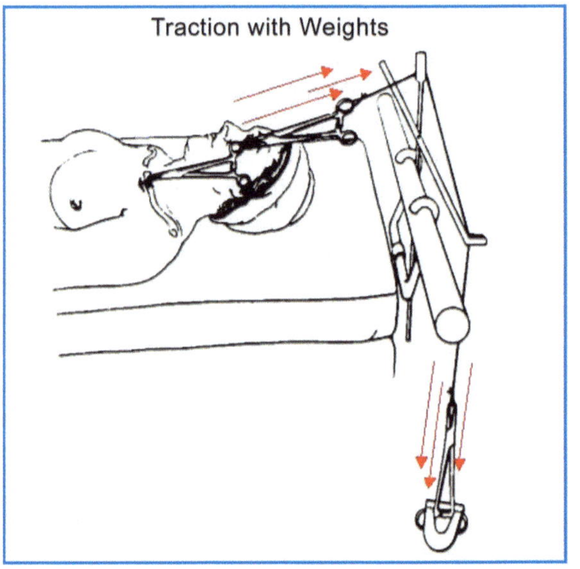

Fig. 4.17 Lead removal using Buck's traction. Figure courtesy of Dr. Belott PH. Reprinted with permission

Table 4.5 Traction effectiveness

	Low ST effectiveness	High ST effectiveness
Characteristics of lead bodies	Small and fragile	Large and strong
Implant duration	Long	Short
Adhesions	Present/widespread	Absent/scanty

ST simple traction

With a longer dwelling time, fibrous encapsulation along the lead/vascular wall/myocardium interface develops [4]. Force applied to the leads during simple traction is either not focused or limited by the tensile strength of the insulation and conductor coils, so the distribution of force to the binding sites is unknown. For these reasons, direct traction was associated either with lead damage and unsuccessful removal or complications such as vein tearing and myocardial wall perforation or rupture. Therefore, lead removal by direct traction is dangerous and often ineffective. The force required can cause cardiac avulsion and tamponade. Moreover, pulling on the lead can cause insulation stretching and lead fracture. The effectiveness of traction is significantly dependent upon length of implant: leads implanted for <6 months can be reasonably removed by simple traction, whereas in leads implanted for >1 year, success rate with traction is low, and a more complex extraction procedure must be performed (see Chapter 6). It is important to apply traction force uniformly over the entire length of the lead. Therefore, additional tools have been developed to increase the success rate and decrease complications of transvenous lead removal. The use of stylets or locking stylets (inserted into the proximal conductor coil and bound to its tip at the distal electrode) has considerably improved the effectiveness of direct traction, but the other complications associated with traction are not eliminated (see Chapter 6).

Locking stylets lock within the lumen of the lead near the distal electrode tip so traction is applied at the lead tip and the rest of the lead body is compressed. As with standard stylets, locking stylets are used to stabilize the lead during dilatation of surrounding tissues, but the force exerted via a locking stylet is almost directly applied at the tip, bypassing most of the conductor and insulation. The Spectranetics Lead-Locking Device stylet, as already discussed, allows traction along the entire length of the lead. Moreover, recently introduced locking stylets can be unlocked and repositioned if necessary. When one considers passing a locking stylet through the inner lumen of the lead, one must expose the inner coil of the lead, test patency of the coil lumen, verify the inner diameter of the lead to choose the appropriate size of locking stylet, advance the locking stylet until it reaches the distal end of the lead, and finally lock the stylet into place. After insertion in the inner coil, a suture is generally used as an additional traction device. It is important to constantly assess the lead's tensile properties during traction. Changes in the tensile response may be due to stylet detachment from the lead, freeing of the lead from binding sites, the inner conductor unravelling, or rupture of the outer insulation. When correctly used, traction with locking stylets allows extraction of a greater number of intact leads. In fact, when using traction with a locking stylet, the chance of lead breakage is minimized, but the other complications associated with traction are not eliminated (see Chapter 6).

There are some limitations to the use of a locking stylet. Once it is inserted into the lead, it may sometimes be difficult or impossible to reverse the locking mechanism and remove the device. Furthermore, if the inner conductor is broken or distorted, it is impossible to introduce or pass the stylet. Excessive force can dislocate the stylet, or the distal conductor coil can still unwind or even disconnect from the electrode.

4.3.2 Counterpressure and Countertraction

Telescoping sheaths (Fig. 4.18) may be used to provide counterpressure and countertraction. Telescoping sheaths are defined as any extraction sheath that can be used as a single sheath or may

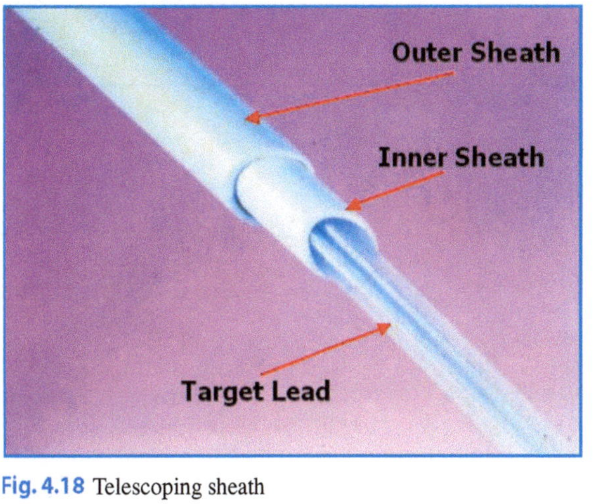

Fig. 4.18 Telescoping sheath

be paired with a second sheath [3]. The use of two sheaths has the advantage of inner sheath flexibility and outer sheath stiffness to prevent kinking and improve the effectiveness of advancement over the lead without overstressing the lead. The outer sheath is usually mechanical, even when the inner sheath uses some other technology, such as laser, electrosurgical, or rotating threaded tip. Sheaths provide counterpressure (forward movement to break adhesions) as they are advanced, countertraction (opposition to movement of the myocardial wall) as the extractors pull to remove the lead, and adhesion dissection when alternatively rotated clockwise and counterclockwise (progressive dissection).

- Counterpressure (Fig. 4.19) is performed by simultaneously applying a forward pressure on the sheath and traction to the lead. Pressure describes the pushing force applied to the sheath that is directed toward the heart, and its objective is to overcome binding sites between lead and vascular system. Traction refers to the pulling force applied to the lead in the opposite direction, and its objective is to allow the sheath to follow the lead around the bends in the vascular system. The goal of counterpressure is to counterbalance the advancement force (pressure) with the retraction force (traction). An imbalance between these two forces can produce failures or complications.
- Countertraction (Fig. 4.20) is performed when the sheath has been progressed to the lead tip-myocardial surface. The traction applied on the lead is counterbalanced by the pressure obtained shoving the outer sheath to support the myocardium; in other words, the force is applied perpendicular and in opposition to the heart wall. This allows centering and limiting the traction force to the binding sites surrounding lead tip, minimizing the risk of myocardial invagination or tear. In countertraction the pulling force applied on the lead (traction) is opposed and counterbalanced by pushing pressure of the overlying sheath on the endocardium (pressure) to limit myocardial invagination or avulsion. Again, an imbalance between these two forces can produce failures or complications.

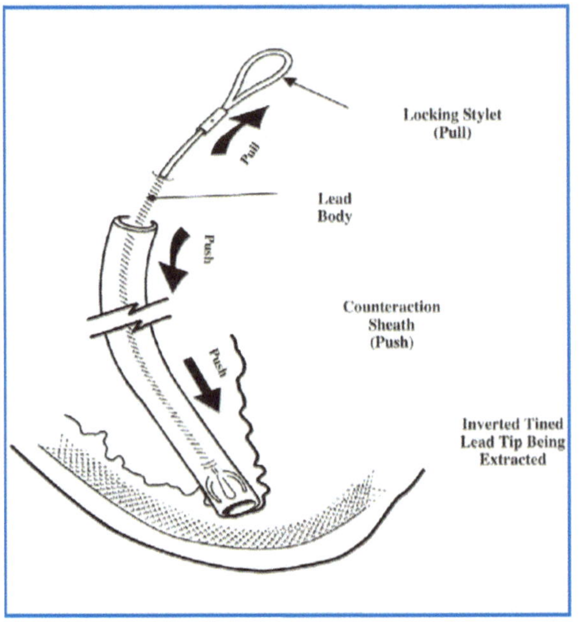

Fig. 4.20 Countertraction. Figure courtesy of Dr. Verma A and Dr. Wilkoff BL [11]. Reprinted with permission

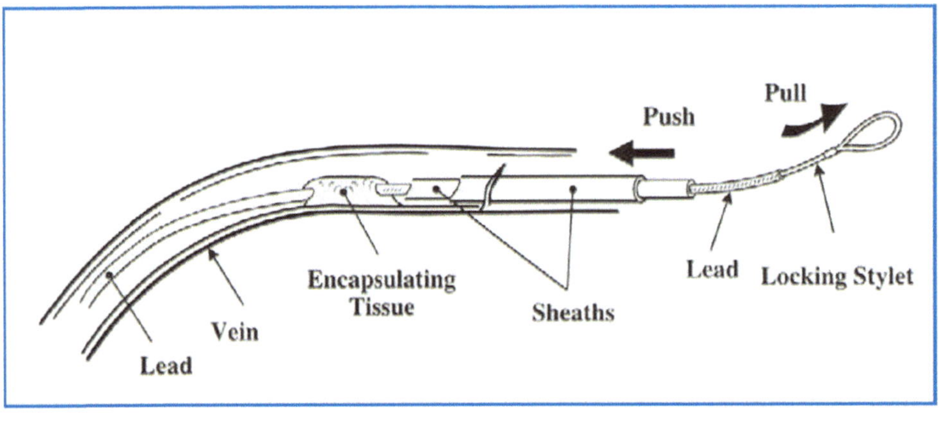

Fig. 4.19 Counterpressure. Figure courtesy of Dr. Verma A and Dr. Wilkoff BL [11]. Reprinted with permission

4.3.3 *Progressive Dissection and Mechanical Dislodgement*

This technique consist of mechanical dissection of adhesions using a single sheath when it is alternatively rotated clockwise and counterclockwise: using this technique, mechanical tip dislodgement is finally achieved. A single-sheath progressive rotational dilatation is performed while maintaining smooth traction on the silk ties (progressive dissection). This rotation is employed uninterrupted until the lead tip is freed by sheath movement (mechanical dislodgement). Therefore, this technique allows lead removal without the use of counterpressure (progressive dissection) and countertraction (mechanical dislodgement). Sheath advancement over the lead is provided by progressive dissection via twisting the single sheath, and the lead tip is freed via mechanical dislodgement. This technique is described more fully in Chapter 5.

When advancing sheaths, it is important to use the sheath technique properly either by maintaining adequate lead tension (via the stylet or directly) or by maintaining alignment between lead and sheath to prevent damage to vessel walls. The appropriate equilibrium between pressure and traction forces is defined as lead control. Imbalance between these two forces can produce failures or complications. If excessive scar tissue or calcification prevents safe advancement of sheaths, an alternative approach must be considered. In fact, excessive force with sheaths used intravascularly may result in damage to the vascular system requiring surgical repair.

4.4 Approaches

Independent of the energy used to free the lead, changing the approach to the lead itself may provide a possible advantage during removal. There are three approaches for transvenous lead extraction (Fig. 4.21):

1. Venous entry approach, also known as the superior approach
2. Transfemoral approach, also known as the inferior approach
3. Internal transjugular approach

It seems more accurate not to use the terms "superior" or "inferior" approach and, instead, to use the terms "venous entry" (implant vein) approach, "transfemoral vein" approach, and "internal transjugular" approach. In fact, the term superior approach can be misleading considering that either venous entry approach or internal transjugular approach can be considered superior approaches.

Most operators begin with a venous entry approach using the implant vein and switch to a transfemoral approach if necessary [30]. Moreover, when leads are broken or free floating, the transfemoral approach is historically performed. Different venous approaches using the mechanical dilatation tech-

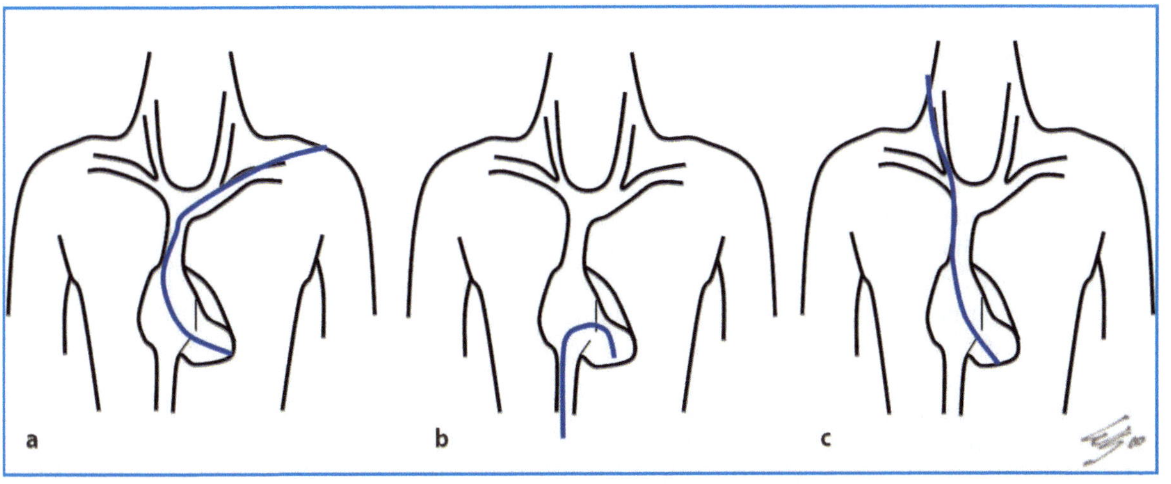

Fig. 4.21 Approaches for transvenous lead extraction: venous entry approach using the implant vein (a), transfemoral approach (b), internal transjugular approach (c)

nique represent the personal contribution to transvenous removal [31–33], with use of the internal jugular vein in case of free-floating leads or difficult exposed leads [31].

4.4.1 Venous Entry Approach

In the presence of leads exposed through tributary veins of the SVC system (cephalic, subclavian, external jugular), the venous entry approach is the first-choice technique (Fig. 4.22). This approach is also known as the superior or SVC approach, even if the term venous entry approach appears to be more correct. The venous entry approach consists of a combination of traction by a stylet, mechanical dilation of binding sites by the dilating sheaths, and countertraction at the tip of the lead by the outer telescopic sheaths. Lead extraction tools necessary to prepare the lead and accomplish the venous entry approach are reported in Table 4.6.

Before starting the extraction procedure, the operator must identify the type and manufacturer of leads submitted to removal. One must identify lead fixation mechanism and type of fixation in case of an active fixation lead; in some active fixation leads, special stylets are needed in order to unscrew the screw. After lead identification, the procedure of lead extraction consists of lead preparation and sheath application when gentle manual traction is unsuccessful.

4.4.1.1 Lead Preparation and Gentle Manual Traction

The first step consists of surgical exposition of the proximal end of the indwelling lead and removal of the lead from its connections. Once all leads are liberated from surrounding tissue and the sleeve is removed, the leads are manifestly free all the way to the venous entry site. In case of active fixation leads, the screw must be unscrewed. At this point, the lead may be prepared. It is important to cut the lead very close to the connector, almost 10–15 cm out of the venous entry site, leaving as long as possible the portion of the indwelling lead to work with. By using lead clippers, the proximal end of the lead is removed, then a short segment of the outer insulation and

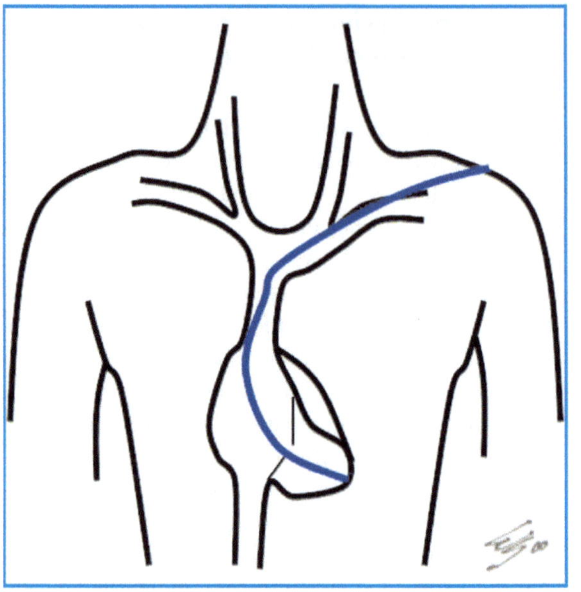

Fig. 4.22 Venous entry approach

Table 4.6 Lead extraction, venous-entry approach

Tools
Stylets
• Standard stylet wires
• Locking stylets
• Wilkoff (Cook Vascular)
• Liberator (Cook Vascular)
• Viper stylet (Vascomed)
• Lead locking device (Spectranetics)
Extraction sheaths
• Mechanical sheaths: Teflon, polypropylene, stainless
• Laser sheaths
• Electrosurgical sheaths
• Rotating threaded tip sheath
Others
• Sutures
• Bulldog lead extender
• Soft-grip hemostat
• Coil expander
• Pin vise
• Lead clippers

outer coil is removed with a scalpel and wire cutters. In a bipolar coaxial lead, inner insulation is exposed using cutters. Closing off the interior lumen (or coil) when cutting the lead must be avoided. A stiff normal stylet supplied by the lead manufacturer, of appropriate length and diameter for the lead, is introduced into the lead body with its tip as close as possible to the lead tip in order to stiffen it. It is important to always check fluoroscopically during stylet insertion. Sometimes it is not possible to advance the stylet inside the lead: at this point, an alternating clockwise/counterclockwise rotation of the stylet can overcome obstruction inside the inner lumen of the leads. Alternatively, if occlusion is proximal enough, it may be possible to pull the lead in order to cut away the occluded section and prepare the lead again for stylet insertion. In this latter case, a soft-grip hemostat and sometimes a Bulldog lead extender can be useful. Moreover, the Bulldog lead extender allows extension and direct traction of lumenless cardiac leads (which incorporate a cable design instead a helical coil). In these cases, the end of the lead and conductors are placed into the metal loop, and the sleeve is advanced over the loop to close it, allowing a firm grasp of the lead components. After stylet insertion, gentle manual traction, limited by the tensile strength of both the lead and tissue, is performed. In this process, either the operator's experience or careful observation of the lead under fluoroscopy are necessary to determine if the lead is beginning to deform or pull apart or if excessive deformation of the heart is occurring.

If success is not achieved when a locking stylet is intended to be used, the normal stylet is used to test coil lumen patency and removal (alternatively, the normal stylet is left in place). After this, the inner diameter of the lead must be verified so that the appropriate size of the locking stylet is chosen. It is important to correctly execute this measure: if the locking stylet is too thin, it will not lock; alternatively, there is risk of withdraw from the lead during extraction. In these cases, the stylet should be removed and a large size tried. Then the appropriate locking stylet is advanced to the distal end of the lead, where the locking stylet is finally locked in place. At this point, pulling the lead and locking stylet, checking fluoroscopically that the locking stylet does not withdraw, ensures that the correct size of locking stylet has been chosen. A standard or locking stylet can be used, with some differences. Standard vs. locking stylets: as dissection of binding sites has to be performed by sheaths, the lead must be as stiff as possible in order to allow a firm hold. A locking stylet allows strong lead traction, but sometimes some locking stylets cannot be removed. However, locking and traction at the lead tip (i.e., locking stylet) is not a key point because binding sites at the tip have to be overcome by dilatation and rotation of the sheath rather than by traction. A standard stylet and a suture, if used with moderate traction, can accomplish the task with a low risk of removing the outer insulation. The other advantage of the standard stylet is that, being easily removable, it is useful when crossovers to an alternative transvenous approach are required.

At this point, either using a standard or a locking stylet, a suture is used as an additional traction device. One or two (in the presence of unipolar or bipolar leads, respectively) ties of nonabsorbable silk suture material are secured, respectively, around the outer and the inner insulation of the lead. Once the lead is freed and secured, gentle manual traction is applied in an attempt to remove the lead. In case of active lead fixation, one should attempt to unscrew the lead by rotating the lead (and locking stylet if used) counterclockwise. As traction is applied, the electrocardiogram should be monitored for atrial or ventricular ectopy, and the patient's blood pressure should also be observed for hypotension. In some cases, even if gentle traction is not initially successful, continued steady traction for 1–2 min may be successful. Fluoroscopic observation during traction may indicate the site and extent of fibrosis holding the lead to the vascular system. Whereas occasionally the lead can be easily removed by traction, more frequently, the lead has multiple binding sites of fibrous scar and requires the application of sheaths. Therefore, when manual traction fails to remove the lead, an extraction sheath is required. Telescopic sheaths are designed to break, cut, and dilate fibrous adhesions; offer countertraction; and help dilate some adhesions. When using a sheath, some precautions must be followed (Table 4.7).

Table 4.7 Indispensable attention required when using sheaths

Precautions during sheath utilization
• A sheath must be large enough to allow its advancement over the lead without causing the lead to buckle or its insulation to brunch up
• Sheaths must not be excessively loose
• No matter which system is used, it is crucial to stay "in line" with the lead at all times
• Sheath advancement must always be monitored fluoroscopically
• During sheath advancement, maintaining adequate tension on the lead to support and properly guide the sheath within the vessel is crucial
• Insufficient tension on the lead could cause vein rupture by the sheath; excessive tension on the lead may cause myocardial avulsion
• Never use sheaths on more than one lead at a time

4.4.1.2 Sheath Application

When performing extraction procedures, either proper lead preparation and lead control or correct use of sheaths by means of counterpressure and countertraction or progressive dissection and mechanical dislodgement is usually necessary.

1. Mechanical sheaths: these are generally used under fluoroscopic guidance to perform counterpressure. With the lead in tension, the inner sheath is advanced along the length of the lead. Then telescopically, the outer sheath is advanced over the inner sheath, keeping it within the vessel. In general, the inner sheath should not be advanced more than 4 cm beyond the outer sheath. Rotating the sheath during advancement may facilitate progress through excessive scar tissue. Therefore, telescopically, the inner and then the outer sheaths are alternatively advanced while maintaining adequate tension on the lead and/or its wire guide or locking stylet until the lead is free of tissue restriction. If the lead has not been freed by the time the sheaths are near the myocardium, it is possible to position the outer sheath so that the blunt end is directed toward the myocardium and the inner sheath is pulled back several centimeters. At this point, countertraction is employed by holding the outer sheath firmly 1 cm from the heart wall and steadily pulling the locking stylet back. The pacing tip will then be pulled into the sheath. Rotation of the sheath may help dislodge the tip. Once freed from tissue attachment, it is possible to completely remove the lead. Following extraction, the sheath allows venous access if a new pacing or defibrillating system is to be implanted. In these cases, proper use of guidewires and introducer sheaths is required to advance the new lead, avoiding obstacles created by fibrodissected tissue. With these objectives, hydrophilic-coated guidewires advanced into the IVC and followed by a long introducer sheath are often required.
2. Laser sheaths: when using a laser sheath, the lead must first be prepared by inserting a locking stylet (the Spectranetics Lead-Locking Device is generally used) and securing the lead and stylet with a suture, which is used as an additional traction device during the removal procedure. Laser sheaths need to be calibrated before use, and during this process, the operator wears protective glasses. Laser is particularly useful in case of dense fibrotic adhesions that may be resistant to counterpressure applied with a mechanical sheath. In fact, laser extraction sheaths reduce the pressure required to dissect through binding sites. Under fluoroscopic visualization, it is important to enter the access vein aligned coaxially with the lead and to maintain coaxial alignment between sheath and lead during sheath advancement. The laser sheath then advances to the binding sites. Once adhesions are reached, the laser is activated and the sheath ablates through the binding sites. After binding sites are cleared, the laser sheath is advanced to the following adhesion (Fig. 4.23). In the event of difficult sheath advancement, it is possible to slightly rotate the bevel tip of the sheath or use the outer sheath to help dissect the binding sites.
   A crucial point is the powered dilatation along the SVC. First, appropriate lead control maintaining light and steady traction must be achieved. Second, the proper alignment between sheath and lead must be obtained and all pressure against the SVC avoided. Finally, it is important to orient the shorter end of the 15° bevelled sheath toward the SVC wall. Lasing is stopped before the tip is reached (about 1 cm

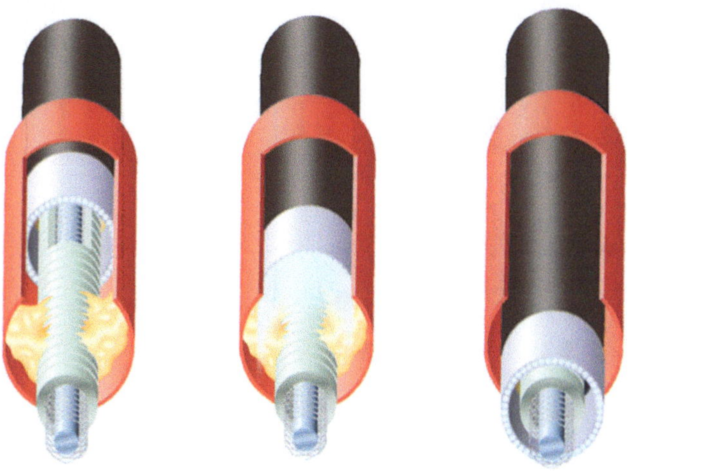

Fig. 4.23 Laser ablation of binding sites

before reaching the myocardium) due to the high risk of wall tears. The tip is then freed by a combination of traction by a locking stylet and sheath advancement. In an ideal situation, the sheath is passed over the lead, dissecting each binding site until the sheath reaches a point about 1 cm from the heart wall. The lead is then removed from the heart wall using countertraction.

Tears in the venous wall of the innominate vein and SVC have been reported with the Excimer sheath [34–39], as has cardiac tamponade due to lasing into the heart [22]. The inability of the laser technique to overcome calcified scar tissue and to perform dilation near the tip of the lead are major limitations [19]. Laser sheaths have a larger diameter compared with mechanical sheaths, and advancing them through the costoclavicular space is often difficult. Another limitation is the consistently higher cost of equipment and sheaths. Despite these disadvantages, this technique spreads rapidly and is today the most commonly used technique in the USA [9, 11]. Whereas earlier studies addressed the efficacy and safety of the initial laser sheath models [36], the recent Lead Extraction in the Contemporary Setting (LExICon) Study [40] showed that laser-assisted extraction is either effective or safe. In this study, the modified SLS II (Spectranetics) sheaths, which have improved mechanical properties to enhance advancement over the lead, were used.

3. Electrosurgical dissection sheaths (EDS): reports about the clinical effectiveness and safety of these sheaths are similar to laser dilation [41, 42]. The removal procedure using ESD is less expensive than laser dilatation, and advantages and limitations between the two appear to be similar. There is a major difference between laser and EDS sheath systems. Whereas the EDS sheath tip is beveled with the electrodes at the leading edge, thus allowing them to be placed on the inner side when turning tight corners (i.e., bending into the SVC), laser sheaths have circumferential cutting capacity that may damage the SVC (Fig. 4.24). On the other hand, the EDS can cause some patient discomfort during the extraction procedure because the phrenic nerve can be transiently stimulated when the sheath passes close to it. This technique is less commonly used in comparison with laser-assisted removal, and only limited experience is reported in the literature [41, 42].

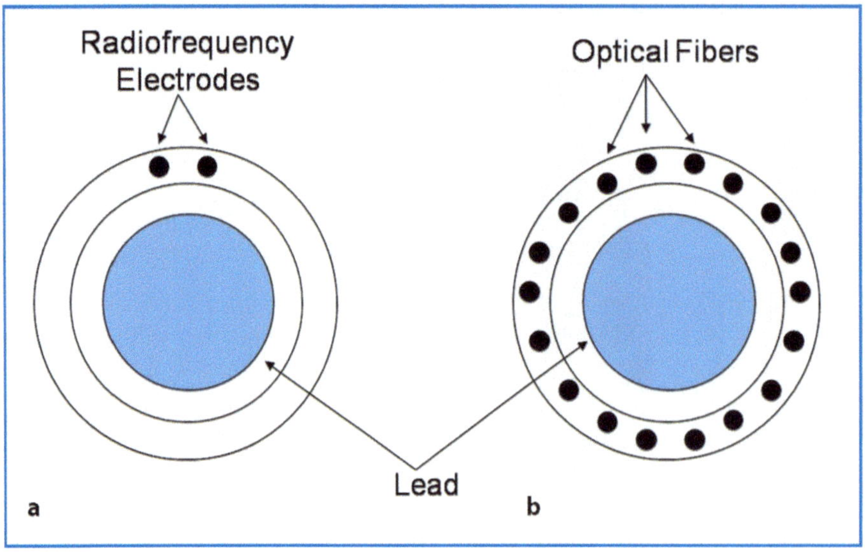

Fig. 4.24 Tips of an electrosurgical dissection sheath (a) and a laser extraction sheath (b)

4. Rotating threaded-tip sheath: this can be used in lead removal through the venous entry approach. Although this sheath has the capability of dissecting through all types of tissues, even calcified adhesions, there are not enough published data about this type of sheath due to its recent development [20, 21]. Nevertheless, there have been no studies comparing the different powered tools to each other.

Authors' Technique

Our technique, developed by Dr. Bongiorni [31], is described fully in Chapter 5. It consists of a modified percutaneous dilatation, defined as a progressive dissection and mechanical dislodgement technique. A standard instead of a locking stylet is used. Dilatation is performed using polypropylene sheaths by Cook Vascular. A progressive dissection with single twisting sheath (rotating alternatively clockwise and counterclockwise) dilatation is performed while maintaining smooth traction on the silk ties. The twisting of the sheath allows the lead tip to be dislodged. In this method, the lead is removed without countertraction. If the venous entry approach is unsuccessful or became difficult or dangerous, then the transfemoral or internal transjugular approaches should be considered.

4.4.2 Transfemoral Approach

A transfemoral approach (Fig. 4.25) using a workstation provided with different remote control tools was introduced in the early 1990s, the same time as mechanical dilatation techniques were introduced [26]. The transfemoral approach is versatile and is used in percutaneous retrieval of car-

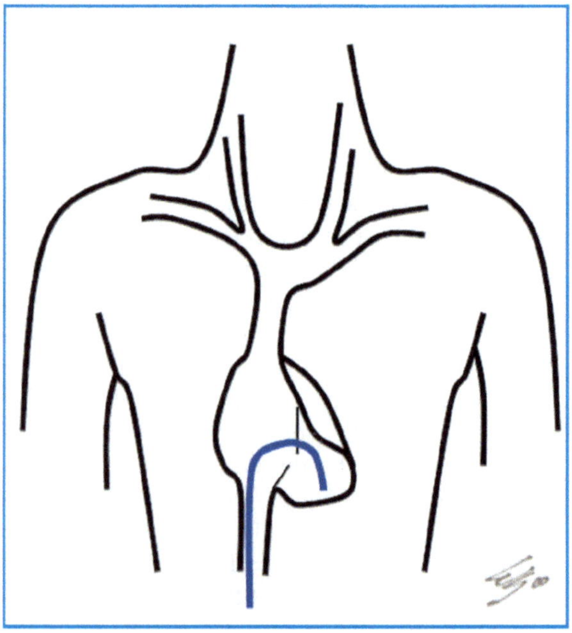

Fig. 4.25 Transfemoral approach

diac leads, indwelling catheters, fragments of catheter tubing or wire guides, and other foreign objects. In particular, the approach through the femoral vein, also known as inferior approach, is useful in the presence of free-floating leads, the proximal end of which cannot be approached at the generator pocket. Lead extraction tools available for the transfemoral approach are reported in Table 4.8. Femoral extraction requires a 16-F (inner diameter) sheath with a hemostatic valve (Byrd Workstation, Cook Vascular). The workstation is inserted through the femoral vein and advanced to the IVC or lower right atrium. Because it acts as a conduit, different positioning and grasping tools, called snares, can be inserted through the workstation so the lead can be grasped and pulled down from the superior veins and then from the heart. The helical loop basket and tip-deflecting wire guide and the Needle's Eye snare (Cook Vascular) are commonly used. Once snared, the lead is pulled into the sheath, which is advanced over the lead to the myocardial interface providing countertraction for lead extraction.

The transfemoral approach is adopted in many centers as a primary approach when free-floating leads are involved and as an alternative approach in case of failed primary approach through the implant vein [23, 43–45]. Some techniques using the transfemoral approach allow grasping and removal of exposed or intravascular leads, fragments of catheter tubing or wire guides, and other foreign objects. Nevertheless, all techniques are based on two general approaches: the first (the one-step approach) is used when free ends of a foreign object are available and requires the combination of a wire loop and catheter to grasp and remove the foreign object; the second (the two-step approach) is used when there is no free end accessible for snaring and grasping and is performed by establishing a reversible loop around the body of the lead in order to pull it, so that the proximal end of the lead is then pulled into the IVC. In fact, pulling often frees the lead from binding sites in the superior veins without exerting traction on the electrode–myocardium interface; in other words, the lead slides inside binding sites. Failure to extract the proximal portion of the lead from the superior veins is rare. Once the proximal end of the lead is pulled into the IVC, a free end is available, so the first approach is then used to remove the leads [43].

The femoral workstation is 16 F with an approximately 30-cm-long sheath equipped with a check-flow valve that serves to irrigate the sheath continuously to prevent clot formation. After the sheath is flushed with saline fluid, the side port is connected with a continuous intravenous line. Once a femoral access using the Seldinger technique is obtained, a guidewire is advanced on fluoroscopic observation to the right atrium. The dilator and sheath are inserted over the guidewire until it extends to the lower right atrium; the dilator is then removed. At this point, several femoral extraction techniques are available for use with the Byrd Workstation [43]: one of these uses the helical loop basket and tip-deflecting wire guide, which are positioned into the right atrium by carefully advancing each one from the 12-F femoral sheath. By deflecting the wire guide >360° around the lead body within the atrium allows the lead to be encircled (Fig. 4.26a). The tip-deflecting wire guide is a long, thin steel cable, the tip of which can be wound around the object to be removed from the heart. It is used with a handle that holds the proximal end of the wire guide, allowing the wire tip to bend around the lead. The role of the wire is to encircle, capture, and stabilize the lead. Once the lead is encircled, the basket is slid forward, and the distal end of the wire guide is captured in the basket, which is then closed over the wire guide by carefully advancing the 12-F sheath,

Table 4.8 Lead extraction: transfemoral approach

Tools
Byrd Workstation • 16-F workstation check-flow introducer sheath set • 12-F straight inner femoral sheath • Helical loop-basket and tip-deflecting wire guide
Needle's Eye snare
Others • Amplatz gooseneck snare (Microvena) • Lassos/catcher (Osypka) • Various angiographic guide catheters • Simple electrophysiology deflectable leads, pigtails, angiographic catheters

creating a strong loop around the body of the indwelling object (Fig. 4.26b). This loop is sometimes irreversible; in fact, it cannot always be released and repositioned on the lead body. At this point, the deflecting wire captured by the basket is pulled into the workstation (Fig. 4.26c). Finally, the workstation is advanced to the lead tip using the principles of both countertraction and counterpressure (Fig. 4.26d).

An alternative to the basket and tip-deflecting wire is the Needle's Eye snare (Fig. 4.27). This extraction tool can be inserted through and used in conjunction with the Byrd Workstation [23]. This, too, is a transfemoral grasping tool that forms a basket snare around the lead body. It is delivered to the vicinity of the lead through a long, flexible, 12-F cannula placed coaxially within a larger outer cannula that has a hemostasis valve at its proximal end. The flush port is continuous with the snare's innermost lumen. The Needle's Eye snare is designed to grasp straight or configured objects with or without free ends, providing quick-release capability by simply retracting the threader mechanism. It is compatible with either the straight or curved (for added positionability) inner femoral sheath.

Once positioned at the site of the indwelling object, the snare is deployed by retracting the12-F inner sheath so that the snare emerges and assumes its preformed curled shape. After positioning the snare loop over the lead body, the threader is advanced (moving the black side knob of the handle fully forward) inside the loop of the snare, closing the open segment of the circle and obtaining the lead engagement. At this point, the 12-F inner sheath is advanced, thus immobilizing the lead body in the snare. Finally, the lead is prepared for removal by advancing the 16-F introducer sheath over the lead and/or retracting the 12-F inner sheath until the lead enters the 16-F sheath.

Whereas free-floating leads with detached tips

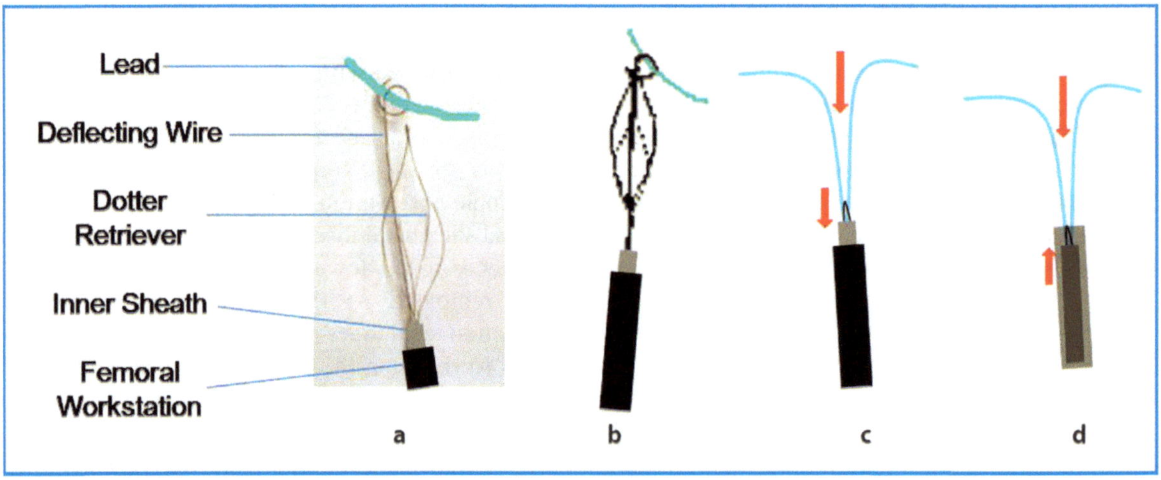

Fig. 4.26a-d Removal of lead using the Byrd Workstation, tip deflecting wire and basket

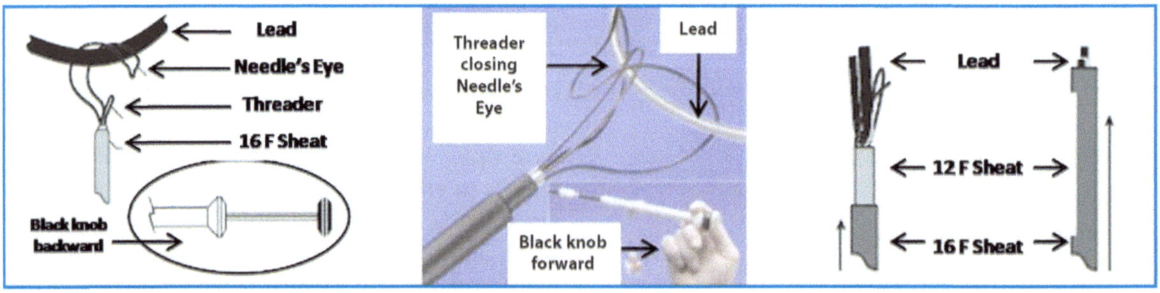

Fig. 4.27 Needle's Eye snare

can be effectively removed, the femoral approach has some limitations, especially when the tip of the lead is fixed to the heart. Femoral extraction techniques may be irreversible, making an open chest extraction necessary. Moreover, dilatation into the right ventricle is challenging and risky. Advancement of the workstation beyond the tricuspid valve is often precluded due to the sharp turn to be navigated. Moreover, due its flexibility, the sheath cuts through tissue poorly and often does not cut through adhesions. In this condition, most of the energy applied to the lead is traction. In addition, the absence of a stylet (either normal or locking) in the lead, generally used to stiffen the lead, does not allow minimization of lead damage during traction. Finally, sometimes the lead is difficult to snare because of its encapsulation on fibrosis, and different fluoroscopic projections are therefore needed (three dimensional heart using two dimensional imaging).

4.4.3 Internal Transjugular Approach

We use the internal transjugular approach (Fig. 4.28) as a first choice for free-floating leads and as an additional step for difficult leads when mechanical dilatation is ineffective or risky [8, 46]. In the presence of free-floating leads, this approach results in removal of all leads submitted to the procedure. In the presence of difficult exposed leads, the internal transjugular approach increases the success rate from 91.1% to 98.5% [31].

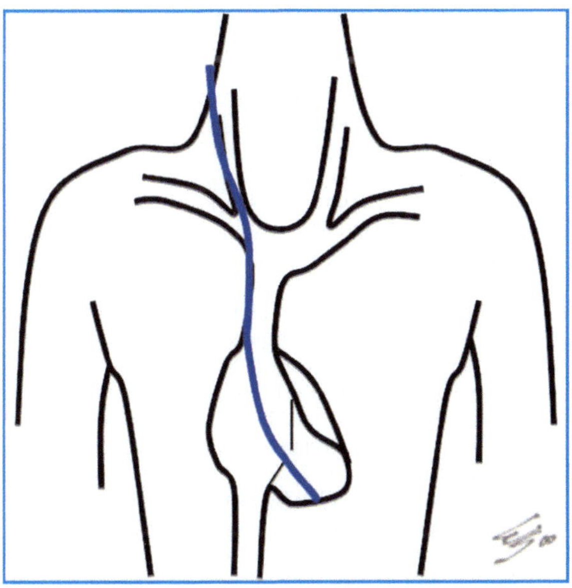

Fig. 4.28 Internal transjugular approach

In the presence of free-floating leads dilatation is often impossible: lead exposure through an SVC tributary, such as the right internal jugular vein, can enhance dilatation by allowing the use of the same technique and tools as used for exposed leads. Actually, once exposed through the internal jugular vein, free-floating leads can be managed in the same way as exposed leads. Difficult conditions for removing leads exposed at the implant site are lead damage (fracture, insulation loss), hard turns in the lead's course (the energy of dilatation may be applied to the venous wall, increasing the risk of tears), very thin costoclavicular space (precluding the use of large dilation sheaths), and the presence of very tight binding sites (sometimes calcified) where dilatation is not effective. A difficult lead can, however, be turned into a free-floating one that can be slipped through some binding sites and then exposed through the internal jugular vein. At this point, there is a "straight-line" course all the way to the tip of the lead. Conventional dilatation of distal binding sites and the tip can be performed. Regardless of the energy used, the straight course of the lead from the jugular vein to the heart facilitates dilatation and allows the use of large sheaths, thus avoiding the use of countertraction. Lead extraction tools used in the internal transjugular approach are reported in Table 4.9, and procedural steps are described in Chapter 5.

Table 4.9 Lead extraction: internal transjugular approach

Tools
Venous entry site
• For lead preparation
Femoral site
• For snaring and grasping (simple electrophysiology deflectable leads, pigtails, snares, etc)
Jugular site
• 11-F introducer
• For snaring and grasping (snares/lassos)
• For lead preparation (sutures and standard stylets)
• For lead extraction (mechanical sheaths)

References

1. WordReference.com Online Language Dictionaries. http://www.wordreference.com/. Accessed 14 Sep 2010
2. Love CJ et al (2000) Recommendations for extraction of chronically implanted transvenous pacing and defibrillator leads: indications, facilities, training. North American Society of Pacing and Electrophysiology Lead Extraction Conference Faculty. Pacing Clin Electrophysiol 23(4 Pt. 1): 544–551
3. Wilkoff BL et al (2009) Transvenous lead extraction: Heart Rhythm Society Expert consensus on facilities, training, indications, and patient management: this document was endorsed by the American Heart Association (AHA). Heart Rhythm 6(7):1085–1104
4. Robboy SJ et al (1969) Autopsy findings with permanent pervenous pacemakers. Circulation 39(4):495–501
5. Smith HJ et al (1994) Five-years experience with intravascular lead extraction. U.S. Lead Extraction Database. Pacing Clin Electrophysiol 17(11 Pt. 2):2016–2020
6. Bongiorni MG et al (2007) Usefulness of mechanical transvenous dilation and location of areas of adherence in patients undergoing coronary sinus lead extraction. Europace 9(1):69–73
7. Bongiorni MG et al (1994) A "step by step" protocol for leads extraction procedures: relation with success rate and complications. Pacing Clin Electrophysiol 17:786 [abstract]
8. Bongiorni MG et al (1999) [Transvenous removal of permanent electrocatheters for heart stimulation and defibrillation]. Cardiologia 44(Suppl 1,Pt. 1):395–398
9. Love CJ (2007) Lead extraction. Heart Rhythm 4(9):1238–1243
10. Love CJ (2000) Current concepts in extraction of transvenous pacing and ICD leads. Cardiol Clin 18(1):193–217
11. Verma A, Wilkoff BL (2004) Intravascular pacemaker and defibrillator lead extraction: a state-of-the-art review. Heart Rhythm 1(6):739–745
12. Rosenheck S et al (2002) Noninstrumental pacemaker and defibrillator lead removal. The importance of the rotation forces. Pacing Clin Electrophysiol 25(7):1029–1036
13. Manolis AS et al (1998) Successful percutaneous extraction of pacemaker leads with a novel (VascoExtor) pacing lead removal system. Am J Cardiol 81(7):935–938
14. Vassilikos VP et al (1999) Percutaneous extraction of transvenous defibrillator leads using the VascoExtor pacing lead removal system. J Interv Card Electrophysiol 3(3):247–251
15. Alt E et al (1996) Three-year experience with a stylet for lead extraction: a multicenter study. Pacing Clin Electrophysiol 19(1):18–25
16. Kennergren C et al (2000) Cardiac lead extraction with a novel locking stylet. J Interv Card Electrophysiol 4(4):591–593
17. Byrd CL et al (1990) Intravascular lead extraction using locking stylets and sheaths. Pacing Clin Electrophysiol 13(12 Pt 2):1871–1875
18. Fearnot NE et al (1990) Intravascular lead extraction using locking stylets, sheaths, and other techniques. Pacing Clin Electrophysiol 13(12 Pt 2):1864–1870
19. Epstein LM et al (1999) Initial experience with larger laser sheaths for the removal of transvenous pacemaker and implantable defibrillator leads. Circulation 100(5):516–525
20. Hussein AA et al (2010) Initial experience with the Evolution mechanical dilator sheath for lead extraction: safety and efficacy. Heart Rhythm 7(7):870–873
21. Dello Russo A et al (2009) Lead extraction: a new effective tool to overcome fibrous binding sites. J Interv Card Electrophysiol 24(2):147–150
22. Hauser RG et al (2010) Deaths and cardiovascular injuries due to device-assisted implantable cardioverter-defibrillator and pacemaker lead extraction. Europace 12(3):395–401
23. Klug D et al (2002) Pacemaker lead extraction with the needle's eye snare for countertraction via a femoral approach. Pacing Clin Electrophysiol 25(7):1023–1028
24. Yue A (2008) System and lead extractions. In: Timperley J et al (eds) Pacemakers and ICDs. Oxford University Press, Oxford, pp 313–331
25. Belott PH (1998) Endocardial lead extraction. Futura, Armonk, p 142
26. Byrd CL et al (1992) Lead extraction: indications and techniques. Cardiol Clin 10:735–748
27. Bilgutay AM et al (1969) Incarceration of transvenous pacemaker electrode. Removal by traction. Am Heart J 77(3):377–379
28. Furman S et al (1987) Retained pacemaker leads. J Thorac Cardiovasc Surg94(5):770–772
29. Furman S, Escher DJ (1968) Retained endocardial pacemaker electrodes. J Thorac Cardiovasc Surg 55(5):737–740
30. Smith MC, Love CJ (2008) Extraction of transvenous pacing and ICD leads. Pacing Clin Electrophysiol 31(6):736–752
31. Bongiorni MG et al (2008) Transvenous removal of pacing and implantable cardiac defibrillating leads using single sheath mechanical dilatation and multiple venous approaches: high success rate and safety in more than 2000 leads. Eur Heart J 29(23):2886–2893
32. Bongiorni MG et al (2005) Pacing and implantable cardioverter-defibrillator transvenous lead extraction. Ital Heart J 6(3):261–266
33. Bongiorni MG et al (2007) Techniques for transvenous leads extraction. Minerva Cardioangiol 55(6):771–781
34. Parsonnet V et al (2001) Laser extraction of entrapped leads. Pacing Clin Electrophysiol 24(3):329–332
35. Moon MR et al (2002) Laser-assist during extraction of chronically implanted pacemaker and defibrillator leads. Ann Thorac Surg 73(6):1893–1896
36. Wilkoff BL et al (1999) Pacemaker lead extraction with the laser sheath: results of the pacing lead extraction with the excimer sheath (PLEXES) trial. J Am Coll Cardiol 33(6):1671–1676
37. Byrd CL et al (2002) Clinical study of the laser sheath for lead extraction: the total experience in the United States. Pacing Clin Electrophysiol 25(5):804–808
38. Kennergren C (1999) Excimer laser assisted extraction of permanent pacemaker and ICD leads: present experiences of a European multi-centre study. Eur J Cardiothorac Surg 15(6):856–860
39. Kennergren C et al (2007) Laser-assisted lead extraction: the European experience. Europace 9(8):651–656
40. Wazni O et al (2010) Lead extraction in the contemporary setting: the LExICon study: an observational retrospective study of consecutive laser lead extractions. J Am Coll Cardiol 55(6):579–586

41. Neuzil P et al (2007) Pacemaker and ICD lead extraction with electrosurgical dissection sheaths and standard transvenous extraction systems: results of a randomized trial. Europace 9(2):98–104
42. Scott PA et al (2009) Extraction of pacemaker and implantable cardioverter defibrillator leads: a single-centre study of electrosurgical and laser extraction. Europace 11(11):1501–1504
43. Belott PH (2007) Lead extraction using the femoral vein. Heart Rhythm 4(8):1102–1107
44. Jarwe M et al (1999) Single center experience with femoral extraction of permanent endocardial pacing leads. Pacing Clin Electrophysiol 22(8):1202–1209
45. Kantharia BK et al (2000) Feasibility, safety, and determinants of extraction time of percutaneous extraction of endocardial implantable cardioverter defibrillator leads by intravascular countertraction method. Am J Cardiol 85(5):593–597
46. Bongiorni MG et al (1998) [The transvenous removal of definitive electrocatheters for stimulation and defibrillation: the indications, methods and results]. Cardiologia 43(10):1105–1109

Personal Technique and Experience: The Pisa Approach

5

Maria Grazia Bongiorni

5.1 Introduction

Technological advances in transvenous lead removal can be achieved by improving the materials and tools for lead extraction or modifying the techniques and approaches. I started the activity of transvenous lead removal in S. Chiara Hospital in Pisa, Italy, in December 1989; since then, with my coworkers, we have managed more than 2,500 pacing and implantable cardioverter–defibrillator (ICD) leads [1]. From the beginning, the technique and approaches have been continuously changed and improved, and by the beginning of 1997, we considered technique maturation to be complete [2]. From 1994 to 1996, we experienced the internal jugular approach to remove free-floating leads, and at the beginning of 1997, we started using it also in case of standard technique failure [3]. The first techniques I learned and applied for lead removal were traction with locking stylet, counterpressure, and countertraction, as described by Byrd et al. [4], using polypropylene sheaths. Very often, we experienced the inability to insert the stylet up to the lead tip because of lead damage or stylet unlocking during traction; moreover, the force necessary to apply counterpressure and countertraction was discouraging. Working with those techniques, I progressively changed the kind of stylets and the way in which polypropylene sheaths were used, performing special knots over the leads. The femoral approach was used in some cases to complete extraction procedures, and in difficult cases, I utilized a different type of venous entry, the jugular approach, making the procedure easier due to the straight line from the right jugular vein to right chambers.

No single tool or technique or approach for transvenous lead removal should be considered perfect and applicable to all cases. Much to the contrary, the different tools and approaches must be tailored to each individual case. Independent of technique, transvenous lead removal is affected by a significant risk of serious complications, including death. Equipment, facilities, well-qualified and trained personnel, and surgical backup are well defined in current guidelines and recommendations [5]. In this chapter, I describe the technique and approaches I routinely use for lead extraction.

5.2 Procedure: Strategic Plan

Before starting an extraction procedure, I always prepare a strategic plan with the team. Preferably, the day before the procedure I check all data described in Chapter 2 regarding perioperative patient management.

5.2.1 Check Phase

First, I verify the indication for removal following current guidelines and recommendations [5]. Patient history, physical examination, comorbidities, cardiac function parameters, echocardiography evaluation, medical therapy (antibiotics and cessation of anticoagulants), laboratory tests, and indications for removal are checked to identify very sick and high-risk patients while planning

M.G. Bongiorni (✉)
2nd Cardiovascular Department AOUP, Santa Chiara University Hospital, Pisa, Italy

M. G. Bongiorni (Ed.), *Transvenous Lead Extraction*.

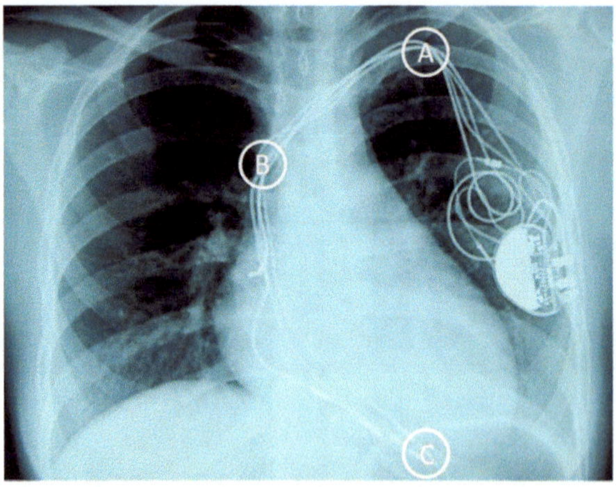

Fig. 5.1 Pacemaker patient, anteroposterior chest X-ray. Two functional bipolar leads (atrial and ventricular) are connected to a device housed in a lower left subclavicular region; there are also two abandoned, nonfunctional bipolar leads (both in the right ventricle). Note the three anatomically crucial lead extraction points: *A*, the subclavicular region where the leads lie between the clavicle and the first rib; *B*, the innominate–superior vena cava junction, noting lead angle at that level; *C*, lead-tip position in the right ventricle

general anesthesia in some cases. The type and number of leads, veins of introduction, lead-tip locations, lead dwelling time, and particular characteristics are noted. Posteroanterior (PA) and laterolateral (LL) chest-X-rays are closely studied to identify lead course and the presence of acute bends, distortions, fractures, and calcifications. Three points are crucial and must be very well observed: (1) the subclavicular region, where the leads lie between the clavicle and the first rib; (2) the innominate–superior vena cava (SVC) angle, noting the angle of the leads at that level; (3) tip position and type of fixation (Fig. 5.1).

5.2.2 Team Phase

A procedural strategy is then developed and discussed with the team regarding anesthesia type (local, heavy sedation, general), technique, and type of venous approach, and all necessary tools are checked in the cath lab or surgical room. The procedure can fail if a particular tool is missing. The surgeon is informed about the procedure to ensure surgical standby.

5.2.3 Patient Phase

A meeting with the patient and someone from her or his family is planned to explain the indication for lead extraction, procedural strategy plan, possible risks and complications for the specific case (showing the performance of the team in similar cases), and pre- and postprocedural preparation and care. At the end of the meeting, a written informed consent is obtained, and the preoperative checklist is completed.

5.3 Patient Preparation

I routinely perform lead extraction in cath lab because of the availability of high-quality fluoroscopy. Cardiac surgery is in the same building as the cath lab, with five surgical rooms, and the surgeon is informed and on call. In very few cases judged at particular risk of cardiac perforation (suspicion of anomalous position of lead tip as shown in Chapter 3, Fig. 3.3) or after a first attempt in the cath lab is stopped because of a high risk of complications, the removal procedure is performed under general anesthesia, in a surgical room, with the patient drafted in case sternotomy is required. After a 12-h fast, the patient is situated on the bed in the cath lab, which must allow the Trendelenburg position in case of hypotension or difficult jugular and subclavian venous punctures. A device programmer is used to verify spontaneous rhythm in pacemaker patients and to turn off ICD therapies. Surface electrocardiogram (ECG) and blood oxygen saturation are continuously monitored. A large-bore intravenous line is placed to administer fluids, medications, and blood products if needed. Moderate sedation is routinely used at the beginning of the procedure and deep sedation during the painful phases. General anesthesia is chosen for younger patients or in cases judged difficult due to the presence of multiple leads or leads with very long dwell time. An arterial line is always placed to monitor beat-to-beat blood pressure measurement because: (1) arterial blood pressure can decrease very quickly if complications arise and it is impossible to monitor arterial pressure in that situation; (2) vagal activation during dilatation of vascular adherences and reduction of cardiac output during traction makes beat-to-beat blood pressure the only parameter to control and thus avoids long-term hypotension. A temporary 5-F pacing lead is placed through a 6-F introducer in the left femoral vein, which can be used for emergency. The right femoral vein is preserved in case the femoral approach is necessary for extraction.

Before starting the procedure, in the presence of a noninfective indication and if an implant of a new lead is planned, I perform a venography through an antecubital vein in order to assess venous patency and visualize the zone where a safe and effective venous puncture can be performed. In the presence of venous patency, I prefer creating a new access into the vein rather than inserting the new lead inside the sheath after lead removal. In this way, it is possible to avoid a risky lead position (in case of subclavian crush, for example), and the positioning of the new lead is easier outside of the fibrous endovascular tunnel. The intraoperative checklist is then completed.

5.4 Lead Removal from Venous Entry Site

5.4.1 Lead Preparation

After the patient has been draped and prepped, the device pocket is cut with a scalpel. The device is freed up and disconnected from the leads. Once exposed, the leads are checked, and in presence of a noninfective indication to removal, electrical testing is carried out to confirm electrical problems. Next, the lead is débrided as close as possible to the venous entry site. In a cephalic insertion, it is very important to remove the suture around the vein. In subclavian insertion, it is important to remove the anchoring sleeve and further sutures around the lead up to where the clavicle edge can be felt with the finger. Debridement is safely done with electrocautery except in the case of insulation failure that exposes the metal conductor and thus could cause high-frequency heart stimulation. When multiple leads or capped and trifurcated ICD leads are present, this operation can be time consuming; fluoroscopy can be useful in identifying leads and visualizing venous insertion. If the pocket is infected, it is mandatory to remove all items, such as sleeves, adaptors, and caps, for a definitive elimination of infection. The connector is cut almost 10–15 cm out of the venous end; the lead insulation is cut with a scalpel to free the inner coil (in connection with the tip) for 2 cm. In bipolar leads, the inner coil is exposed by pulling and unravelling the outer coil and cutting the excess outer coil away.

5.4.2 Simple Traction

A nonlocking, standard-stiffness stylet is inserted up to the lead tip or as far as possible. It is important to always monitor stylet insertion fluoroscopically. Sometimes, it is difficult to insert the stylet inside the lead: an alternating clockwise or counterclockwise rotation of the stylet while pushing can improve its introduction. In case of over-the-wire left ventricular (LV) leads, fluoroscopic observation is necessary to avoid the stylet from coming out, thus preventing venous or heart perforation. If there is a retractable screw mechanism, a counterclockwise rotation is performed on the inner coil under fluoroscopy to retract the fixation screw. In order to hold the lead securely, the outer insulation (as well as the inner in the presence of bipolar leads) is tied using a special "low-profile" knot with a nonabsorbable suture (Fig. 5.2). This special knot does not exceed the external lead circumference, which is important particularly if dilating sheaths are necessary. Simple traction on the suture – or two sutures in the case of bipolar leads –is performed using fluoroscopy to observe movement of the lead tip. Fluoroscopic observation may also indicate the extent of fibrosis holding the lead to the cardiovascular structures. During traction, which is applied with progressive force to feel the heart contraction, ECG should be monitored for ectopies and invasive blood pressure for hypotension. Traction should be continued for several minutes, causing minimal changes in blood pressure and few ectopies. For beginners, it is useful to insert a spring balance between the fingers and the lead to become confident in measuring traction force. Recently implanted leads (<6 months for atrial and ventricular leads; <3 months for ICD leads; unpredictable for LV leads) are removed with this technique (see Chapter 6) [6–8].

Complications such as cardiac perforation and tamponade are also possible using this technique,

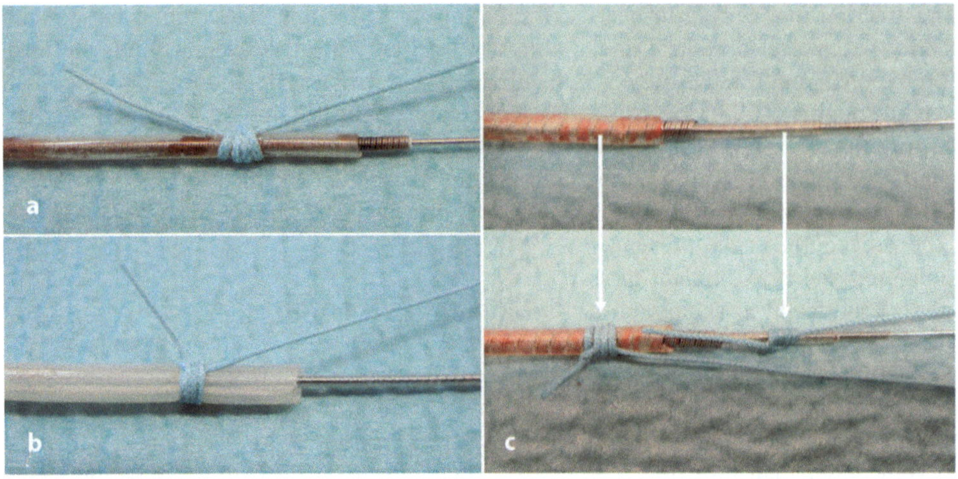

Fig. 5.2 Low-profile knot performed with a nonabsorbable suture over the insulation of each conductor present in the lead: (a) unipolar pacing lead; (b) implantable cardioverter–defibrillator (ICD) integrated lead; (c) bipolar pacing lead. The *arrows* show at which level the low-profile knot should be performed

and the risks obviously increase with heavy traction forces. I do not use the locking stylet for three fundamental reasons: (1) traction force is applied directly on the tip, and the risks of tears in the vasculature or atrial or ventricular wall are higher. (2) During traction on the tip, the lead diameter (especially ICD leads) increases and, as a consequence, the lead embeds into the adherences, making extraction more difficult. If dilating sheaths are needed, the adherences must be extracted with the lead, which creates a major risk of vascular and heart damage. (3) If it was impossible to withdraw the locking stylet, the internal transjugular approach, if needed, will be challenging or impossible.

5.4.3 Dissection of Areas of Adherence with a Single Sheath

Adherence dilatation and dissection start by using a single polypropylene sheath, with the diameter as close as possible to that of the lead body. The sutures are passed inside the sheath and are taken in the left hand. Under fluoroscopic monitoring, the sheath is gently pushed, maintaining the same direction as that of the lead, as parallel as possible to the clavicle in order to smooth the angle. Sheath advancement is facilitated by rotating the sheath two or three turns clockwise and then counterclockwise with a handle. When the device pocket is far from the venous entry, a second skin incision at the venous entry level must be performed to correctly and successfully perform this procedure.

Adherence dilatation and rupture around the lead are performed by advancing the single sheath, simultaneously rotating it alternatively clockwise and counterclockwise using the handle. During dilatation, smooth traction on the suture(s) is performed to keep strain on the lead and thus use it as a rail. When sheath advancement is difficult, it is pulled back a few millimeters and advanced again, resuming dilatation. When sheath rotation is difficult, the sheath is replaced with one of larger diameter, and in some cases, a little modification with a scalpel of the bevelled tip is required to enlarge the orifice (being careful not to modify the rounded distal part of the end of the sheath). Then, it is possible to move to the previous sheath to resume dilatation and dissection with greater ease. During sheath advancement and rotation, three aspects are of crucial importance: (1) continuous fluoroscopic monitoring to verify sheath advancement, keeping strain on the lead; (2) avoiding excess traction to prevent lead lengthening and damage; (3) advancing the stylet all the way to the lead tip, reinserting it if withdraws (during sheath advancement, the stylet tends to withdraw, and on fluoroscopy, the lead becomes less radio opaque, with more body mobility).

Adherence dilatation using the single sheath with a normal stylet inside is, in my opinion, not dangerous, because the sheath penetrates the space between the lead and the adherences. When traction on the sutures is maintained, the lead decreases in circumference and can separate from the adherences enough to allow sheath penetration (Fig. 5.3). When dilatation is correctly performed, adherences break and remain attached to the vascular wall, with no risk of complications. This is very important at the SVC level (Fig. 5.4). Intravascular echocardiography documents the rupture of an SVC adherence during dilatation when using this technique (Fig. 5.5). If adherences are calcified, the single sheath technique is often successful, but rotational movement must be performed for a considerable length of time while the right hand feels for rupture of the calcium. In ICD leads, dilatation of coil adherence is possible, although very often using a larger sheath is necessary to avoid coil disruption. When dilating coil adherence, sheath progression is visible at fluoroscopy at each turn.

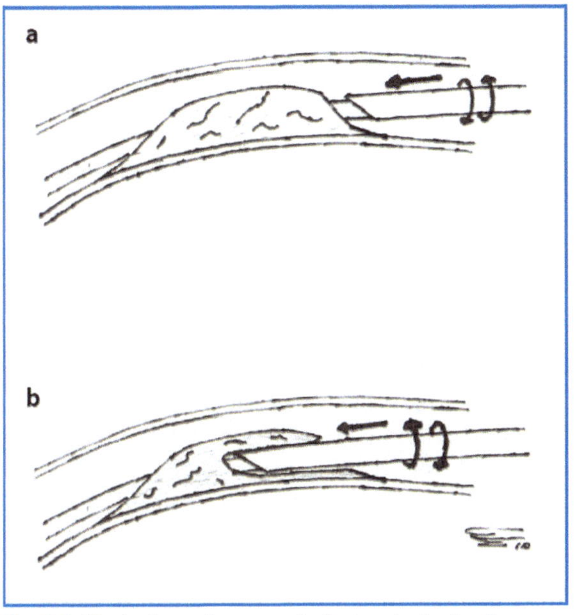

Fig. 5.3 Clockwise and counterclockwise single-sheath movement (**a**) before entering the adherence and (**b**) inside it. In the latter case, maintaining traction on the sutures over the conductor's insulation, the lead decreases its circumference and so can separate from the adherence enough to allow sheath penetration

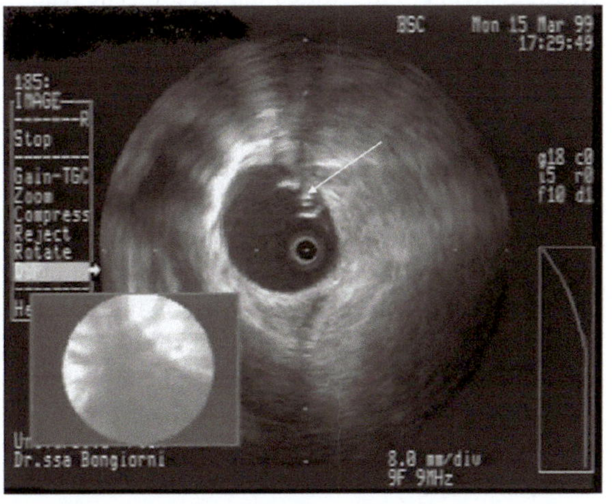

Fig. 5.5 Intravascular echography at the left innominate vein level during lead extraction. The *arrow* indicates rupture of the adherence around the lead

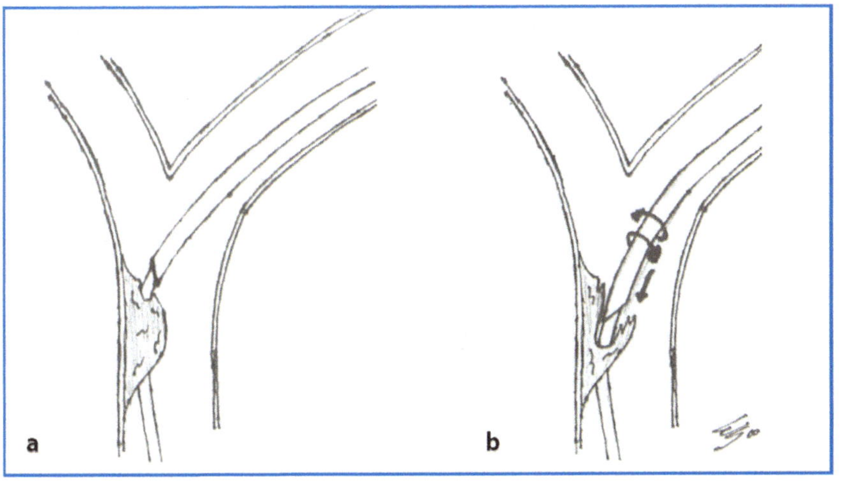

Fig. 5.4 Clockwise and counterclockwise single-sheath movement: (**a**) before entering the adherence and (**b**) inside it at the superior vena cava level. At this point, correctly performing the dilatation, the adherence breaks and remains attached to the wall, with no risk of complications. During dilation, smooth traction on the suture(s) is performed to maintain strain on the lead and thus use it as a rail

5.4.4 Mechanical Tip Dislodgement

While maintaining strain on the lead and after checking stylet insertion to the lead tip, rotational advancement of the sheath is continued under fluoroscopic, ECG, and blood pressure monitoring. If there is a large amount of fibrosis, sheath movement creates a tunnel all the way to the tip. Once the tip is reached, movement of the tip, like a swing, is observed. At that point, it is crucial to maintain the sheath at the base of the tip, avoiding sheath advancement over the tip. Once the distal binding site around the base of lead tip is disrupted, the lead comes out abruptly and enters the sheath. Sheath advancement, tunneling, and tip dislodgement are illustrated in Fig. 5.6. The lead is then removed through the vein of insertion. Fluoroscopic images of sheath advancement to the lead tip are shown in Chapter 7, Fig. 7.2.

During the process of adherence dilatation and dissection, the sheath may be torn or become buckled; if this happens, it should be replaced by a new one. In some cases, when a piece of fibrous tissue remains around the lead tip, the lead does not enter into the sheath and stops at level of the SVC or innominate or subclavian vein. In these cases, to complete the procedure, it is sufficient to insert telescopically a larger sheath to include the tip; in other cases, a transfemoral approach may be necessary to complete the procedure and remove the lead through the femoral vein. When, despite the use of a larger sheath, lead-tip detachment is not obtained or sheath rotation or advancement is difficult at any level and progression of the procedure is stopped for more than 5 min, the transjugular approach is to be considered.

5.5 Lead Removal from Internal Jugular Vein (Pisa Approach)

The internal jugular venous approach is used as (1) a first choice in the presence of free-floating leads with attached tip; (2) in case of an unsuccessful approach from the venous entry site.

5.5.1 Free-Floating Leads with Attached Tip

The right internal jugular vein is percutaneously cannulated using an 11-F introducer. A lasso is advanced via the jugular vein, and the proximal end of the lead is grasped and then exposed. Lead exposure from the right internal jugular vein allows insertion of a stylet and sheaths as described for a standard approach through the venous entry site. When the lead length does not allow lead exposure, the lasso is used as an extension of the lead itself, and dilatation is performed by a dilating sheath that was previously inserted over the lasso. The technique to remove free-floating leads is extensively described in Chapter 10. In our experience, this approach resulted in removal of all leads submitted to the procedure without complications.

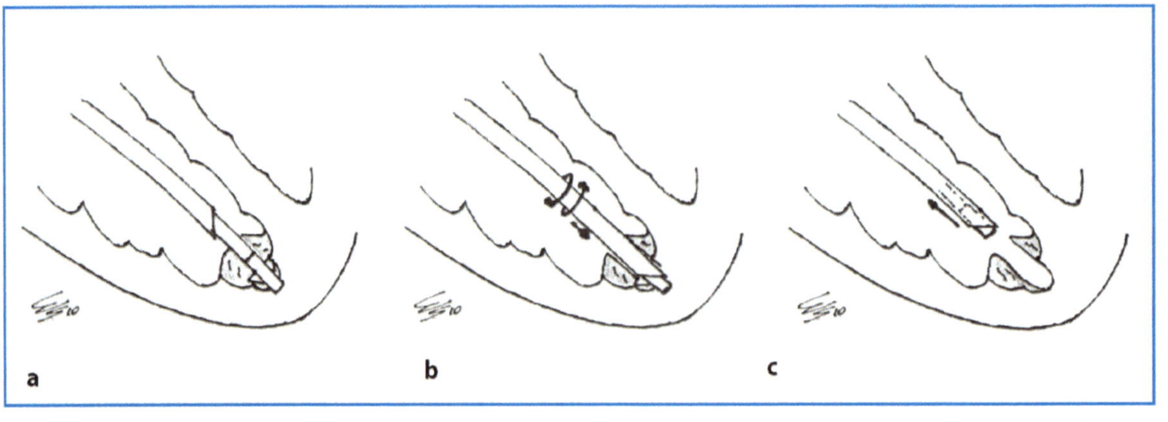

Fig. 5.6 Clockwise and counterclockwise single-sheath movement: (a) before entering the adherence and (b) inside it at the apex of the right ventricle. Once the distal binding site around the base of the tip is disrupted (by tunnelling and tip dislodgement), the lead comes out abruptly and (c) enters into the sheath

5.5.2 Unsuccessful Approach from Venous Entry Site

The venous-entry-site approach can be troublesome and risky in presence of: (1) tight space between clavicle and first rib (as in medial access to the intrathoracic subclavian vein); (2) tenacious adherences in some critical points, such as at the innominate vein–SVC junction, SVC–right atrium spring, right atrium, tricuspid valve, and right ventricle.

The approach through the internal jugular vein presents some advantages in these conditions. The straight course of the lead from the jugular vein to the SVC, right atrium, and right ventricle allows dilatation of adherences along the longitudinal axis of the lead. Using this technique, narrow bends (in case of leads inserted through the right site) and tight binding sites at the SVC are bypassed or safely dilated. In case of tight binding sites in the right chambers and tricuspid valve, the internal jugular approach allows better dilatation of adherences than through the insertion vein because it avoids the long turns associated with the venous entry access. Chapter 10 provides further solutions using the internal jugular approach to problems that occur during lead extraction.

5.5.2.1 How to Perform Internal Transjugular Approach if Venous Entry Approach Fails

Preliminary conditions for this approach are: (1) patency of right internal jugular vein (or left internal jugular vein if the right one is occluded) and absence of obstacles to reach the leads (checked by pulling the temporary lead or a hydrophilic guide wire or a tip-deflecting wire into the internal jugular vein); (2) sliding of leads inside the adherences (checked by pushing leads with a stylet inside), as showed in Fig. 5.7; (3) grasping the leads above the adherences (checked by pushing leads with a short stylet), as showed in Fig. 5.8. If occluded

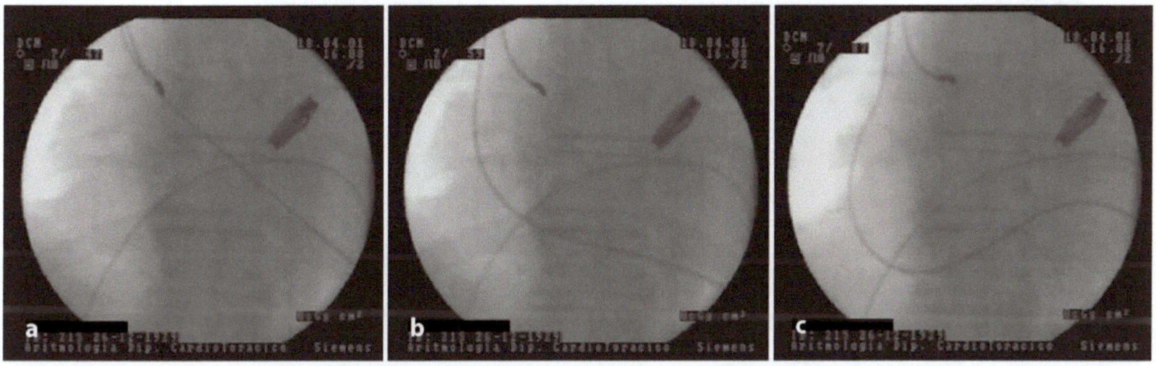

Fig. 5.7a–c Temporal-sequence fluoroscopic images showing a ventricular lead being slid inside the adherences (checked by pushing the lead with a stylet inside)

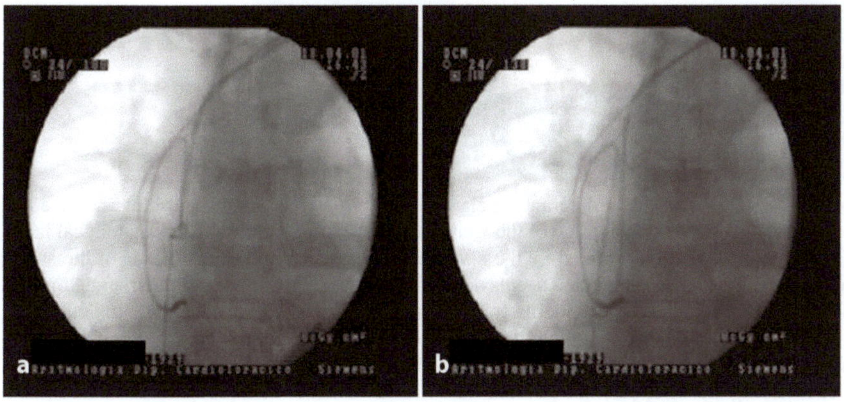

Fig. 5.8 Temporal-sequence fluoroscopic images showing: (**a**) the atrial lead being grasped by a tip-deflecting wire inserted through a transfemoral approach, (**b**) proximal end of the lead now intravascular

internal jugular veins or obstructions preclude access to the right chambers through the superior venous circulation, the internal transjugular approach is impossible. Consecutive steps of the internal transjugular approach if crossover from the venous entry approach is necessary are described below:

1. Percutaneous cannulation of internal jugular vein with an 11-F introducer with continuous saline solution perfusion (Fig. 5.9).
2. Preparing the proximal end of the lead. The stylet is removed, and the lead is cut to allow an excess of 1 cm of insulation to prevent venous damage during intravascular lead movement and to allow the possibility of doubling the lead and pulling it through the internal jugular vein introducer (Fig. 5.10). A normal stylet is then inserted to close and push the lead, and then removed when the lead is made free-floating.
3. Transfemoral approach with a tip-deflecting wire or steerable catheter in order to catch the lead in the region where the lead is free (in the right atrium if the lead slips through the adherences; in the innominate vein if the lead does not slip into the adherences) and to make the proximal end intravascular and free floating. It is important to catch the lead as near as possible to the proximal end, where only insulation is present (Fig. 5.11).
4. Inserting a lasso or loop retriever through the internal jugular vein in order to catch the free-floating proximal end of the lead and pull it toward the internal jugular vein, doubling the insulation inside the 11-F introducer (Fig. 5.12).
5. Exposing the lead through the introducer into the internal jugular vein (Fig. 5.13a).
6. Restarting a procedure described for the venous entry approach after introducer removal. A nor-

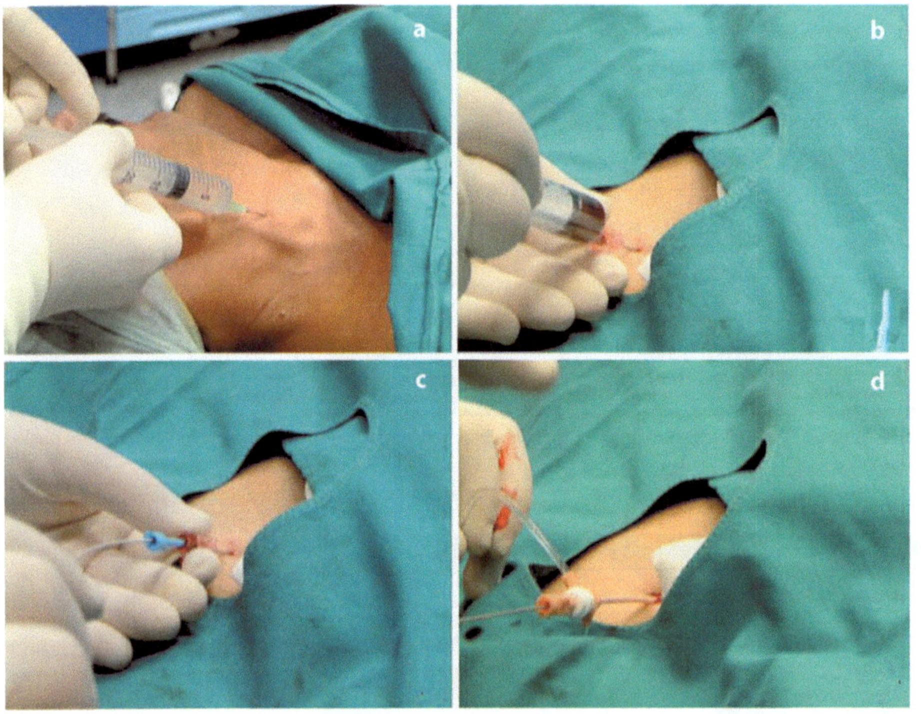

Fig. 5.9 Procedural steps for percutaneous cannulation of the internal jugular vein. Using sterile clothes and gloves, place the patient in a supine position, turning the head 45° to the opposite side of the vein access. (**a**) After identifying the anatomical landmarks, introduce 0.5% lidocaine at the apex of the triangle formed by the clavicle and clavicular and sternal heads of the sternocleidomastoid muscle. (**b**) Attach a 20-ml syringe to the cannulation needle and insert the needle in the apex of the triangle formed by the clavicle and the clavicular and sternal heads of the sternocleidomastoid. The needle must be advanced in a sagittal plane 30º posterior, toward the ipsilateral nipple. Advance and aspirate gently until there is free return of venous blood. (**c**) Without moving the needle, pull back the syringe and insert the wire. (**d**) Then, introduce the cannula (11-F introducer is preferred) over the wire into the internal jugular vein and after removing the wire, flush the cannula

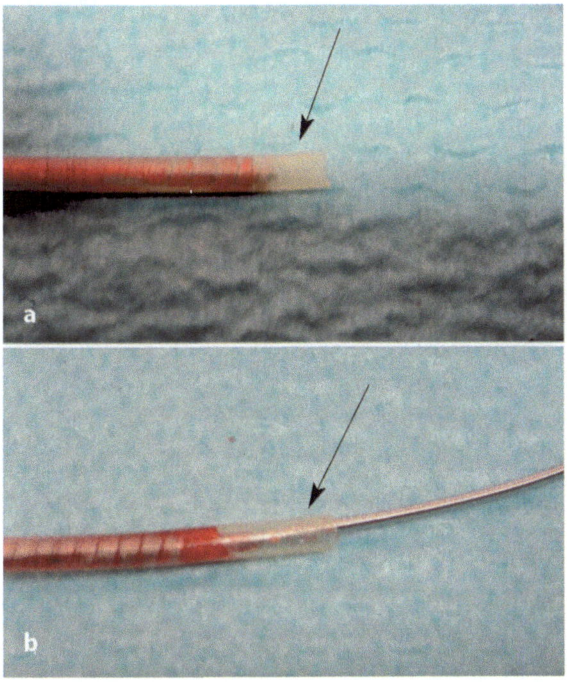

Fig. 5.10 Preparing the proximal end of the lead. (**a**) After removing the stylet, the lead is cut to allow an excess of 1 cm of insulation (*arrows*) to prevent venous damage during the intravascular lead movement and to have the possibility of doubling the lead to pull it through the internal jugular vein introducer. (**b**) A normal wire is then inserted to close and push the lead

mal stiff stylet is inserted, one or two low-profile knots are tied, and a single-sheath dilatation is started, facilitating entry through the skin by creating a small incision with scalpel (Fig 5.13b).

Fluoroscopic guidance facilitates sheath introduction, advancement, and movement to the binding site (Fig. 5.14). When extracting a single

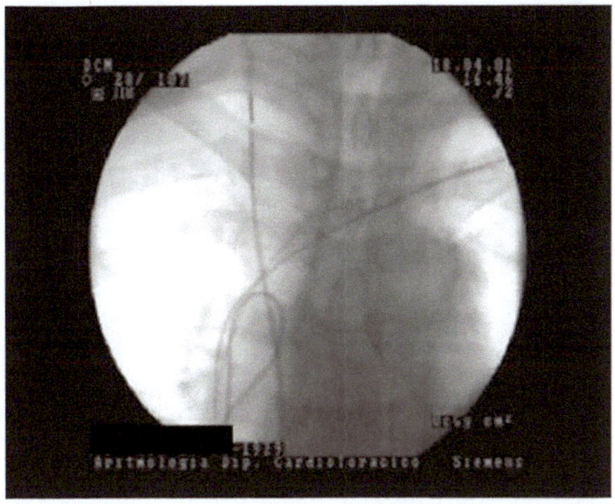

Fig. 5.12 Fluoroscopic image of step following those in Figure 5.11: the lead is pulled toward the internal jugular vein, doubling the insulation inside the 11-F introducer

sheath, if a larger sheath is required, it is important to keep the larger sheath over the single (inner) sheath to avoid air embolism. Clockwise and counterclockwise rotation allows the physician to feel disruption of the binding sites as the sheath is advanced to the lead tip, where mechanical tip dislodgement is performed, followed by complete lead removal. In the experience at our center, using the transjugular approach if the venous entry approach fails increases the success rate from 90.3% to 98.3% without increasing the complication rate. Other authors confirmed the efficacy of internal transjugular approach, calling it the Pisa approach [9]. The technique is schematically presented in Fig. 5.15.

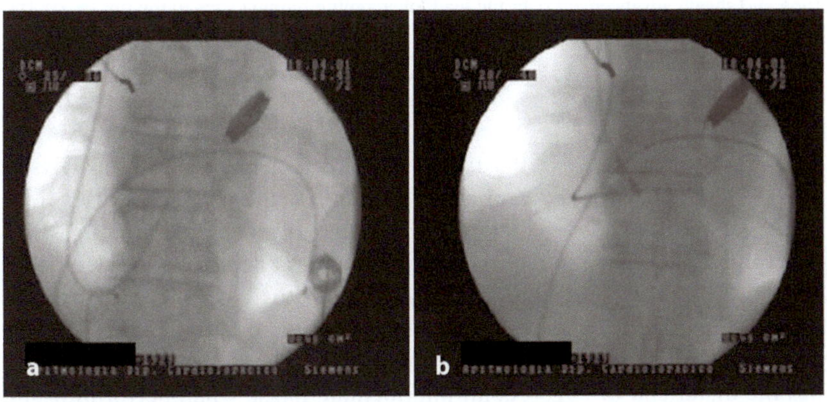

Fig. 5.11 Fluoroscopic images showing the next two steps in the case in the Figure 5.8: (**a**) atrial-lead-grasping maneuver using a tip-deflecting wire inserted via the transfemoral approach; (**b**) proximal end of the lead, now intravascular, is then caught by a lasso

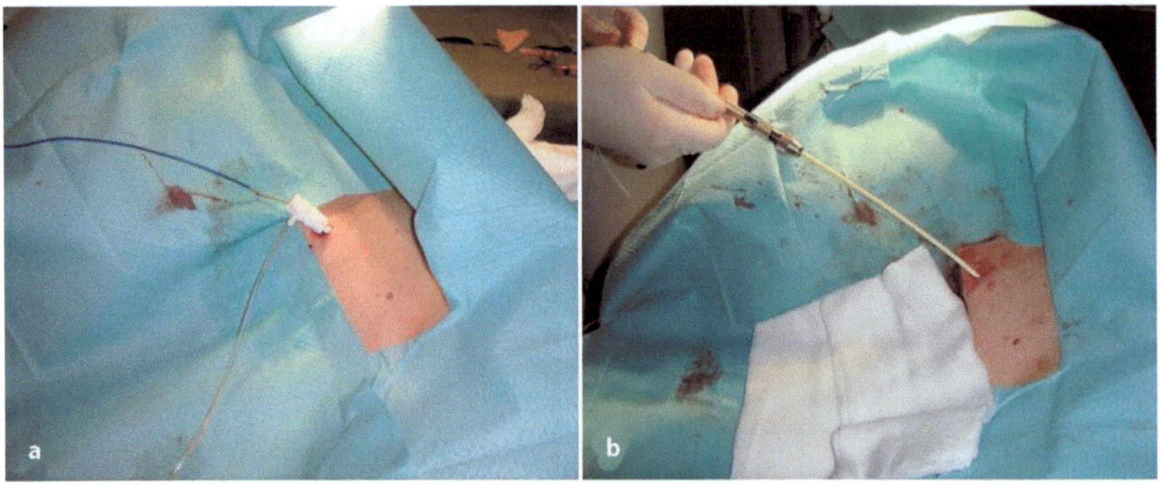

Fig. 5.13 (a) The pacing lead is exposed through the introducer into the internal jugular vein and prepared as described before (with the stylet inside and a knot over each present insulation). (b) The dilatation maneuver is begun. While the right hand moves the sheath in the clockwise and counterclockwise direction in order to dilate adherences, the left hand keeps the lead in tension using the strings

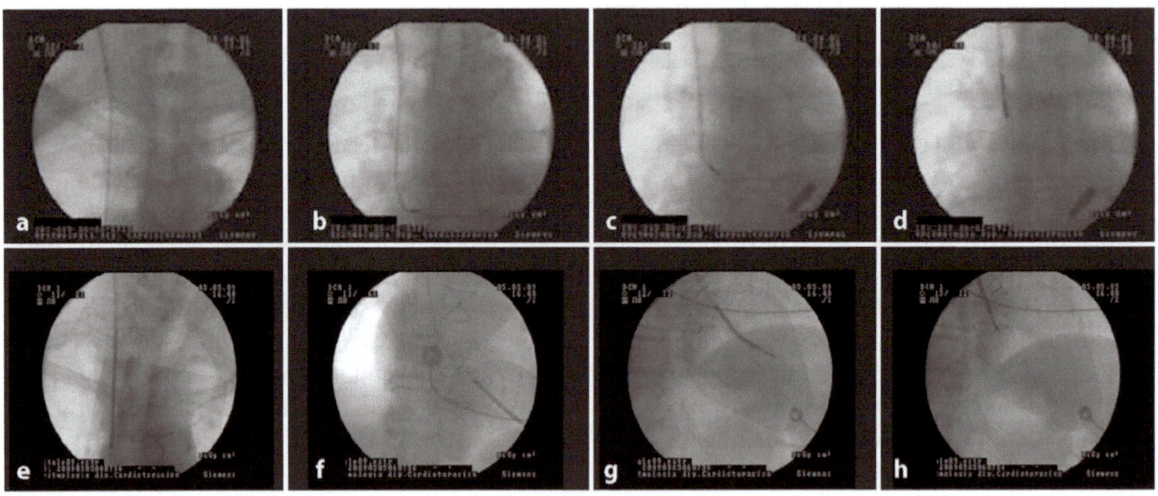

Fig. 5.14 (a-d) Temporal-sequence fluoroscopic images (same patient as in Figure 5.8) after exposure of the atrial lead from the internal jugular vein showing introduction and sheath advancement over the lead, overcoming binding sites to the tip. (e–h) The same maneuver on an implantable cardioverter–defibrillator (ICD) ventricular lead

5.6 Lead Removal from the Femoral Vein

I use the femoral approach in the following situations:

1. Incomplete extraction from the venous entry site: the lead tip is freed by traction and dilatation before the sheath reaches the distal end of the tip or if there is a piece of fibrous tissue around the lead; in these cases retrieval is impossible because of unablated binding sites. Using the transfemoral approach and dedicated tools, it is possible to grasp the lead tip and remove it by slipping it through the binding sites (further described in Chapter 10).
2. As an intermediate phase when performing the

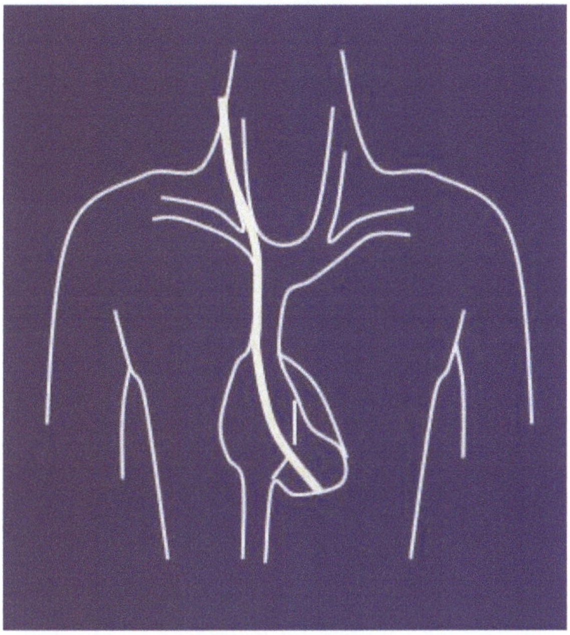

Fig. 5.15 Internal transjugular approach (Pisa approach). Note the straight course of the sheath over the lead, increasing efficacy and safety of adherence dilatation

internal transjugular approach.

3. When removing free-floating leads (see Chapter 10).
4. In the presence of adherences located in the coronary sinus or right ventricular outflow tract (also described in Chapter 10).

5.7 Closure and Sutures

After lead extraction for a noninfective indication, I reimplant a new pacing or ICD system. Details for reimplantation are described in Chapter 9. A check for bleeding is essential to prevent hematoma, and appropriate care of the pocket is essential to prevent recurrent infection. In the majority of infected pocket, extensive debridementand sutures are required, following the rules and techniques of plastic surgery. If the pocket is infected, I place a small drain to prevent hematoma formation, which may lead to reinfection. In many patients with infective indications, the procedural time for lead preparation, closure, and suture is greater than for lead extraction.

5.8 Personal Experience

Between January 1997 and December 2009, 1,469 consecutive patients, (1,111 men, mean age 65.4 years) were considered for transvenous removal of 2,615 leads. These leads had been implanted for a mean period of 69.1 (range 1–336) months. There were 2,254 pacing leads removed (912 atrial, 1,205 ventricular, 137 coronary sinus), 361 ICD leads (342 ventricular, 13 SVC, six atrial). Of the free-floating leads replaced, 73 were pacing leads (28 atrial, 44 ventricular, one coronary sinus) and five ICD leads (all ventricular). Population and lead data are summarized in Table 5.1. Indications for removal were mostly due to infection and are reported in Table 5.2. Among the 2,615 leads considered for transvenous removal, eight intravascular leads were judged not suitable for transvenous techniques because they were completely included into the venous wall, with an absence of any site where grasping the lead was possible. The remaining 2,607 pacing and ICD leads were submitted to the removal procedure. Procedural outcome for all leads is shown in Fig. 5.16.

5.8.1 *Leads Exposed at the Venous Entry Site*

The venous entry approach was performed on 2,529 leads (2,234 pacing and 295 ICD leads). Manual traction was effective in 397 leads; in the remaining 2,132, mechanical dilatation was attempted. The procedure was completely successful in 1,886 leads and partially successful in 13. Among the remaining 233, removal was completed by the transfemoral approach in 15 leads, the tips of which were freed while performing dilatation. The crossover to the internal transjugular approach was performed in 187 leads. In the remaining 31 leads, the procedure was stopped due to class II indications or impossibility of performing the jugular approach (six cases), and the procedure was judged ineffective.

5.8.2 *Free-Floating Leads*

Seventy-eight free-floating leads were approached via the femoral vein. Grasping the lead allowed

Table 5.1 Patient and lead characteristics

	Number	Lead type		
		Atrial	Ventricular	CS
Patients	1,469			
Men/women	1,111/358			
Mean age (years)	65.4			
Range (years)	6–95			
Leads	2,615			
Mean implant time (months)	69.1			
Range (months)	1–336			
Pacing leads	2,254			
Exposed		884	1,161	136
Free-floating		28	44	1
Total		912	1,205	137
ICD leads	361			
Exposed		6	337	13
Free-floating		0	5	0
Total		6	342	13

CS, coronary sinus; *ICD*, implantable cardioverter–defibrillator

Table 5.2 Indications for lead removal

Indications	Leads
Infection	
Class I (level of evidence B)	2,188
Chronic pain	
Class IIa (level of evidence C)	4
Thrombosis or venous stenosis	
Class I (level of evidence C)	45
Functional leads	
Class I (level of evidence B)	30
Nonfunctional leads	
Class I (level of evidence B)	9
Class IIa (level of evidence C)	339
Total	2,615

direct removal of 19 leads; 59 were exposed through the internal jugular vein and then submitted to dilatation. In one case, the lead was too short to be exposed; a dilating sheath was positioned over the lasso, and this tool was used as an extension of the lead. Complete removal was achieved in all leads.

5.8.3 Internal Transjugular Approach

The internal transjugular approach was successful in 59 free-floating and 187 exposed leads as crossover from the venous entry approach. In two patients, due to failure to cannulate either the right or the left internal jugular vein, we used the right subclavian vein. Using this approach, 246 leads were completely removed. The procedure was partially successful in seven leads and unsuccessful in two. In the group with exposed leads, the approach increased the success rate from 90.3% to 98.3%.

5.8.4 Overall Results

For the overall population treated at our center, 2,563 leads were completely (success rate 98.3%) and 23 partially (0.9%) removed, as shown in Table 5.3. We totally removed 2,202 of 2,254 pacing leads and 361 of 361 ICD leads. The venous entry approach was effective in 2,283 of 2,529 leads (90.3%). In the overall population, mean extraction time was 21 ± 48 (range 1–360) min.

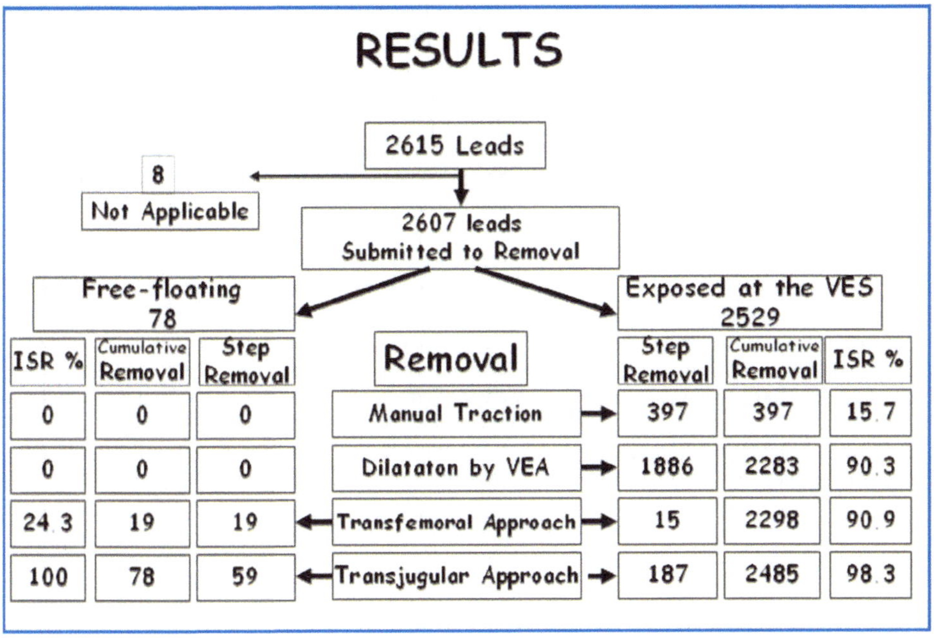

Fig. 5.16 Procedural outcome in lead extractions performed from January 1997 to December 2009. *VEA*, venous entry approach; *VES*, venous entry site; *ISR*, incremental success rate

Table 5.3 Procedural patients and leads outcome overall

Removal	A & RV PL	LV PL	ICD L	Total	Percent
Complete	2066	136	361	2563	98.31
Partial	23	-	-	23	0.88
Failed	20	1	-	21	0.81
TLR not applicable	8	-	-	8	0.30
Complications		**Tamponade**	**Hemothorax**		
Major		8	1	9	0.61
Fatal		2	1	3	0.20
Not Fatal		6	-	6	0.41

TLR, transvenous lead removal; *A*, atrial; *RV*, right ventricular; *LV*, left ventricular; *PL*, pacing leads; *ICD*, implantable cardioverter defibrillator; *L*, leads

5.8.5 Complications

Perioperative complications were observed in 101 patients. Major complications requiring interventional treatment were observed in nine patients (0.6%). Cardiac tamponade occurred in eight patients, seven during venous entry and one during internal transjugular approach. Pericardial drainage was successfully performed in three patients, and surgical repair was necessary in three; one patient died despite drainage and subsequent surgical intervention. In one patient, who was transferred to another hospital after the procedure, tamponade and death occurred 12 h later. Intraoperative hemothorax occurred in one patient during removal of a fractured subclavian crush lead. Despite medical treatment and lung drainage, the patient died due to hemorrhagic shock. Massive bleeding followed vessel damage due to a fractured exposed coil. Undesired dislodgement of chronic pacing leads not submitted to removal occurred in five patients. In all cases, implant of a new lead was performed prior to hospital discharge. Minor complications not requiring intervention were observed in 92 patients. No complications directly related to the transfemoral and internal trans jugular approaches (venous access to the femoral and jugular veins) were observed.

References

1. Bongiorni MG, Soldati E, Zucchelli G et al (2010) Transvenous removal of pacing and defibrillating leads: 13 years of experience in a single center. Heart Rhythm 7(Suppl 5) pp 36–42
2. Bongiorni MG, Soldati E, Grana M et al (1997) The internal transjugular approach: a new technique for transvenous lead removal. Proceedings of Third International Symposium on Pacing Leads Sept 11–13, 1997, Vol 1. Monduzzi Editore, Italy, pp 487–490
3. Bongiorni MG, Soldati E, Gherarducci G et al (2002) Percutaneous extraction of infected pacemaker/ICD leads: what are the current technological advances and result? In: Raviele A, ed. Cardiac arrhythmias 2001, Springer-Verlag Italia, Milan pp 623–630
4. Byrd CL, Schwartz SJ, Hedin NB et al (1990) Intravascular lead extraction using locking stylets and sheaths. Pacing Clin Electrophysiol 13:1871–1875
5. Wilkoff BL, Love CJ, Byrd CL et al (2009) Transvenous lead extraction: Heart Rhythm Society Expert Consensus on Facilities, Training, Indications, and Patient Management. Heart Rhythm 6(7):1085–1104
6. Eckhard A, Neuzner J, Binner L (1996) Three year experience with a stylet for lead extraction: a multicenter study. Pacing Clin Electrophysiol 19(1)18–25
7. De Martino G, Orazi S, Bisignani G et al (2005) Safety and feasibility of coronary sinus left ventricular pacing leads extraction: a preliminary report. J Interv Card Electrophysiol 13(1):35–38
8. Bongiorni MG, Zucchelli G, Soldati E et al (2007) Usefulness of mechanical transvenous dilatation and location of areas of adherence in patients undergoing coronary sinus lead extraction. Europace 9:69–73
9. Kennergren C (2008) European perspective on lead extraction. Part II. Heart Rhythm 5(2):320–323

Clinical Experiences in Lead Extraction

6

Ezio Soldati and Maria Grazia Bongiorni

6.1 Introduction

Since the development of effective techniques for transvenous removal of permanent pacing leads, a large volume of experience regarding clinical results of these techniques has been published [1]. The development of different techniques, mainly differing due to the type of energy used for dilatation, raised the debate about their relative superiority. As always happens when clinical results have to be analyzed, evaluated, and compared with different experiences, it is difficult to assess the relative importance of the technique itself, operator skill and experience, and how those procedures and their results are applicable to physicians and clinical practice in their particular field of interest. This general observation is particularly important with regard to transvenous lead extraction.

In order to evaluate different techniques and experiences surrounding lead extraction, we first need clear definitions of success and procedure-related complications. Standard definitions were included in the North American Society of Pacing and Electrophysiology (NASPE) Lead Extraction Conference Faculty policy statement in 2000 [2]. The radiographic outcome considered for each single lead, including complete success, partial success (a fragment of less than 4 cm not removed), and failure was distinguished by the clinical outcome: success was considered the achievement of all clinical goals associated with the indication to lead removal (elimination of infection, access for the implant of new leads, removal of risk related to the leads) in the absence of major complications and in the presence of control of the pacing status. These definitions of results were revised in the last expert consensus document of the Heart Rhythm Society (HRS) in 2009 [3]. In this document, the clinical outcome was described: complete procedural success was defined as complete removal of all targeted leads in the absence of major complications; clinical success was defined as removal of all targeted leads or retention of small parts (tip, conductor coil, insulation) when fragments did not affect the desired clinical outcome and major complications were absent. Failure was defined as the inability to achieve procedural as well as clinical success, or the occurrence of significant complications. Despite the fact that a favorable clinical outcome is the aim of treatment, in patients with device-related infections, the results of transvenous lead removal (combined with antibiotic therapy) is assessed after a lengthy period. Therefore, radiological assessment of the procedure seems to be more useful for determining extraction outcome. Most results reported in this chapter used radiological outcome to evaluate procedure effectiveness.

To evaluate results, another key point is to define complications. The HRS expert consensus document defined a major complication as any outcome related to the procedure that is life threatening or results in death. Major complications include the development of persistent or significant disability and conditions requiring significant surgical intervention to prevent unfavorable outcome [3].

The use of implantable cardiac devices significantly increased over recent years. However, pacing and implantable cardioverter–defibrillator (ICD) lead-related complications are not rare in

E. Soldati (✉)
2nd Cardiovascular Department AOUP, Santa Chiara University Hospital, Pisa, Italy

M. G. Bongiorni (Ed.), *Transvenous Lead Extraction*.

clinical practice, and consequently, treating these complications is becoming an important clinical issue [4–8]. The need to effectively manage device-related complications and to perform successful transvenous extraction procedures is felt by most implant centers. Regardless of techniques and tools used, transvenous lead extraction is a complex and risky procedure requiring appropriate tools and facilities and significant operator training and experience with experienced surgical backup. Each procedure is different, and many different conditions in relation to leads and patient anatomy occur. All these features suggest that most currently used techniques and tools are difficult to compare and must be evaluated in the contest of each center's experience. Aim of this chapter is to report data regarding different extraction techniques and related tools, as well as results of extraction techniques with different leads. Distinguishing between tools and techniques is difficult, and a detailed description of tools appears in another chapter. Most extraction techniques share at least some similar tools, and these are generally discussed here, with the type of energy used to overcome lead-binding sites being the most global feature. Tools usually used in complex techniques are discussed separately only with regard to their use in the absence of subsidiary tools.

6.2 Traction Devices

Since the beginning of transvenous techniques for lead extraction, lead traction has been assumed to play a significant role in the procedure's success. Simple traction of the distal end of the lead is relatively ineffective, even after a short implant period, usually resulting in coil lengthening and lead damage. Attention then focused on systems allowing application of traction energy at the tip of the lead or on a long tract of it to free the tip and avoid coil lengthening. Stylets locking at the lead tip were included in the original technique by Byrd et al. and used in combination with mechanical dilatation [9]. The effectiveness of traction with locking stylets was also poor, ranging between 10% and 25% and mainly depending on implant time. Traction effectiveness was also related to the possibility of reaching the lead tip and locking the stylet there. The stylet makes the lead stiffer, thus helping scar tissue dilatation independently of the type of energy used. On the other hand, once the stylet was locked, it was impossible to unlock and withdraw. This was a significant problem in the event of failed extraction. A new stylet model was developed, following the suggestions of an operator. The locking system allowed the styled to be fixed and unlocked; traction was not affected. Other traction devices were developed in the subsequent years; the VascoExtor was introduced at the end of the 1990s [10, 11].

Together with laser-powered sheaths, different models of locking stylets were introduced. The lead locking device (LLD) can be expanded into the coil lumen over a long portion of the lead, thus delivering traction energy all along the lead. Reports on the use of the LLD suggest that simple traction is not highly effective. Bracke et al. [12, 13] reported the results of a stepwise approach using traction directly or with a locking stylet and laser-assisted extraction in case of failure. A total of 145 leads (including 16 ICD leads) with a mean implant period of 71 months were extracted [12]. Forty-nine (34%) leads were extracted by traction; in 96 (66%) leads, a laser sheath was necessary. All leads implanted for less than 6 months could be removed with traction alone. In a multivariate logistic regression model, time from implant was the main factor determining traction success ($p < 0.001$), but in case of infection, the success rate increased ($p = 0.004$).

Marijon et al., in 2009, published the results of using traction devices in two experienced high-volume centers [14]. In a population of 311 consecutive patients undergoing removal of 250 atrial, 318 right ventricular (RV), and 22 left ventricular (LV) leads with a mean implant time of 85 months, traction was effective in complete removal of 27%, whereas complementary tools and techniques, including mechanical and laser sheaths and transfemoral tools were necessary to remove the remaining 73%. Overall success rate was 89.7%; there was one procedure-related death (0.3%). The results of traction are similar in these last two experiences (Table 6.1); data confirm that the success rate of this approach can be estimated at about 30% overall. These results support the opinion of some experienced centers that suggest the key point of transvenous extraction is freeing the lead from binding fibrous tissue more than applying

Table 6.1 Traction devices

Author	Year	Type of report	No. leads	Complete removal (%)
Bracke [12]	2002	Single center	145	34
Bordachar Marijon [14]	2009	Multicenter	580	27

traction to pull the lead out and slip it back to the insertion site. Traction effectiveness is significantly dependent on implant time: leads implanted for less than 6 months can be reasonably removed by simple traction, whereas for leads with an implant time longer than 2 years, success rate is low, and traction must be considered one of the possible approaches to a complex extraction technique.

6.3 Mechanical Sheaths

6.3.1 Early Experiences

At the end of the 1980s, Byrd et al. developed and introduced into clinical practice the first effective technique for transvenous extraction of chronic pacing leads [9]. The mainstays of this technique were the use of locking stylets and mechanical dilatation of fibrotic binding sites by means of dilating sheaths [15]. The stylet, introduced into the coil's lumen and locking the coil itself at the tip of the lead, or as far as possible into the lead, was thought to provide effective traction while avoiding coil lengthening and lead disruption. As the major obstacle was judged to be the presence of binding sites due to fibrous tissue surrounding and entrapping the lead in its intravascular portion, the other component of the technique was the use of dilating sheaths to advance over the lead's body all the way to the tip, thus dissecting by mechanical force the binding sites. If, despite the use of traction by stylet and dissection by sheath, the tip of the lead were still anchored to the myocardial wall, an outer sheath of larger diameter was advanced over the inner one telescopically. Once the outer sheath had reached the tip, it could be forced against the myocardial wall (countertraction) to enhance the effect of the traction as well as prevent myocardial invagination and damage. Finally, the technique included a transfemoral approach by means of a transvenous workstation and several different tools (retrieval basket, snares) to approach the lead's fragment or a free-floating lead [15]. This brief summary of the original technique clearly suggests that it was complex, requiring skill with different operations and tools and was significantly influenced by operator experience. According to these observations, the results in clinical practice could be very different in different centers and situations.

6.3.2 Large Clinical Results

After some reports related to limited experiences, the clinical results of mechanical dilatation using the original approach described by Byrd et al. [9] were provided by the US Lead Extraction Database [16]. A large amount of data about transvenous lead removal procedures performed in most of centers in the USA were collected in a database and subsequently analyzed. The first report, published in 1994, was related to early experience and included a significant percentage of procedures performed during operator learning curve. As usual in the presence of multicenter experiences using newly developed and complex techniques, the results are often difficult to evaluate and translate to clinical practice. In particular, when the learning curve seems to be long and operator experience may play an important role in determining results as well as complications, the result of similar experiences do not reflect the real effectiveness and safety of the technique used.

From December 1988 to April 1994, the extraction of 2,195 intravascular pacing leads from 1,299 patients was attempted at 193 centers. Leads had been implanted for 0.2 months to 24 years (mean 56 months). Indications were infection (54%, including 10% septicemia), removal of nonfunctional or incompatible leads (40%), and other causes (6%). Extraction was attempted via the implant vein using locking stylets and dilator sheaths; via the femoral vein using snares, retrieval baskets, and sheaths; or using both approaches. With this technique, 86.8% of leads were completely removed, 7.5% were partially removed, and 5.7% were not removed [16].

As previously emphasized, the impact of operator experience on final results was investigated. In the presence of physicians performing their first case, 12% of leads were not removed; for physicians who had performed more than ten cases, only 2% of leads were not removed. Previous attempts at removal decreased the success rate. Of the 189 leads for which extraction attempts had previously failed, 75.1% were completely removed, 14.8% were partially removed, and 10.1% were not removed. This observation suggested that lead damage is a factor decreasing the procedure's effectiveness. Scar tissue entrapping the lead increased in severity with implant duration was the most important complicating factor and found to be the main cause of failure. The femoral approach increased with implant duration (5% of leads implanted 12 months or less, 11% 13 months to 3 years, 20% 4–7 years, and 31% 8–24 years), primarily due to increasingly abundant scarring and prior lead damage. Fatal and near-fatal complications occurred in 2.5%, including eight (0.6%) deaths. The incidence of serious complications was found to be acceptable, particularly when compared with surgical removal techniques.

In 1999, a new release by the US Lead Extraction Database was published [17]. In comparison with the previous paper, it showed an increase in the number of procedures and in success rate. This experience was during a period when extraction techniques were fairly stable and most operators were trained and experienced in removal procedures. On the other hand, a significant number of leads being removed were Accufix or Encor Telectronics leads; the particular characteristics of these models could have affected both results and complication rates.

From January 1994 through April 1996, extraction of 3,540 leads from 2,338 patients (mean age 64 years, range 5–96) was attempted at 226 centers. Indications for removal were infection (27%), nonfunctional or incompatible leads (25%), Accufix or Encore leads (46%), or other causes (2%). The leads were implanted for a mean of 47 ± 41 months (maximum 26 years); 53% were atrial leads, 46% ventricular leads, and 1% superior vena cava (SVC) defibrillating coils. The conventional technique for mechanical dilatation with Cook extraction-kit tools (Cook Vascular Inc., Leechburg, PA, USA) was used. Extraction was attempted via the implant vein using locking stylets and dilator sheaths; and/or transfemorally using snares, retrieval baskets, and sheaths. Complete removal was achieved for 93% of leads, partial for 5%, and 2% were not removed. Major complications were reported for 1.4% of patients (<1% at centers with >300 cases) and minor for 1.7%. Statistical analysis of results was useful to elucidate predictors of failed extraction and complications. Risk of incomplete or failed extraction increased with implant duration ($p < 0.0001$), less experienced physicians ($p < 0.0001$), ventricular leads ($p < 0.005$), noninfected leads ($p < 0.0005$), and younger patients ($p < 0.0001$). The experiences collected suggested that a long lead dwell time induced more extensive growth of fibrous tissue entrapping the lead in tight binding sites; a longer portion of ventricular leads needed to be freed, and intraventricular dilatation was often difficult. Most noninfected leads have to be removed after a long implant period or else they are damaged, thus complicating the procedure and reducing the success rate. Younger patients were found to be more likely to develop scar tissue encapsulating the lead.

The incidence of major complications was slightly less compared with early experiences but did not significantly differ from previous reports. Risk of complications increased with number of leads removed ($p < 0.005$) and with less experienced physicians ($p < 0.005$); risk of major complications was higher for women ($p < 0.01$). The higher incidence of complications in women may be due to the higher fragility of the venous and myocardial wall in these patients, increasing the possibility of tears leading to significant bleeding or cardiac tamponade. In the presence of multiple leads, the extraction procedures are usually complex and the risk of extraction is multiplied for the number of leads to be removed. It was emphasized that operator experience plays a key role either in achieving a high success rate or in reducing the occurrence of major complications.

After these reports, many other single-center experiences were published, but no significant contribution about technique or results was added but in a few cases. In 2003, Mathur et al. [18] published their clinical experience about the removal of 165 leads in 80 patients using traction and/or locking stylets and dilator sheaths (89.7%), Byrd workstation (6.1%), and open thoracotomy (4.8%). Complete removal was achieved for 143 leads

(86.7%), partial for 12 (7.3%) and ten (6.1%) could not be removed. A shorter lead dwell time was associated with extraction success; there was a trend for a higher rate of success in atrial rather than ventricular leads (93.2% vs 80.9%, p = 0.052). Major complications occurred in three patients (3.2%); there were no deaths.

6.3.3 Latest Additions

In recent years, the development by Bongiorni and colleagues of a new transvenous approach through the internal jugular vein using mechanical sheaths for free-floating and difficult exposed leads provided a significant contribution. In 2005, these authors reported their experience with extracting 1,330 consecutive leads, including pacemaker (PM), ICD and LV leads, using a modified mechanical dilatation technique [19]. The success rate of the standard approach (85.4% complete success; 0.9% partial success) was raised by using the internal jugular vein approach for free-floating or difficult leads, which was performed in 164 PM and 16 ICD leads. Major complications occurred in four cases (0.3%). After this approach, the final results were total extraction 98.88%, partial extraction 0.90%, unextracted 0.15%, and not applicable 0.07%; one patient died. No complications were directly related to the jugular approach.

Modification of the technique of mechanical dilatation by polypropylene sheaths and the use of the jugular approach lead to a significant improvement in results. In 2008, this group published the results of a very long and large single-center experience [20] demonstrating the effectiveness of both the use of a single sheath technique and of the transjugular approach to difficult leads. Transvenous extraction was attempted in 2,062 leads (1,825 PM and 237 ICD leads, including 73 free-floating leads) in 1,193 consecutive patients. The technique for mechanical dilatation was modified to avoid using locking stylets, counterpressure and countertraction; a detailed description is provided in another chapter. A single sheath was advanced over the lead, and scar tissue dilatation was performed mainly by rotating the sheath, moving to a larger size sheath when dilatation did not progress and then going back to a smaller one when a binding site was overcome. This approach by mechanical dilatation at the venous entry site was effective in 1,799 leads (90.4%). The transjugular approach to free-floating leads or after failure of the conventional approach allowed complete removal of 2,032 leads (98.4%) and partial removal of 18 (0.9%); removal failed in 12 (0.6%). Major complications were observed in eight patients (0.7%), causing three deaths (0.3%). These results suggest that, independent of the development of powered dilatation, mechanical dilatation techniques are very effective and acceptably safe, particularly when different approaches are used for difficult cases and operators are highly experienced. The reported results of different experiences using polypropylene sheaths are summarized in Table 6.2.

6.4 Laser Sheaths

During the early experience with mechanical dilation, one of the most important determinants of failed extraction was judged to be the presence of scar tissue entrapping the lead. Freeing the lead at these binding sites was difficult and time consuming. The possibility of ablating scar tissue by delivering energy at the distal edge of a sheath seemed to increase the possibility of effectively removing pacing leads.

Table 6.2 Mechanical dilatation

First author, reference no.	Year	Type of report	No. leads	Complete removal (%)	Partial removal (%)	Complications (%)	Deaths (%)
US Extraction Database [16]	1994	Multicenter	2,195	86.8	7.5	2.5	0.6
US Extraction Database [17]	1999	Multicenter	3,540	93	5	2.7	0.5
Mathur [18]	2003	Single center	165	86.7	7.3	3.2	0
Bongiorni [20]	2008	Single center	2,062	98.4	0.9	0.7	0.3

In the early 1990s, an extraction system using dilating sheaths powered by excimer laser was developed and introduced into clinical practice [21]. The system consists of large sheaths connected to a laser generator; pulses of laser energy are delivered at the edge of the sheath, destroying scar tissue and disrupting binding sites. This new technique was favorably welcomed, particularly in the USA, and its use rapidly spread in subsequent years. Dilatation using laser sheaths seemed more effective than mechanical dilatation, and procedural time was reduced. On the other hand powered dilation has some disadvantages. The technique seems to be intrinsically more dangerous than mechanical dilatation, and no feedback on its aggressiveness is provided to the operator. Also, the materials are significantly more expensive.

The first report on the clinical use of laser sheaths was published by Wilkoff et al. at the end of the 1990s. A randomized trial [21] of lead extraction was conducted in 301 patients with 465 chronically implanted pacemaker leads. Patients in the laser group had leads removed with identical tools as those in the nonlaser group, with the exception that the inner telescoping sheath was replaced with the 12-F excimer laser sheath. Complete lead removal rate was 94% in the laser group and 64% in the nonlaser group (p = 0.001); failed nonlaser extraction was completed with the laser tools in 88% of cases. In addition, the mean time to achieve successful lead extraction was significantly reduced for patients randomized to the laser tools (10.1 ± 11.5 min compared with 12.9 ± 19.2 min). Potentially life-threatening complications occurred in none of the nonlaser and three of the laser patients, including one death (p = NS).

After this initial report, results of the multicenter experience were released in 2002 [22]. From October 1995 to December 1999, 1,684 patients (2,561 pacing and defibrillator leads) were treated with laser sheaths at 89 sites in the USA. Complete removal was achieved in 90% of leads, 3% were partially removed, and 7% were failures. The large number of procedures and increasing number of centers using the procedure reduced the difference in success rate in comparison with mechanical dilatation. Major perioperative complications (tamponade, hemothorax, pulmonary embolism, lead migration, death) were observed in 1.9% of patients with in-hospital death in 13 (0.8%). Minor complications were observed in an additional 1.4% of patients. These results support the observation of higher risk of complications related to powered dilatation. Multivariate analysis showed that implant duration was the only preoperative independent predictor of failure (as observed for mechanical dilatation); female gender was the only multivariate predictor of complications.

Similar results were shown by the European multicenter experience [23]. Kennergren et al. published the final report of the Pacing Lead Extraction Surveillance Study in Europe (PLESSE) trial in 2007 [24]. From August 1996 to March 2001, 383 leads (170 atrial, 213 ventricular; mean implant time 74 months) implanted in 292 patients (mean age 61.6 years; range 13–96) were extracted at 14 European centers. Complete extraction was achieved in 90.9% of leads and partial extraction in 3.4%; extraction failed in 5.7%. Median extraction time was 15 min. Total complication rate, including five minor complications (1.7%), was 5.1%. Cardiac tamponade occurred in ten cases, but no in-hospital mortality occurred.

In the subsequent period, results of single-center experiences were published; in most cases, the new models of laser sheaths were used (described in another chapter). Among this large number of papers, Moon et al. [25] reported a series of 128 consecutive patients undergoing extraction of 229 leads (138 PM, 91 ICD; mean dwell time 61 months). Using powered sheath extraction was complete in 88%, near complete (retained tip) in 10%, and failed in 2%. Major complications were observed in five cases; there were no procedure-related deaths. Powered dilatation was necessary in 56% of leads implanted for >1 year (16% in leads with <1 year implant time) and only in 3% of patients affected by sepsis. The results at this center are nearly the same as previously published experiences and can be assumed to be a representative sample of clinical practice with laser sheaths. Another paper exemplifying the clinical practice of laser-assisted extraction was published by Roux and colleagues in 2007 [26], who reported on 200 lead extraction procedures performed at the Montreal Heart Institute between September 2000 and August 2005. The extraction technique consisted in traction by locking stylets and excimer laser sheath dilatation. In the overall population, success rate was 89%, partial removal 3%, and failure 8% of leads. Acute complications were observed in 7.9%: eight (4.5%) minor and six (3.4%) major, with one death. Predictors of failed extraction were longer time from implant and history of hypertension; predictor of complications was the use of laser from both right and left sides.

In recent years, the results of transvenous removal in high-volume single centers have been published. In 2008, Jones et al. reported their experience between 2000 and 2007 [27]. A total of 975 chronic leads (median implant duration 5.7 years; range 0.5–32.7) were removed from 498 patients using laser-assisted dilatation. Overall, 97.5% of leads were completely removed. Major complications occurred in two (0.4%) patients, and no deaths occurred. Laser assistance for extraction was more likely to be necessary with leads implanted >3.4 years compared with <3.4 years and with ICD compared with PM leads. Kennergren and colleagues published another large single-center experience in 2009 [28] reporting data from 1,032 leads (mean implantation time 69 months) and 647 procedures. The technique consisted of laser-assisted extraction and a step-by-step approach using different techniques. Laser was used to extract 60% of leads (implanted for a mean of 91 months), 29% were manually extracted, 6% were extracted with mechanical tools, 4% surgically removed, and 0.6% extracted by a femoral approach. Failure rate was 0.7% (4.7% including surgical removal), and major complication rate was 0.9%. No extraction-related mortality occurred. The results of the Lexicon Study presented during the 2009 HRS convention reported the analysis of laser-assisted removal of 2,405 leads in 1,449 patients at 13 centers between January 2004 and December 2007 [29]. Data showed a 97.7% clinical success rate and a 96.5% complete lead removal success rate. There was also a 1.4% major adverse event rate, which was a 26% relative reduction compared with a previous multicenter study evaluating the original laser sheath [22]. Results of laser-assisted extraction are summarized in Table 6.3.

The above-mentioned results demonstrate the high effectiveness of the laser-assisted technique. Although no clearly significant improvement in success rate was observed compared with mechanical dilatation, procedural time was reduced. Concern was raised by the slightly higher incidence of major complications, mainly due to venous or myocardial wall injury, but mortality was very low. The latest reports suggest that highly experienced centers and operators increase the safety of laser-assisted lead extraction.

6.5 Radiofrequency Sheaths

After the development of laser-assisted dilatation, a different source of energy was used to power sheath dilatation. Cook Vascular developed a powered sheath using electrosurgical dissection in the 1980s. This Teflon sheath has a dipole at its bevelled edge, and when connected to an electrosurgical unit, radiofrequency (RF) energy is delivered at the edge in the same manner as in bipolar cutting, thus disrupting fibrous tissue and freeing the lead from binding sites. The depth of the lesion induced by electrosurgical dissection seems to be larger

Table 6.3 Laser-assisted dilatation

Author, reference no.	Year	Type of report	No. leads	Complete removal (%)	Partial removal (%)	Complications (%)	Deaths (%)
PLEXES [22]	2002	Multicenter	2,561	90	3	3.3	0.8
PLESSE [24]	2007	Multicenter	383	90.9	3.4	5.1	0
Roux [26]	2007	Single center	347	89	3	7.9	0.6
Epstein Jones [27]	2008	Single center	975	97.5	-	0.4	0
Kennergren [28]	2009	Single center	1,032	95.3	4.7	0.9	0
LexiCon [29]	2009	Multicenter	2,405	96.5	-	1.4	-

PLEXES Pacemaker Lead Extraction with the Laser Sheath, *PLESSE* Pacing Lead Extraction Surveillance Study in Europe than that of laser-assisted sheaths, but it is delivered only near the cutting dipole and not over the entire circumference of the edge of the sheath. The dipole and the limited area of tissue ablation allows the cutting energy to be directed toward the lead at the inner side of the vein, thus avoiding tissue disruption near the venous wall and reducing the risk of bleeding.

This type of dilatation was supposed to be as effective as laser dilatation but significantly less expensive, so interest in this new technique increased. After its introduction into clinical practice, its use did not spread as the use of the laser technique did. Although its use is reported in a consistent number of centers, particularly in the USA, only few experiences have been published in the literature, mainly preliminary reports [30]. In 2007, Neuzil and co-workers published the only report comparing electrosurgical dissection (ESD) and mechanical dilatation [31]. In their study, 120 consecutive patients were randomized to RF-current-powered extraction or standard countertraction lead removal. One hundred and sixty-one leads included 17 ICDleads, and mean implant time was 73 months. Success rate for complete extraction was 93% in the RF group and 73% with the standard transvenous lead extraction system by countertraction ($p < 0.01$); successful removal of ICD leads was 90% (9/10) in the RF group and 57% (4/7) in the standard group. Dilatation time was significantly shorter in the ESD group, whereas serious complications (pulmonary embolism, bleeding; in 5/120 patients) showed no significant difference between techniques. The major limitation of the study seems to be a very low success rate using standard mechanical dilatation techniques, significantly lower in comparison with most reports about this method [16, 17, 18–20]. It is then difficult to assess whether and how much RF-powered sheaths are superior to mechanical sheaths. Success rate among the RF group only (93%) was slightly less than either mechanical or laser-assisted dilatation in the majority of the reports. This may be due to the learning curve using the different techniques, but further data are lacking.

In conclusion, few data are available regarding RF-assisted dilatation; this technique does not appear to add a significant advantage when compared with other dilatation techniques, and its clinical use seems to be restricted to a small number of centers.

6.6 Rotating Threaded Tip Sheath

A new extraction tool was introduced in recent years by Cook Vascular. Due to the observation that rotation of the mechanical polypropylene sheath was one of the most important determinants of the technique's effectiveness, a system for rotating a mechanical dilator was introduced. The Evolution mechanical dilator sheath is a rotationally powered telescoping device with by a steel inner sheath. The rotation mechanism is manually operated, allowing rotation of the steel sheath, and is provided with small winglets near the distal end. This technique combines counterpressure, rotation, and movement of the threaded end of the sheath to enhance dilatation effectiveness at binding sites.

Preliminary experiences using this device are reported in the literature; evaluation of the effectiveness is affected by the small number of patients in single-center and single-operator experiences [32, 33]. Results suggest effectiveness similar to powered sheaths in overcoming binding sites; further data are necessary to determine possible advantages of using this technique. Some concern has been raised about the aggressiveness of the mechanism, which can lead to tissue disruption induced by the rotation of the treaded tip, particularly in the absence of any feedback for the operator. In the survey of major complications related to transvenous lead extraction, Hauser et al. reported six fatal events and two serious injuries in 2008 using this tool, mainly due to tears to innominate vein and SVC [34]. Hussein et al. recently reported a success rate of 86% in 29 patients, with the absence of mortality or significant complications [35]. These results, related to a relatively small number of cases, suggest that safety of the mechanical dilator sheath should be further investigated.

6.7 Transfemoral Approach

The possible different approaches used for transvenous extraction are discussed in a separate section; in this chapter, results of the approaches are evaluated in respect to their use as a separate technique, not as part of complex procedures. The usefulness of a transvenous approach in extracting of free-floating leads or lead fragments was recognized from the time techniques for transvenous extractions were introduced into clinical practice. A transfemoral kit consisting of a transfemoral workstation and several remote-control tools (basket retriever, tip-deflecting wire) was included in the Cook Vascular extraction system [15, 36]. In the presence of free-floating leads, the transfemoral approach can be used to directly attempt removal; in addition, it can be helpful to complete the extraction procedure in combination with the superior approach, particularly when the lead tip was not anchored to the myocardial wall. As the use of transvenous removal techniques spread, several intravascular tools were developed and used, alone or in combination with the others. Different snares and a loop retriever were introduced, as were other retrievers, such as the Needle's Eye catcher. Most of these tools proved useful in different procedural conditions.

A primarily transfemoral approach in situations different from free-floating leads arouses little enthusiasm in most operators. Some key points of the technique were criticized [37]. First, traction with tools, even when combined with a transvenous workstation, was found to be poorly effective and unsafe; anchored-tip lead dilatation of binding sites using the transfemoral sheath appeared difficult, particularly for ventricular leads. Concern was raised by the possibility of lead entrapment (e.g., in the event of an exposed coil in damaged leads) into the retrieving tool, which would require surgical removal following failed extraction. Regardless of the criticisms, the technique was accepted and used in some centers.

Jarwe et al. reported experience with the transfemoral approach [38]. In 1999, the authors published the results of extraction using a snare (lasso) via the femoral vein as a first approach in 116 leads and an alternate approach – after extraction from the original site of implantation had failed – in another 12 leads. Mean implant time was 62 months. Of the 128 leads, 122 (95%) were completely removed, two (2%) were partially extracted (distal electrode remaining attached to the myocardium), and four (3%) could not be removed. Complications occurred in four cases. In the same period, they reported their experience with ICD lead removal using the same technique [39]. In 11 patients, they removed five leads using a superior approach, whereas eight leads were removed by a femoral approach using a lasso alone or added to a pigtail catheter. There was no failure of explantation.

Some years later, a new report by the same group evaluated results of different tools using the transfemoral approach [40]. Among 222 leads removed in 99 patients, Klug et al. analyzed the use of the Needle's Eye snare using the femoral approach. Attempted extraction was performed in 70 leads implanted for a mean of 113 months. Sixty-one (87.2%) leads were successfully extracted; extraction was incomplete in three (4.3%) cases and failed in six (8.5%). Failures were due to leads totally excluded from the venous flow in four cases, the impossibility of advancing the 16-F-long sheath through the femoral veins for one case, and intolerable ventricular arrhythmia induced by traction in one case. Complications included two deaths.

Most papers about large experiences report the use of the transfemoral approach and intravascular tools mainly as an aid in complex procedures and in combination with other techniques [37]. The use of intravascular tools may be helpful for completing an extraction procedure started with dilatation, when extracting free-floating fragments, or cross to an alternative transvenous approach, such as the transjugular approach [19, 20]. A recent multicenter study compared laser-assisted extraction with the transfemoral approach, reporting similar success rates and incidences of complications [41]; regardless of this report, all available data to date seem to suggest that a primary attempt to remove transvenous leads with an anchored tip using this technique results in a lower success rate and may increase the risk of complications.

6.8 Transjugular Approach

A significant contribution to transvenous removal techniques was made by Bongiorni et al. [19]. In the presence of free-floating leads, the impossibility of performing dilatation using a dilating sheath may affect the results of transvenous techniques. If the free-floating proximal end of the lead can be exposed through the internal jugular vein, the lead is suitable for a standard dilatation with a high success rate. After an initial experience limited to free-floating leads, the approach was extended to exposed leads whose removal with standard techniques failed. The leads to be removed are grasped using a deflecting wire advanced through the femoral vein, thus creating a free-floating lead. After percutaneous cannulation of the right internal jugular vein, a lasso is advanced to catch the proximal end of the lead and retrieve it through the jugular vein. Once the lead is exposed, dilatation can be performed. The transjugular approach provides several significant advantages: first, it allows dilatation with sheaths, even in the presence of free-floating leads. In addition, the course of the lead from the tip to the jugular vein is usually straight, which can help dilatation of scar tissue at the binding sites and near the tip; the absence of turns and the ability to avoid the costoclavicular space permits the use of larger dilators. Finally, during the procedure of making the lead free floating, the lead itself can be slipped through many binding sites, thus avoiding further dilatation. Potential disadvantages are the complexity of the approach or the impossibility of cannulating the jugular vein.

After a paper published in 2005, in 2008, Bongiorni and co-workers reported their experience in consecutive patients over a period of about 10 years [20]. During extraction of 2,062 leads (1,753 PM, 237 ICD, 72 LV) using mechanical dilatation technique, the transjugular approach was attempted in 205 leads. In 73 free-floating leads, it was used as the first approach, whereas in 148 difficult exposed leads, the transjugular approach was performed after the ineffectiveness of dilatation at a binding site for more than 5 min. The transfemoral approach used for the crossover to the jugular approach allowed removal of 16 free-floating leads; dilatation through the jugular vein was performed in the remaining 57 free-floating and 156 exposed leads. The transjugular approach was effective in that it allowed complete removal of 205 out of 213 (96.2%) leads, thus leading to a success rate of 98.4% in the overall study population. One case of cardiac tamponade during mechanical dilatation at the tip of a ventricular lead occurred during the transjugular procedures, whereas complications strictly related to the approach were never observed.

No other author has published further experiences about this approach, even though some author mention its use (named the Pisa approach) and the satisfactory results obtained [42]. Mazzetti et al., in 2008, reported the removal of 22 leads through the jugular vein using a similar approach [43]. In this experience, however, the operators performed a surgical approach to the internal jugular vein and used different tools to remove the leads.

The transjugular approach seems to be a very effective solution in the presence of complex extraction procedures and difficult leads. The basic concept of moving the lead to the place where the best conditions for extraction can be found makes the transjugular approach very useful. Potential limitations of the technique are internal jugular vein patency, complexity of subsequent manoeuvres to move the lead to this position, and the possibility of grasping the lead and slipping it into the venous system. Conversely, the advantages are reduced number of binding sites to be ablated and the increased effectiveness of dilatation from the jugular approach, particularly in the presence of free-floating leads. Advantages of the approach are not related to the energy used for freeing the lead of scar tissue. Even if the largest experience was performed using mechanical dilatation with polypropylene sheaths, the technique appears to be even more helpful when using powered dilatation due to the larger size of the sheath and the higher potential for complications in comparison with mechanical dilatation.

6.9 Results of ICD Lead Extraction

Since their introduction into clinical practice, ICD leads were supposed to be significantly more troublesome than conventional pacing leads [4, 5]. The larger size of these leads was considered a disadvantage in the case of transvenous removal due to the need to use larger dilating sheaths that are more difficult to handle. In particular, defibrillating coils seemed to make extraction more complex and challenging. The coil consists of metallic material, and its surface is not smooth due to the spiral or net design of conductors. These characteristics significantly raise the potential to induce irritation and damage of the venous and myocardial walls and subsequently the growth of fibrous tissue. In addition, the scared surface of defibrillating coils and the different diameters of coils and lead body, creating a step-like transition at their connecting site, appear to increase the difficulty of dilatation. In addition to all these potential obstacles to transvenous removal, the problem of ICD lead extraction was worsened by the observation of higher complication rates due to either infection or lead failure. With respect to the rate of lead malfunction, it must be emphasized that the long-term clinical performance of ICD leads, even today, proved to be significantly lower than PM leads [44]. Independently of single models, submitted to recall because of unacceptable failure rates, long-term ICD lead reliability is still unsatisfactory. Considering that lead damage or malfunction may have dramatic consequences and that in most cases these complications require lead removal in order to implant a new one, it is easy to understand that ICD lead extraction becomes an important issue for implanting centers.

The concern about ICD extraction using conventional equipment was averted by clinical results. Even if extraction procedures were complex and time consuming, the final outcome showed no outstanding differences in comparison with results of PM lead extraction. Results of ICD lead extraction using mechanical sheaths were included in the US Lead Extraction Database published in 1999 [17], and early trials on laser-assisted sheaths were performed for both PM and ICD leads [21, 23, 45]. In 2000, Kantharia et al. reported their experience with transvenous extraction of 47 transvenous high-voltage leads implanted in 42 patients [46]. All leads were extracted – 11 by traction and 36 by mechanical dilatation – in the absence of serious complications. Extraction time was related to time from implant and degree of fibrosis; nevertheless, no statistically significant difference was found for leads with implant durations of 12, 24, or 48 months. In 2003, Saad et al. reported on a larger population [47]. Mainly using laser-assisted sheaths, extraction of ventricular transvenous defibrillating leads was completely achieved in 96.9% of attempts in a population of 161 consecutive ICD recipients. Including partial success, clinical success was achieved in 98% of patients, whereas failure occurred in three. Major complications were observed in 2/161 patients, including one death. Many further reports, including those relating to a significant number of ICD leads submitted to transvenous removal, demonstrated a success rate for extraction at least the same as conventional PM leads. In some large experiences, as reported by Bongiorni et al. [20], Jones et al. [27], and Kennergren et al. [28], success rate approximated 100% (Table 6.4).

In our opinion, it is possible that the disadvantages of the ICD leads in regard to transvenous extraction, as described, were counterbalanced by other factors. First, ICD leads submitted to removal usually have an implant period shorter in comparison with the overall population of PM leads. In addition, the larger size and the greater stiffness of most ICD leads were proved in clinical practice to facilitate dilatation, independent of the energy used to free the lead from scar tissue. The need for larger sheaths is counterbalanced by the characteristics of the ICD lead, and it is likely to be not important for the final outcome of extraction procedures. It is possible that different ICD lead materials and the presence of only one inner coil, usually endowed in significant insulation, may play a favorable role in scar tissue dilatation. On the other hand, the presence of defibrillating

Table 6.4 Implantable cardioverter–defibrillator lead extraction

Author	Year	Type of report	No. leads	Technique	Complete removal (%)	Partial removal (%)	Complications (%)	Deaths (%)
Kantharia [46]	2000	Single center	47	Mechanical	100	-	-	-
Wilkoff, Saad [47]	2003	Single center	161	Laser	96.9	1.2	1.2	0.6
Bongiorni [20]	2008	Single center	237	Mechanical	100	0	0	0
Epstein, Jones [27]	2008	Single center	215	Laser	98.3	1.7	0	0
Kennergren [28]	2009	Single center	165	Laser	98.2	1.8	1.7	0

coils was proved to induce a more extensive growth of scar tissue surrounding and entrapping the lead. All experiences reported a high rate of binding sites related to the coils, into the ventricle as well as in the SVC, where dilatation can be challenging and risky.

In conclusion, even if in the presence of ICD leads extraction is more complex and time consuming, ICD leads can be transvenously extracted with results similar or even superior in comparison with PM leads.

6.10 Results of LV Lead Extraction

The development of cardiac resynchronization therapy (CRT) as an effective treatment for end-stage heart failure in the late 1990s increased the number of implanted cardiac devices and the complexity of implanting interventions. The use of an additional lead inserted in a coronary sinus branch, the increased number of tools necessary to accomplish the intervention, and the longer time required for CRT implant raised the number of related complications. Most studies published in the literature suggest a significant percentage of CRT recipients undergoing infective complications; furthermore, complications related to lead dislodgement or malfunction were estimated to be at least 6% in the overall population [48].

In the presence of local or systemic infection, no significant difference in management can be found between PMs for antibrady pacing and ICDs and CRT devices. Conversely, malfunctioning or dislodged LV leads may prevent a new lead implantation; in these cases, transvenous removal is required. The completely different site of implant – usually into a small branch of the coronary sinus – in the absence of any fixation mechanism, in comparison with leads implanted in large chambers and anchored with fixation mechanisms, raised some concern about transvenous removal of LV leads. If binding sites due to fibrous tissue around the lead were frequent in the Coronary Sinus (CS), most experienced operators believed that dilatation at this site would be very difficult and significantly risky. Fortunately, clinical experience demonstrated that transvenous removal of LV leads can be performed effectively and safely in most patients. A significant number of small experiences with LV lead extraction was published that demonstrated a success rate near 100% and an absence of a significant percentage of serious complications [49–53]. Most LV leads were completely removed by simple manual traction, whereas sheath dilatation of binding sites was required only in a few cases. Bongiorni and colleagues [53] reported that in 37 LV procedures, scar tissue entrapping the lead in the CS occurred in only a few patients and represented 10% of the overall number of binding sites to be dilated in order to free and remove the LV leads.

Even if infrequent, the presence of CS adhesions requiring dilatation may be challenging. The size of the CS and branches in which the LV leads are positioned are usually too small for the dilating sheath, particularly when powered sheaths are used, thus increasing the difficulty of sheath advancement and increasing the risk of bleeding. The use of large sheaths and lasing in the CS seems to be unsafe [52]. In addition, it is difficult to insert the sheath into the CS, as there are several significant turns to maneuver in order to reach the distal part of the lead. This may prevent sheath advancement to the distal part of the lead. In their experience, Bongiorni and colleagues [53] reported in one case the need to perform a different transvenous approach. In the presence of a tight binding site into the CS, after creating a free-floating lead and exposing it through the femoral vein, successful mechanical dilatation was performed using an extra-long (XL) mechanical polypropylene sheath. Most recent reports include a significant number of LV leads and results of successful transvenous extraction close to 100% [14, 20, 27, 28] (Table 6.5).

The shorter implant time, different characteristics of lead insulation, and absence of a fixation mechanism can explain the substantial ease of transvenous removal of LV leads. Regardless of the ease of lead removal by simple traction, binding sites into the CS are present in most patients as evidenced by findings during LV lead reimplantation. These include CS stenosis, presence of thrombi, and obliteration of venous branches. These observations suggest that, due to their different characteristics, it may be easier to slip LV leads through adhesions than the other leads. On the other hand, these observations and clinical experiences suggest that the use of fixation mech-

Table 6.5 Left ventricular lead extraction

Author, reference no.	Year	Type of report	No. leads	Technique	Complete removal (%)	Complications (%)	Deaths (%)
De Martino [49]	2005	Single center	12	Mechanical	100	0	0
Kasravi [50]	2005	Single center	14	Mechanical	100	0	0
Tyers [52]	2003	Single center	14	Laser	100	7.1	7,1
Bongiorni [53]	2007	Single center	37	Mechanical	100	0	0

anisms for LV leads can significantly reduce extractability. The retractability of any fixation mechanism after a lengthy implant time is never certain, and this condition can make transvenous removal complex, or even impossible, as described recently by Bongiorni et al. [54]. The use of stents [55–57] to fix the lead should be considered a contraindication to transvenous extraction.

6.11 Determinants of Results and Complications

Since the development of transvenous lead extraction techniques, efforts have addressed the individuation of factors affecting results and incidence of complications. The aim of these efforts was the possibility of evaluating the risk–benefit ratio in individual patients to improve results and reduce possible risks. Many clinical and technical factors may play significant roles in transvenous extraction [2, 37, 58]; characteristics of the material to be extracted (lead design, implant site, fixation mechanism, coils, polarity, thickness, insulation), of the patient (sex, age, underlying diseases), and of clinical history (implant time, implant vein, number and position of leads, lead failure or damage) must be evaluated to help predict the outcome of the extraction procedure and to forecast possible complications. A brief summary follows.

6.11.1 Predictors of Results

Early experiences with extraction were essentially by traction, and they evidenced the important role of lead implant time [1, 4]. It was a foregone conclusion that dwell time since implantation would decrease the possibility of lead removal. Reports of autopsy findings [59] in PM recipients showed that implanted leads induce fibrous reaction and scar-tissue growth, encapsulating at least part of the lead body. This process is time dependent; the longer the implant time, the higher the degree of scar-tissue fixing the lead. It is difficult to predict the time required for development of a significant growth of scar tissue in an individual patient or a cutoff period to determine the presence or absence of binding sites. Most data suggest that after a period of about 12 months, effectiveness of traction, even using traction devices, is significantly reduced [13, 14]. An important role may be played by the age of the recipient due to the higher degree of fibrous reaction in young people in comparison with older patients. Another important factor may be lead design; for example, most experiences report a higher incidence of binding sites induced by defibrillating coils in ICD leads [45–47]. Pacing site may also be a factor. Most analyses report that extraction failure is significantly higher for RV leads [16, 17], even though the report by Mathur et al. [18] showed no statistically significant difference between atrial and ventricular leads. Lead length, the tricuspid valve, and entrapment of the lead tip may explain this different result in comparison with atrial leads.

Autopsy reports in PM patients [58] highlight the possibility of tricuspid valve leaflet perforation and abundant scarring due to ventricular leads. In 2005, Lin et al. [60] reported that in 41 PM or ICD patients undergoing tricuspid valve repair or replacement, a perforation of the tricuspid valve leaflet by the permanent PM (PPM) or ICD lead was found in seven patients. Lead entanglement in the tricuspid valve occurred in four patients, lead impingement of the tricuspid valve leaflets in 16, and lead adherence to the tricuspid valve in 14. Damage to the tricuspid valve by PPM or ICD leads is not rare and may result in severe symptomatic tricuspid regurgitation, even if it may be not overtly visualized by echocardiography.

Younger patients are more likely to develop a significant fibrous reaction leading to abundant scar tissue surrounding the lead. This condition may affect the result of transvenous extraction techniques. A concomitant factor complicating extraction in young patients is implantation in the pediatric period, when lead positioning is influenced by the predictable growth of the patient and congenital heart disease and subsequent surgery. Data in the literature report a lower success rate for mechanical dilatation in younger patients. Younger age was identified as a predictor of lower success rate from the time of publication of the first databases in the 1990s [16, 17]. Recently, Roux et al. [26] confirmed that younger age is a predictor of failure in lead extraction.

Results of large databases suggest that indications for removal may play a role in the outcome of transvenous extractions. Since the first reports were published [16, 17], leads undergoing transvenous removal for indications other than infectious complications were found to have a less favorable outcome in comparison with infected leads. Many factors may play a role in this situation. One may be that uninfected leads may undergo extraction procedures for indications different than class I, and this factor may affect either the aggressiveness or the outcome of the procedure. The different outcome was not observed in other reports. In 2006, Gaynor et al. [61] analyzed 283 consecutive patients in whom a total of 500 leads (302 PM and 198 ICD) were extracted over a 5-year period. Laser-assisted dilatation was used whenever moderate traction failed and was used as a marker of scar growth and difficult extraction. A total of 203 leads in 128 patients was removed for noninfectious indication; infective indication was present in 155 patients (297 leads), including sepsis, pocket infection, and erosion. Even though overall results were similar, laser assistance was required for 6% of septic leads, 51% of leads associated with erosion or pocket infection, and 60% of uninfected leads ($p = 0.001$). Laser assistance was necessary more often for leads implanted >12 months (53% vs 6%) and for ventricular compared with atrial leads (52% vs 35%). No clear and unquestionable explanation can be found regarding these findings; nevertheless, the presence of systemic infection may play a role. In his report regarding ICD lead removal, Kantharia et al. [46] found no statistically significant difference in leads with infective or noninfective indications, and extraction time was similar in both groups.

Another significant factor affecting the outcome of extraction procedures is related to lead damage. Most extraction tools and techniques may not be applicable or may prove useless if the lead is severely damaged. Stylets cannot be inserted for free-floating leads or in the presence of a break of the conductor coil; broken leads cannot be submitted to traction and resist strongly to aggressive dilatation. Damaged insulation or defibrillating coils may require a very large sheath, and even then, the procedure may be very risky [37]. The extraction procedure may induce significant damage to the lead; in case of failed extraction, the possibility of removing the lead in a second attempt is significantly reduced.

The final factor affecting the results of transvenous lead extraction procedures is operator experience. As discussed in the introduction to this chapter, transvenous extraction procedures require operator training, experience, and ability to find solutions to complex and different situations. Most of these conditions are acquired after a long period of training and significant personal experience using transvenous techniques. All data in the literature emphasize that results, as well as complications, are heavily influenced by the experience of both operators and staff. In the US Lead Extraction Database, operator experience affected the outcome of extraction in a statistically significant manner [17]. It is critically important that before starting clinical activity of transvenous extraction, each center compiles a complete program for operator and staff training.

6.11.2 Predictors of Complications

Most factors discussed above can influence the incidence of complications in transvenous extraction procedures. Regardless of technique and tools used, transvenous extraction is affected by a significant risk of serious complications, including fatal events. Many conditions may be managed by the experienced operator and by training to immediately and effectively treat life-threatening complications, including open-chest surgery. Nevertheless, the possibility of fatal complications is intrinsic to transvenous extraction and must always be considered. In the survey recently published by Hauser et al., deaths and major complications with all available techniques are reported [34].

Most data regarding risk factors for complications are derived by the large, multicenter experiences performed in the 1990s [16, 17, 21–23]. The most important predictors of undesired events were found to be the number of leads requiring removal, female gender, and operator experience. The importance of other factors, such as lead design (for example, Accufix or Encor leads) or lead fracture or damage, is clear, as previously discussed. The presence of multiple leads can impact the risk of complications in many ways. The risk related to removal is multiplied for the number of lead submitted to extraction; in addition, multiple leads are more likely to induce fibrous tissue growth and venous occlusion, particularly if implanted in both the left and right sides. Multiple leads are frequent in patients with a long clinical history of cardiac pacing, so it is likely that implant time for some of these leads was significantly long at the time the patient underwent lead extraction. Roux et al. [26], in a 270 leads submitted to laser-assisted extraction, found that at multivariate analysis the only predictor of complications was laser-lead extraction from both the right and left sides during the same procedure. Agarwal et al., in 2009 [62], analyzed data from 212 consecutive patients (456 leads; ICD 49%) and reported 26 (11.8%) complications in 25 patients, including nine (4.2%) major (one death) and 17 (8.0%) minor. Independent predictors of complications included a higher number of explanted RV leads. Extraction of ICD as opposed to a PM device showed a strong trend toward significance. Limitation of this study was the high incidence of complications as compared with many other reports; furthermore these observations emphasize the higher risk related to leads in the ventricular position, multiple leads, and ICD leads.

Major complications are statistically more frequent in the female gender. The possible explanation of this observation is that in women, particularly the elderly, the venous and myocardial walls are more fragile than in men. The smaller vein size and thinner venous wall may induce a higher rate of complications. Heart size is normally related to body surface area and is therefore smaller in women; the myocardial wall is usually thinner in women than in men, so that the possibility of inducing a tear in the wall is higher. Franceschi et al. [63] recently evaluated the possibility of significant tricuspid regurgitation induced by transvenous extraction procedures of chronically implanted PM and ICD leads. After removal of 237 ventricular leads in 208 patients, a new tricuspid regurgitation was observed in 19 patients (9.1%), requiring surgical repair in two cases. This finding suggests that traumatic injury to the tricuspid valve is not uncommon during transvenous lead removal. Three independent risk factors of traumatic tricuspid regurgitation were found: use of laser sheath, use of both laser sheath and lasso, and female gender. Whereas the tools used suggest the difficulty of lead extraction and the approximate degree of scar tissue ablation in order to remove the lead, the impact of gender suggests that women are more prone to complications from mechanical devices during aggressive extraction manoeuvres.

Another important issue is the presence of infective vegetations linked to the leads or infective endocarditis. In PM or ICD patients, vegetations are frequent in the presence of septicemia. The risk of transvenous extraction procedures is related to the possibility of vegetation detachment and subsequent embolism. Small vegetations are not usually considered dangerous; vegetation embolism into the lung is most frequent, but it has no clinical relevance in most cases. Large vegetations may be significantly dangerous if embolism occurs. Concern regarding lead removal in the presence of large vegetations – due to the risk of fatal or near-fatal embolism – led to surgical removal of leads as well as vegetations. Despite all these considerations, the size of vegetation contraindicating transvenous extraction cannot be defined. Experts agree that in the presence of vegetations >2 cm, transvenous extraction must be considered as very risky [2]; furthermore prospective data about this issue are lacking. Reports in the literature suggest that the outcome of vegetations during transvenous extraction is better than expected. In 2003, Meier-Ewert et al. [64] reported the presence of vegetations ranging in size from 10 mm to 38 mm in their largest dimension on endocardial leads or right-sided cardiac structures in nine patients. All patients underwent successful transvenous removal of endocardial leads. Five of the nine patients (55%) had late evidence of pulmonary embolism; however, all these patients made a full recovery with antibiotic and anticoagulation treatment. Ruttmann et al. reported the presence of vegetations >1 cm in 23 patients [65]. Perioperative mortality was 5.7% (three patients); all of these patients underwent primary surgical removal and had severe endocarditis of the tricuspid valve. None of the patients who underwent transvenous lead removal died, and there were no further complications in the follow-up. All these finding suggest that even if vegetation embolization during transvenous lead removal using sheath dilatation is fairly common, life-threatening complications are not likely to occur. Further data are required to identify the conditions in which the risk of the transvenous procedure is too high.

As discussed regarding factors affecting success rate, operator experience plays a key role in the risk of procedural complications [35, 66]. In the U.S. Lead Extraction Database [17], high volume centers (>300 extraction procedures overall) were found to have about half the number of complications in comparison with less experienced centers. The learning curve for transvenous extraction is very important due to the intrinsic risk associated with removal procedures. As every case is different from the previous ones, only lengthy training and a great deal of experience will reduce the risk of serious complications and obtain the highest success rate.

Regardless of procedural complications, it must be emphasized that patients affected by systemic infection related to an implantable cardiac device are at high risk because of the infective disease and overwhelming sepsis. Hamid and colleagues [67] recently reported their experience with 183 patients referred for transvenous lead extraction. The incidence of death due to sepsis was as high as 2.7%; predictor of unfavorable outcome was a significant increase in inflammatory markers.

References

1. Byrd CL, Schwartz SJ, Hedin NB et al (1990) Intravascular lead extraction using locking stylets and sheaths. Pacing Clin Electrophysiol 13:1871–1875
2. Love CJ, Wilkoff BL, Byrd CL et al (2000) Recommendations for extraction of chronically implanted transvenous pacing and defibrillator leads: indications, facilities, training. North American Society of Pacing and Electrophysiology Lead Extraction Conference Faculty. Pacing Clin Electrophysiol 23(4 Pt 1):544–551
3. Wilkoff BL, Love CJ, Byrd CL et al (2009) Transvenous lead extraction: Heart Rhythm Society expert consensus on facilities, training indications and patient management. Heart Rhythm 6:1086–1104
4. Love CJ (2000) Current concepts in extraction of transvenous pacing and ICD leads. Cardiol Clin 18:193–217
5. Verma A, Wilkoff BL (2004) Intravascular pacemaker and defibrillator lead extraction: a state-of-the-art review. Heart Rhythm 1:739–745
6. Furman S, Behrens M, Andrews C, Klementowicz P (1987) Retained pacemaker leads. J Thoracic Cardiovasc Surg 94:770–772
7. Parry G, Goudevenos J, Jameson S et al (1991) Complications associated with retained pacemaker leads. Pacing Clin Electrophysiol 14:1251–1257
8. Zerbe F, Ponizynski A, Dyszkiewicz W et al (1985) Functionless retained pacing leads in the cardiovascular system. Br Heart J 54:76–79
9. Byrd CL, Schwartz SJ, Hedin NB et al (1990) Intravascular lead extraction using locking stylets and sheaths. Pacing Clin Electrophysiol 13:1871–1875
10. Eckhard A, Neuzner J, Binner L (1996) Three-year experience with a stylet for lead extraction: a multicenter study. Pacing Clin Electrophysiol 19:18–25
11. Vassilikos VP, Maounis TN, Chiladakis J et al (1999) Percutaneous extraction of transvenous defibrillator leads using the VascoExtor pacing lead removal system. J Interv Card Electrophysiol 3(3):247–251
12. Bracke F, Meijer A, Van Gelder B (2002) Extraction of pacemaker and implantable defibrillator leads: patient and lead characteristics in relation to the requirement of extraction tools. Pacing Clin Electrophysiol 25(7):1037–1040
13. Bracke FA, Meijer A, Van Gelder LM (2004) Lead extraction for device related infections: a single centre experience. Europace 6:243–247
14. Marijon E, Boveda S, De Guillebon M et al (2009) Contribution of advanced techniques to the success and safety of transvenous lead extraction. Pacing Clin Electrophysiol 32(Suppl 1):S38–S41
15. Byrd CL, Schwartz SJ, Hedin NB (1991) Intravascular techniques for extraction of permanent pacemakers leads. J Thoracic Cardiovasc Surg 101:989–997
16. Smith HJ, Fearnot NE, Byrd CL et al (1994) Five-years experience with intravascular lead extraction. U.S. Lead Extraction Database. Pacing Clin Electrophysiol 17(11 Pt 2): 2016–2020
17. Byrd CL, Wilkoff BL, Love CJ et al (1999) Intravascular extraction of problematic or infected permanent pacemaker leads: 1994–1996. U.S. Lead Extraction Database, Med Institute. Pacing Clin Electrophysiol 22(9):1348–57
18. Mathur G, Stables RH, Heaven D et al (2003) Cardiac pacemaker lead extraction using conventional technique: a single centre experience. Int J Cardiol 91(2–3):215–219
19. Bongiorni MG, Giannola G, Soldati E et al (2005) Pacing and implantable cardioverter–defibrillator transvenous lead extraction. Ital Heart J 6:261–266

20. Bongiorni MG, Soldati E, Zucchelli G et al (2008) Transvenous removal of pacing and defibrillating leads using single sheath mechanical dilatation and multiple venous approaches: high success rate and safety in more than 2000 leads. Eur Heart J 29(23):2886–2893
21. Wilkoff BL, Byrd CL, Love CJ et al (1999) Pacemaker lead extraction with the laser sheath: results of the pacing lead extraction with the excimer sheath (PLEXES) trial. J Am Coll Cardiol 1999; 33:1671–1676
22. Byrd CL, Wilkoff BL, Love CJ et al (2002) Clinical study of the laser sheath for lead extraction: the total experience in the United States. Pacing Clin Electrophysiol 25:804–808
23. Kennergren C (1997) Initial European experience with excimer laser assisted extraction of permanent pacemaker leads. Pacing Clin Electrophysiol 20:``4(Pt. II): 1111 [abstract]
24. Kennergren C, Bucknall CA, Butter C et al (2007) PLESSE investigators group. Laser assisted lead extraction: the European experience. Europace 9(8):651–656
25. Moon MR, Camillo CJ, Gleva MJ (2002) Laser-assist during extraction of chronically implanted pacemaker and defibrillator leads. Ann Thorac Surg 73:1893–1896
26. Roux JF, Pagé P, Dubuc M et al (2007) Laser lead extraction: predictors of success and complications. Pacing Clin Electrophysiol 30(2):214–220
27. Jones SO, Eckart RE, Albert CM, Epstein LM (2008) Large, single-centre, single-operator experience with transvenous lead extraction: outcomes and changing indications. Heart Rhythm 5(4):520–525
28. Kennergren C, Bjurman C, Wiklund R, Gabel J (2009) A single-centre experience of over one thousand lead extractions. Europace 11(5):612–617
29. Wazni O, Epstein LM, Carrillo RG et al (2010) Lead extraction in the contemporary setting: the LExICon study: an observational retrospective study of consecutive laser lead extractions. J Am Coll Cardiol 55(6):579–586
30. Wilkoff BL (2000) Transvenous leads extraction with electrosurgical dissection sheaths. Initial experience. Pacing Clin Electrophysiol 23:679–684
31. Neuzil P, Taborsky M, Rezek K et al (2007) Pacemaker and ICD lead extraction with electrosurgical dissection sheaths and standard transvenous extraction systems: results of a randomized trial. Europace 9(2):98–104
32. Schaerf R, Norlander B, Goode L (2008) Clinical experience with the Evolution mechanical dilator sheath set for intravascular lead extraction at a single center. Heart Rhythm 5:S338
33. Dello Russo A, Biddau R, Pelargonio G et al (2009) Lead extraction: a new effective tool to overcome fibrous binding sites. J Interve Cardiac Electrophysiol 24:147–150
34. Hauser RG, Katsiyiannis W, Gornik C (2010) Deaths and cardiovascular injuries due to device-assisted implantable cardioverter–defibrillator and pacemaker lead extraction. Europace 12:395–341
35. Hussein A, Wilkoff B, Martin D (2010) Initial experience with the Evolution mechanical dilator sheath for lead extraction: safety and efficacy. Heart Rhythm 7(7):874–875
36. Byrd CL, Schwartz SJ, Hedin NB (1992) Lead extraction: indications and techniques. Cardiol Clin 10: 735–748
37. Love CJ (2007) Lead extraction. Heart Rhythm 4(9):1238–1243
38. Jarwe M, Klug D, Beregi JP et al (1999) Single center experience with femoral extraction of permanent endocardial pacing. Pacing Clin Electrophysiol 1999;22:1202–1209
39. Le Franc P, Klug D, Jarwe M et al (1999) Extraction of endocardial implantable cardioverter-defibrillator leads. Am J Cardiol 84(2):187–191
40. Klug D, Jarwe M, Messaoudène SA et al (2002) Pacemaker lead extraction with the needle's eye snare for countertraction via a femoral approach. Pacing Clin Electrophysiol 25:1023–1028
41. Bordachar P, Defaye P, Peyrouse E et al (2010) Extraction of old pacemaker or cardioverter defibrillator leads by laser sheath versus femoral approach. Circ Arrhythm Electrophysiol 3(4):319–323
42. Kennergren C (2008) European perspective on lead extraction. Part II. Heart Rhythm 5(2):320–323
43. Mazzetti H, Cichero CF, Tentori MC, Mascheroni O (2008) Transjugular approach for lead extraction. Europace 10(2):156–160
44. Kleemann T, Becker T, Doenges K et al (2007) Annual rate of transvenous defibrillation lead defects in implantable cardioverter–defibrillators over a period of >10 years. Circulation 115(19):2474–2480
45. Epstein LM, Byrd CL, Wilkoff BL et al (1999) Initial experience with larger laser sheaths for the removal of transvenous pacemaker and implantable defibrillator leads. Circulation 100:516–525
46. Kantharia BK, Padder FA, Pennington JC 3rd et al (2000) Feasibility, safety, and determinants of extraction time of percutaneous extraction of endocardial implantable cardioverter defibrillator leads by intravascular countertraction method. Am J Cardiol 85:593–597
47. Saad EB, Saliba WI, Schweikert RA et al (2003) Nonthoracotomy implantable defibrillator lead extraction: results and comparison with extraction of pacemaker leads. Pacing Clin Electrophysiol 26:1944–1950.
48. McAlister FA, Ezekowitz J, Hooton N et al (2007) Cardiac resynchronization therapy for patients with left ventricular systolic dysfunction: a systematic review. JAMA 297(22):2502–2514
49. De Martino G, Orazi S, Bisignani G et al (2005) Safety and Feasibility of Coronary Sinus left ventricular pacing leads extraction: a preliminary report. J Interv Card Electrophysiol 13(1):35–38.
50. Kasravi B, Tobias S, Barnes M, Messenger J (2005) Coronary sinus leads extraction in the era of cardiac resynchronization therapy: single centre experience. Pacing Clin Electrophysiol 28(1):51–53
51. Bracke F (2008) Complications and lead extraction in cardiac pacing and defibrillation. Neth Heart J 16(Suppl 1):S28–S31
52. Tyers GF, Clark J, Wang Y et al (2003) Coronary sinus leads extraction. Pacing Clin Electrophysiol 26(1 Pt 2):524–526
53. Bongiorni MG, Zucchelli G, Soldati E et al (2007) Usefulness of mechanical transvenous dilatation and location of areas of adherence in patients undergoing coronary sinus lead extraction. Europace 9:69–73
54. Bongiorni MG, Di Cori A, Zucchelli G et al (2010) A modified transvenous single mechanical dilatation technique to remove a chronically implanted active-fixation coronary sinus pacing lead. PACE 2010 33:1376-1381
55. Makaryus AN, Boutis L, Goldner B, Park CH (2007) Coronary sinus angioplasty and stenting for biventricular pacemaker left ventricular lead implantation. J Invasive Cardiol 19(5):E128–E130

56. Kowalski O, Lenarczyk R, Prokopczuk J et al (2006) Effects of percutaneous intervention within the coronary sinus on the success rate of implantations of resynchronization pacemakers. Pacing Clin Electrophysiol 29(10):1075–1080
57. Cesario DA, Shenoda M, Brar R, Shivkumar K (2006) Left ventricular lead stabilization utilizing a coronary stent. Pacing Clin Electrophysiol 29(4):427–428
58. Bongiorni MG, Soldati E, Arena G et al (1999) Transvenous removal of permanent electrocatheters for heart stimulation and defibrillation. Cardiologia 44(Suppl 1 Pt 1):395–398
59. Robboy SJ, Harthorne JW, Leinbach RC et al (1969) Autopsy findings with permanent pervenous pacemakers. Circulation 39:495–501
60. Lin G, Nishimura RA, Connolly HM et al (2005) Severe symptomatic tricuspid valve regurgitation due to permanent pacemaker or implantable cardioverter-defibrillator leads. J Am Coll Cardiol 45(10):1672–1675
61. Gaynor SL, Zierer A, Lawton JS et al (2006) Laser assistance for extraction of chronically implanted endocardial leads: infectious versus noninfectious indications. Pacing Clin Electrophysiol 29(12):1352–1358
62. Agarwal SK, Kamireddy S, Nemec J et al (2009) Predictors of complications of endovascular chronic lead extractions from pacemakers and defibrillators: a single-operator experience. J Cardiovasc Electrophysiol 20(2):171–175
63. Franceschi F, Thuny F, Giorgi R (2009) Incidence, risk factors, and outcome of traumatic tricuapid regurgitation after percutaneous ventricular lead removal. J Am Coll Cardiol 53(23):2168–2174
64. Meier-Ewert HK, Gray ME, John RM (2003) Endocardial pacemaker or defibrillator leads with infected vegetations: a single-center experience and consequences of transvenous extraction. Am Heart J 146(2):339–344
65. Ruttmann E, Hangler HB, Kilo J et al (2006) Transvenous pacemaker lead removal is safe and effective even in large vegetations: an analysis of 53 cases of pacemaker lead endocarditis. Pacing Clin Electrophysiol 29(3):231–236
66. Wilkoff BL (2007) How to treat and identify device infections. Heart Rhythm 4(11):1467–1470
67. Hamid S, Arujuna A, Ginks M et al (2010) Pacemaker and defibrillator lead extraction: predictors of mortality during follow-up. Pacing Clin Electrophysiol 33(2):209–216

Utility of Imaging Techniques

7

Andrea Di Cori, Giulio Zucchelli and Francesco Bandera

7.1 Introduction

The clinical use of cardiac devices (CDs) has grown considerably over the past two decades, producing the subsequent increased need for lead removal [1, 2]. The major barrier to lead removal is fibrosis that progressively grows around the lead body and electrode tip, securing leads to the venous endothelium and myocardium. Freeing the lead from these binding sites safely is the goal behind the design of tools and techniques that have been developed for this purpose. In the past, open heart surgery became a useful but invasive option for lead extraction, allowing direct lead visualization and dissection. Standard surgical techniques through a midline sternotomy, lateral thoracotomy, or limited atriotomy were developed as solutions for lead removal. However, they remain an option of last resort given their invasiveness, longer patient recovery time, and a reported mortality rate of 0–12.5% [3, 4].

The need for safe extraction techniques, performed via the implant vein and compatible with the pectoral-pocket transvenous implant method, led to the development of transvenous percutaneous techniques [5, 6]. By using telescoping sheaths made of polymer and/or steel material that slide over the lead body, a countering force is applied to the intravascular fibrotic overgrowth that resists the traction force applied to the lead. This technique of intravascular counterpressure localizes shear stress on the fibrotic tissue and aids in blunt dissection or dilation of the tissue away from the lead circumference. In transvenous techniques, thoracic imaging plays an important role in pacing and defibrillating system removal. Many available contemporary modalities, including radiography, fluoroscopy, venography, echocardiography, scintigraphy, and computed tomography (CT), are frequently applied before, during, and after lead extraction. Historically, critical tools for device removal are X-ray, including radiography and fluoroscopy. More recently, echocardiography (transthoracic, transesophageal, intracardiac) has been developed for widespread applications, ranging from diagnostic purposes to intraprocedural monitoring. In addition to mastering clinical, pharmacologic, and technical knowledge, an interventional cardiologist must also have a good working knowledge of the physical, engineering, and radiobiologic principles underlying ultrasonographic and fluoroscopic–cineangiographic equipment.

In this chapter, we review imaging facilities used in modern-day lead extraction for pre-, intra-, and postprocedural assessment.

7.2. X-Ray and Cineangiographic Imaging

7.2.1 Basic X-Ray Physics

X-rays are a form of electromagnetic radiation, like their longer-wavelength cousins, radio waves and visible light. By virtue of its very short wavelength and related very high frequency, each X-ray photon contains thousands of times the energy of a photon of visible light. This explains why X-ray photons can pass through solid matter and why dif-

A. Di Cori (✉)
2nd Cardiovascular Department AOUP, Santa Chiara University Hospital, Pisa, Italy

M. G. Bongiorni (Ed.), *Transvenous Lead Extraction*.

ferent and more potent biologic effects occur when an X-ray photon is absorbed or scattered from living tissue. The goal of producing a usable X-ray image requires a number of tradeoffs. Ideal X-ray imaging parameters must appropriately balance the requirements for sharpness (needed to characterize it, including image noise) and patient dose. The dose must be chosen at the minimum level that will generate an image with an acceptable degree of noise to minimize patient exposure.

7.2.2 Chest X-ray

Radiographs provide essential information about location, type, and integrity of the pulse generator and leads of both pacing and defibrillating systems. They also provide basic details of patient anatomy. They represent an essential imaging tool before lead extraction and should be approached in a focused and systematic fashion, consisting of examination of bony structures, cardiac silhouette, lung fields, trachea, and aorta, as well as determining the presence and location of all preexisting intracardiac protheses. Posteroanterior (PA) and lateral chest radiographs (Fig. 7.1a, b) should be performed in every patient before the procedure. The aim is to evaluate:

1. Generator: type and location
2. Number of leads (including abandoned)
3. Lead location:
   - Vascular: intra- vs extravascular
   - Site [atrial, ventricular, coronary sinus (CS), left chamber]
4. Site(s) of lead venous access:
   - Lead entry site: right vs left
   - Venous entry site: cephalic, jugular, subclavian
5. Lead course (fracture, adhesions, calcifications)
6. Method used for lead retention (e.g., sleeve)
7. Lead features:
   - Type: pacing vs defibrillating
   - Polarity and coil: unipolar vs multipolar, single coil vs dual coil
   - Fixation: active vs passive

Preprocedural X ray evaluation is important to plan and guide the procedural approach. In our experience, extravascular leads are approached from the venous entry site and intravascular ones

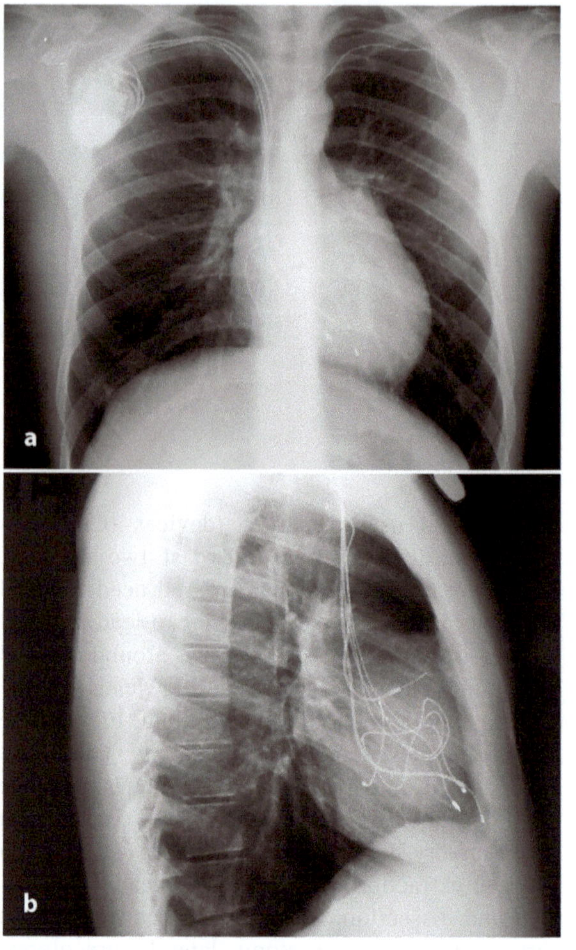

Fig. 7.1 Posteroanterior (**a**) and laterolateral (**b**) chest radiograph of a man referred for lead-related endocarditis. The patient has a dual chamber pacing system in the right pectoral region and three additional abandoned leads, for a total of two atrial and three ventricular leads

from the right femoral or right internal jugular vein [7]. Similarly, extraction starts from the younger lead and, preferably, from CS or atrial leads. Moreover, the presence of a screw-in lead should be determined because of the need of withdrawing the screw before starting dilatation.

7.2.3 Cinefluoroangiography

Fluoroscopy is the gold standard imaging modality by which to perform transvenous lead extraction, and an excellent cinefluorographic system is critical for safe lead removal. Lead extraction may be performed in an electrophysiology (EP) laboratory, catheterization laboratory, or operating room. Most operators perform the procedure in the pacemaker laboratory when cardiovascular surgical support is available if needed. Some surgeons prefer to do the procedure in an operating room to address potential complications immediately or to revert to a thoracotomy if attempts to remove the lead percutaneously are unsuccessful. In any case, adequate fluoroscopy must be available. EP and catheterization labs are therefore superior due to their high-quality fluoroscopy as opposed to portable C-arm units in operating rooms.

The main functions of an X-ray cinefluorographic system are to produce a collimated X-ray beam of appropriate intensity and quality, to project that beam through the patient at a desired angle, to detect the modulated X-ray beam after it passes through the patient, and to transduce the modulated X-ray beam into a usable, visible light image. Through a pair of foot pedals, the operator instructs the generator to initiate beam generation at either fluoroscopic or cinefluorographic levels. X-ray cinefluorographic units operate in two modes: fluoroscopy and acquisition (cine or image recording). The purposes and X-ray generator operating parameters of the two modes are different, particularly in terms of input X-ray dose delivered and image quality.

7.2.3.1 Fluoroscopy

Fluoroscopy provides a real-time X-ray image with adequate quality for guiding manipulations. The physiology of vision effectively integrates several frames; this reduces perceived image noise, so greater image noise can be tolerated, allowing fluoroscopic X-ray input dose rates that are significantly lower than those used for acquisition. Many systems offer variable fluoroscopic frame rates. Decreasing the frame rate saves dose at the expense of visual smoothness of transition between frames. Because of persistence of vision effects, lowering frame rates does not linearly lower required dose rates. Many operators find 15–25 frames per second (fps) to be satisfactory for digital cardiac fluoroscopy.

7.2.3.2 Acquisition (Cine)

The acquisition mode generates images of sufficient quality for single-frame viewing. Higher X-ray input dose rates are needed to reduce image noise and optimize clinical visualization, and most X-ray cinefluorographic units are calibrated such that the per-frame dose for acquisition is approximately 15 times greater than for fluoroscopy.

For the interventional staff, radiation exposure is a product of the procedure, and the occupational dose received during all such procedures should be minimized to the extent possible without compromising appropriate patient care, a precaution referred to as ALARA (as low as reasonably achievable). Relevant aspect to minimize radiation exposure is reducing the amount of fluoroscopy and cine time to the clinically required minimum. It is important to avoid the "lead-foot syndrome"; the operator must learn to press the fluoroscopy pedal briefly, when it is necessary to confirm the sheath position, and to reflexively take his or her foot off the pedal whenever looking away from the television monitor [8].

7.2.3.3 Cinefluoroangiography During Lead Extraction

Pulsed fluoroscopy may be considered the "gold standard" intraprocedural imaging modality during lead extraction. Cineangiography is rarely required for therapeutic purposes but may be a useful option to image acquisition and storage. Although C-arm, U-arm, and biplane varieties provide multiple views [postero-anterior (PA), right anterior oblique (RAO), left anterior oblique (LAO)], the procedure is usually performed using the standard PA projection. Because the principal impediment to lead extraction is intravascular fibrosis that causes the lead to adhere to the endocardium, the objective of imaging is to monitor the sheath while the lead is freed from fibrous bonds to minimize damage to the cardiovascular structures [5]. For this reason, fluoroscopy should ever be used during tool introduction (stylet, sheath, wire, lasso, catcher, snare), particularly during:

1. Stylet introduction: the stylet should be advanced carefully to reach the lead tip (Fig. 7.2a, b). If the stylet is pushed too hard, the lead (especially if damaged) can be easily perforated from the inside with the risk of vascular damage.
2. During unscrewing active lead tips and before starting lead traction or dilatation.
3. During sheath advancement: polypropylene sheaths are commonly visualized as slightly radiopaque devices around the lead (Fig. 7.2), whereas powered sheaths often show a radiologically distal marker. During sheath advancement (Fig. 7.2c–g), mechanisms of counterpressure, countertraction, and counterrotation are involved. Counterpressure is the pressure applied by a sheath that disrupts fibrous tissue-binding sites along the lead as it progresses toward the endocardial contact of the lead tip. The sheath is pushed along the lead and applies a shearing force tangentially; this force shears the fibrous tissue off the vessel wall and other leads. Contemporary, sufficient countertraction must be applied to the lead, usually with a stylet, so that the sheath can follow the lead around the bends in the vein. The objective is to almost exactly counterbalance the advancement force with retraction force on the lead body using the stylet. The lead is kept straight during sheath advancement, and too much traction on the locking stylet and suture is to be avoided. If too much tension is applied to a lead, it will easily damage the insulation and stretch the coils. If too much pressure is applied or if the lead has insufficient traction, the sheath may tear through the vascular wall, resulting in a life-threatening complication. Operator experience in knowing the correct amount of lead tension and counterpressure to apply is vital. Fluoroscopic visualization must be used during advancement of any type of sheath to ensure the sheath follows an intravascular course and that its angle is maintained parallel with the lead. Finally, a limited clockwise and counterclockwise rotation movement should be monitored to avoid lead and vessel torsion.
4. During tip debridement: once the sheath has been advanced to the lead tip, fluoroscopy should be used to avoid sheath advancement over the myocardial interface. According to our single-sheath technique, standard countertraction (i.e., opposing the traction placed on the lead by bracing the myocardium with the overlying sheath) is not utilized. Once the tip is reached, while exerting a mild traction and maintaining the stylet inserted till the tip, dilatation is performed by continuous clockwise and counterclockwise sheath rotation to

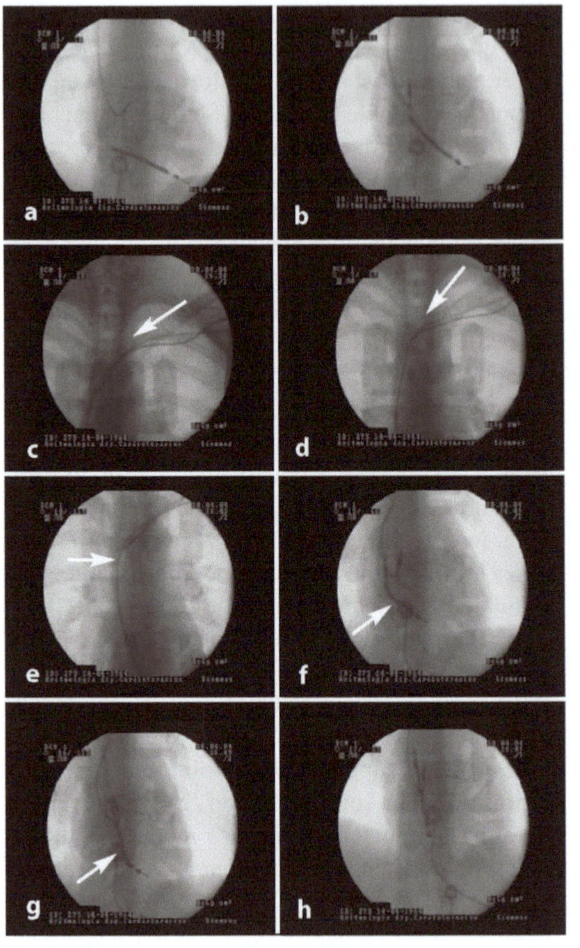

Fig. 7.2 Serial anteroposterior fluoroscopic images taken during transvenous removal of a left-sided dual-chamber implantable cardioverter-defibrillator (ICD) system. After placement of a temporary right-ventricular (RV) pacing system (**a**) and introduction of a standard stylet, manual traction of the RV defibrillating lead was attempted but was ineffective (**b**), with crossover to transvenous mechanical lead removal. The end of the polypropylene sheath (*arrow*) can be seen passing over the lead at the subclavian vein entry site (**c**) and then advancing through the innominate vein (**d**), superior vena cava (**e**), proximal defibrillating coil (**f**), and distal coil up to the tip (**g**). Further traction is effective in obtaining tip detachment from the ventricular endocardium (**h**) and subsequent removal

dissect the distal binding site and by fluoroscopically checking that the sheath does not overcome the lead tip. Rather than perpendicularly to the heart wall, this action focuses the force to the scar tissue immediately surrounding the lead tip. Therefore, the lead can be torn out of the scar tissue while minimizing the risk of myocardial invagination or a large tear [9].

5. After tip detachment: once the tip is freed (Fig. 7.2e), fluoroscopy is used to confirm that the lead is completely introduced inside the sheath and is then removed through the vein of insertion [10].

7.2.3.4 Complication Monitoring

In addition to monitoring vital signs (oxygen saturation and blood pressure), fluoroscopy is useful to monitor potential complications, such as:

- Hemothorax: usually observed after sheath advancement inside the venous district with vessel tear, hemothorax results from blood accumulating in the pleural cavity. Typical X-ray signs include blunting of the costophrenic angles and increased opacification of the hemithorax.
- Cardiac tamponade: usually observed after lead-tip detachment with subsequent myocardial tear. Fluid accumulates in the pericardium, elevates pressure on the heart, and prevents the heart's ventricles from filling properly. The diagnosis of cardiac tamponade is usually made clinically from a constellation of findings, including hypotension, pulsus paradoxus, and electrical alternans. On fluoroscopy, dimensions and configuration of the cardiac silhouette and sudden obliteration of the angle between the right cardiac border and the right hemidiaphragm should be followed closely to enable prompt recognition of cardiac tamponade. Development of a "double shadow" on the cardiac silhouette with visualization of an inner, contracting cardiac border surrounded by a noncontractile pericardial shadow suggests perforation or laceration with pericardial effusion. A normal cardiac picture may be seen in patients with rapid accumulation of fluid or blood [11, 12].

7.3 Ultrasonography

Permanent pacing is achieved by introducing leads through a number of veins (subclavian, cephalic, and internal or external jugular) into the right chambers. Therefore, ultrasonography examination in patients with pacing and implantable cardioverter-defibrillator (ICD) leads are mainly, but not exclusively, directed toward the upper veins and the right heart. Ultrasonographic techniques include three complementary modalities: transthoracic (TTE), transesophageal (TEE), and intracardiac (ICE) echocardiography. Any technique has both advantages and disadvantages in the assessment and may be used complementarily to investigate lead course before, during, and after lead extraction.

7.3.1 Systematic Echocardiographic Examination

The echocardiographic examination in cardiovascular implantable electronic devices (CIED) is based on examination of the right heart, great venous vessels, and venous lead entry site.

7.3.1.1 Transthoracic Echocardiography (TTE) Examination

The complex three-dimensional shape of the right heart and the position of the right ventricle (RV) beneath the sternum preclude complete right heart examination from any one transthoracic window, and examination from multiple windows is required. RV inflow view is obtained from anterior and medial angulation of the transducer from the standard parasternal long-axis view (Fig. 7.3a, b). Structures visible in this view are the free and diaphragmatic RV walls, the anterior and posterior tricuspid leaflets, and the right atrium (RA) with the orifice of the inferior vena cava (IVC). Associated structures are the CS orifice adjacent to the tricuspid annulus, eustachian valve at the IVC orifice, Chiari network (a vestige of the right valve of the sinus venosus), tricuspid annulus, and tricuspid chordae. Clockwise rotation of the probe

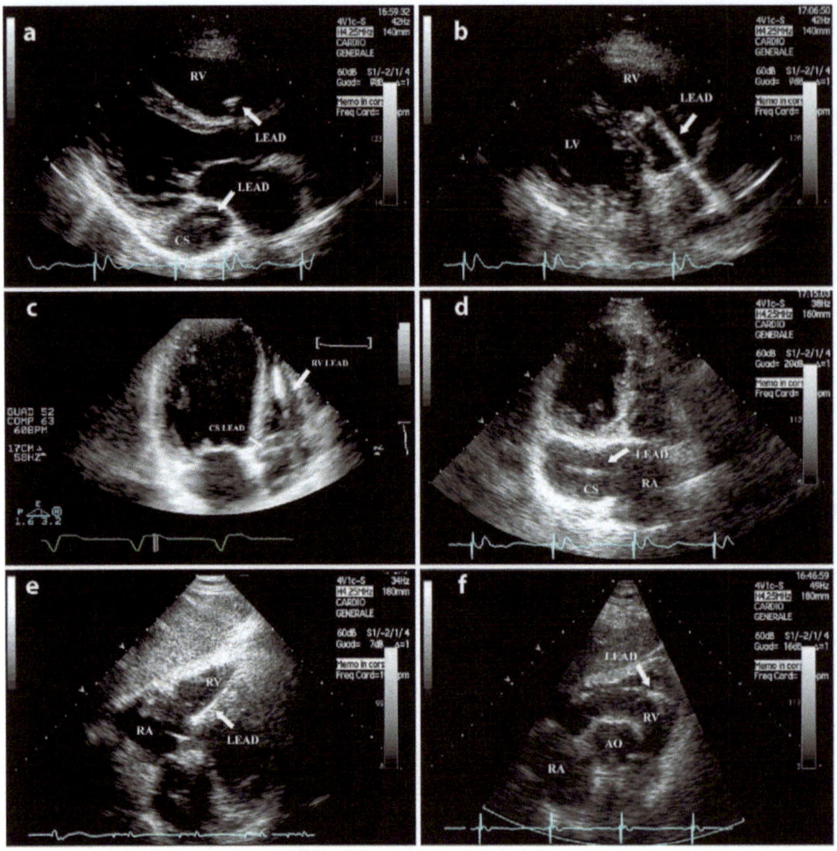

Fig. 7.3 Serial transthoracic echocardiographic (TTE) views in patients with pacemaker (PM) and implantable cardioverter-defibrillator (ICD) leads. Parasternal long-axis view showing an RV pacing lead in a patient implanted through a left persistent superior vena cava (SVC) (**a**). Modified parasternal long-axis projection highlights an RV pacing lead (**b**). Four-chamber long-axis view showing an RV ICD lead and pacing LV lead entering the CS (**c**). Four-chamber long-axis view showing an RV pacing lead introduced from a left persistent SVC through the CS into the right chambers (**d**). Subcostal long-axis (**e**) and short-axis (**f**) views of a patient with a single-chamber VVI PM. *AO*, aortic valve; *CS*, coronary sinus; *RA*, right atrium; *RV*, right ventricle; *LV*, left ventricle

to an orthogonal plane produces images in the parasternal short-axis view. At the base of the heart, the RA, interatrial septum, septal and anterior tricuspid leaflets, RV outflow tract (RVOT), pulmonary valve (PV), and main pulmonary artery (MPA) and its bifurcation can be seen. Geometry and motion of the RV, RA, and septum are well visualized from the apical four-chamber view (Fig. 7.3c). Doppler interrogation of tricuspid flow is often optimal in this view. The tricuspid annulus is well visualized and is located more apically than the mitral valve. In this view, the septal and posterior tricuspid valve leaflets are visualized, as is the moderator band, which can be seen traversing the RV near the apex. The CS can be seen to enter the RA by posterior angulation of the transducer (Fig. 7.3c, d). Inspection of the right heart may be improved by moving the transducer medially from the true apex. The subcostal window may be of particular value in patients with increased lung volume (Fig. 3e, f) [13].

7.3.1.2 Transesophageal Echocardiography (TEE) Examination

Examination of the right chambers begins with the midesophageal four-chamber view (Fig. 7.4a). Image depth is adjusted to include the tricuspid annulus and RV apex. The midesophageal RV inflow–outflow view (Fig. 7.4b) is developed by rotating the multiplanar angle forward to between 60° and 90°, keeping the tricuspid valve (TV) visible until the RVOT opens up and the PV and MPA come into view. This cross-section shows the RVOT to the right side of the display and the inferior (diaphragmatic) portion of the RV free wall to the left. Further multiplanar angle rotation to 120° displays the aortic valve long-axis projection, where the RV is seen to the right side of the display (Fig. 7.4c).

Examination of the RA is initiated from the midesophageal four-chamber view, with the image depth adjusted to maximize the size of the RA in

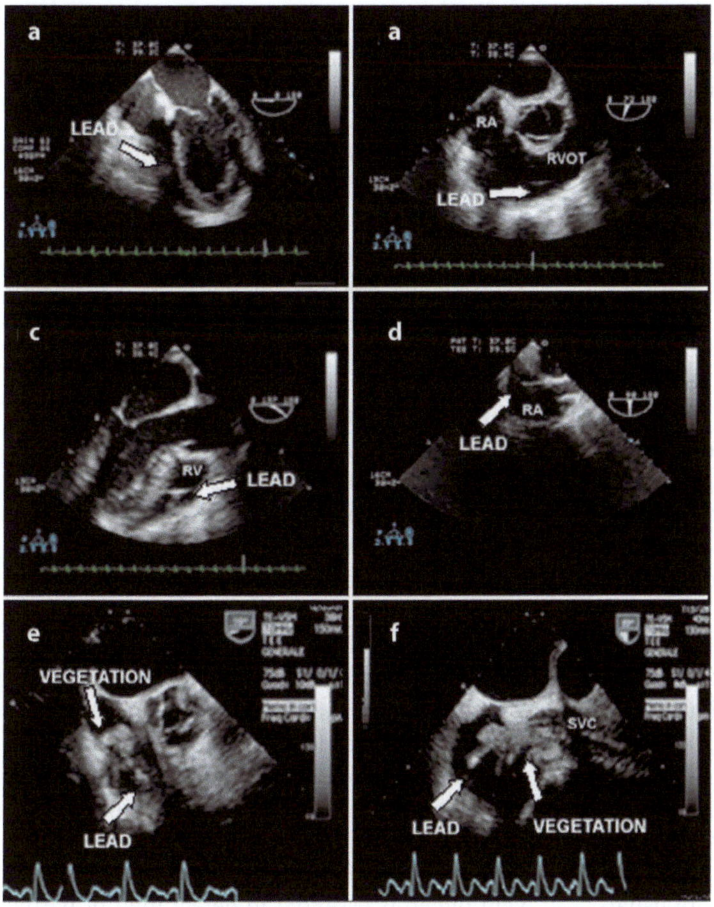

Fig. 7.4 Transthoracic echocardiographic (TEE) sessions showing several common views for pacing and implantable cardioverter-defibrillator (ICD) leads: midesophageal four-chamber view (**a**); midesophageal aortic valve short-axis view (**b**); midesophageal aortic valve long-axis view (**c**); midesophageal bicaval view (**d**). Large lead-related vegetation is seen using **b** and **d** projection (**e, f**). *RA*, right atrium; *RV*, right ventricle; *RVOT*, right ventricular outflow tract; *SVC*, superior vena cava

the display. The probe is then advanced and withdrawn to examine its entire inferior to superior extent. The midesophageal bicaval view (Fig. 7.4d) is next developed by rotating the multiplanar angle forward to between 80° and 110° until the SVC appears in the right side of the display and the IVC in the left. This view also provides good images of the right atrial appendage, seen to emanate from the superior anterior aspect of the RA. The Eustachian valve, a normal structure of variable size, is seen at the junction of the IVC and RA. It is formed by a fold of endocardium that arises from the lower end of the crista terminalis and stretches across the posterior margin of the IVC to become continuous with the border of the fossa ovalis. Occasionally, the Eustachian valve has mobile, serpiginous filaments attached to it, termed the Chiari network, which is considered to be a normal variant. If present, central venous catheters, pacemaker electrodes (Fig. 7.4d), or lead-related vegetation (Fig. 7.4e, f) entering the RA from the SVC (Fig. 7.4d–f) can be clearly seen [14].

7.3.1.3 Intracardiac Echocardiography (ICE) Examination

Intracardiac echocardiography is emerging as an ideal real-time modality to guide intracardiac interventional procedures. ICE allows accurate appreciation of cardiac anatomy and detailed visualization of specific anatomic structures, the most important factors in planning and guiding catheter-based interventional techniques [15–17]. In our daily practice, ICE is performed using a commercially available 9-F/9 MHz ultra-ICE catheter-based ultrasound transducer (EP Technologies, Boston Scientific, San Jose, CA, USA). The Ultra ICE catheter is introduced percutaneously into the right femoral vein through a 55° long, precurved, polyethylene venous sheath (Convoy, EP Technologies) and advanced under limited fluoroscopy. Examination starts with the ultra-ICE catheter positioned initially in the left or right subclavian vein, depending on the cardiac lead venous-entry site. Subsequently, the ultra-ICE catheter is withdrawn through the body of the RA to the IVC in order to obtain the so-called axial imaging planes. Several slice sections on the axial plane are achieved by applying an ideal perpendicular angle of incidence of the ultrasound beam to the vessels and RA wall in the center of their cavity. Full interrogation includes modified tomographic imaging planes at the vessel plane [subclavian vein, innominate vein, superior vena cava (SVC)], atrial, tricuspid, and ventricular plane (Fig. 7.5). By convention, this image is electronically rotated and presented in a consistent and familiar orientation identical to that of a magnetic resonance imaging (MRI) format, with left-sided structures on the operator's right, anterior-sided structures at the top of the image, and so forth [18]. In our experience, ICE is highly feasible, and image quality is adequate to assess all structures involved in transvenous lead extraction [19]. In particular, the following structures may be detected:

1. Cardiac leads: pacing and ICD leads are usually visualized as circular (lead transversal view) (Fig. 7.5a, c) or linear (lead longitudinal view) (Fig. 7.5e, i), echodense structures (depending on ICE position and lead direction), highlighted by an echocardiographic shadow. ICE can also easily distinguish between free-floating leads or leads adherent to the venous wall or to endocardium. Using a 55° sheath, atrial lead course may be followed clearly up to the RA appendage; conversely, it is often impossible to advance the probe into the RV apex and follow ventricular leads. For this purpose, a 120° precurved sheath is necessary.
2. Areas of fibrous adherence: areas of fibrous adherences (i.e., scar tissue) are visualized as echodense structures along the lead, often highlighted by a linear shadow. Scar tissue may be encountered along the leads in multiple locations. Usually, where the lead appears adherent to the venous wall or endocardium, a scar tissue is noted; in the presence of multiple leads, they are usually fibrosed together.
3. Vegetations: ICE is able to show infective vegetations as hyperechogenic structures. Vegetations can appear as variably shaped areas, differently adherent to catheter or cardiac structures even if located at atypical intravascular locations (i.e., subclavian vein, innominate vein, SVC) (Fig. 7.6).
4. Vein permeability: direct visualization of the vein lumen is essential to detect total or partial obstruction and to check permeability of other veins (in order to plan subsequent lead reimplantation).

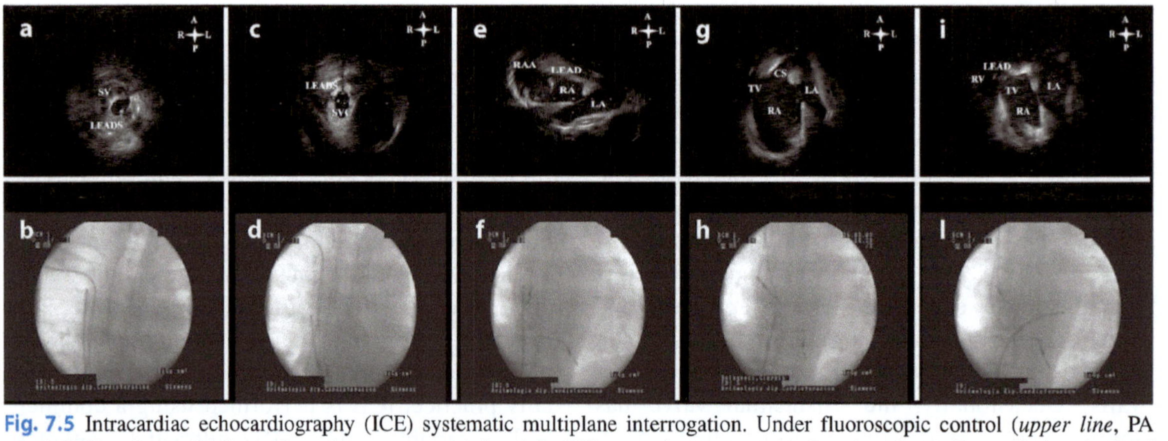

Fig. 7.5 Intracardiac echocardiography (ICE) systematic multiplane interrogation. Under fluoroscopic control (*upper line*, PA view), ICE probe is withdrawn from the venous entry site to the RV to acquire tomographic imaging planes (*lower line*) at the level of the SV (**a, b**), SVC (**c, d**), upper (**e, f**) and lower (**g, h**) RA, TV, and RV inflow tract (**i–l**). *CS*, coronary sinus; *LA*, left atrium; *RA*, right atrium; *RAA*, right atrium appendage; *TV*, tricuspid valve; *RV*, right ventricle; *SV*, subclavian vein; *SVC*, superior vena cava

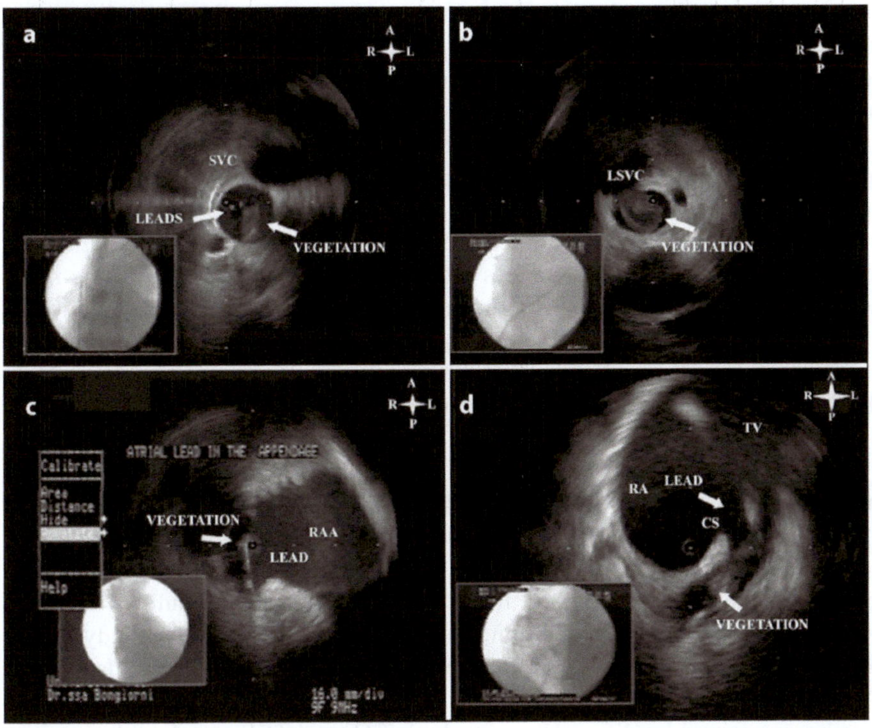

Fig. 7.6 Intracardiac echocardiography (ICE) imaging showing pacing-lead-related vegetation with atypical localization: at the SVC level (**a**); at the LSVC level in a patient with a lead implanted through a persistent left SVC (**b**); at the atrial lead-tip level inside the RAA (**c**); at the CS level around a pacing lead for cardiac resynchronization therapy (**d**). Note that the vegetation was difficulty diagnosed by other echocardiographic approaches (i.e., trans-thoracic and transesophageal examination). *SVC*, superior vena cava; *LSVC*, left superior vena cava; *RAA*, right atrial appendage; *RA*, right atrium; *CS*, coronary sinus

7.3.2 Echocardiography and Timing Assessment

Echocardiography plays a number of roles in evaluating candidates for lead extraction. First, echocardiography permits direct assessment of lead-related vegetations, the hallmark of infective endocarditis (IE), and provides prognostic information concerning risk of embolization related to vegetation size, with implications for cardiac surgery. Second, it may be useful as additional intraprocedural imaging for complication monitoring complementary to fluoroscopy. Finally, it may allow identification of intracardiac remnant vegetations, offering additional data for planning the reimplantation procedure.

7.3.2.1 Preprocedural Assessment: IE Diagnosis and Sizing

Infection of intracardiac devices is a severe condition associated with high mortality rates, and CIED-associated infections are the strongest indications for complete system removal. Theoretically, local device infection (LDI) (i.e., infection limited to the pocket) should be distinguished from a cardiac-device-related IE (CDRIE), defined as an infection extending to the electrode leads, cardiac valve leaflets, or endocardial surface. However, patients can present with a broad range of clinical scenarios, and differentiating LDI and CDRIE is frequently difficult. However, when infection is identified, this indicates that the removal of all components of the CIED system (including the device, lead, adapters, caps, sutures, and as much of the infected tissue as possible) is required to obtain consistent cure [20]. CDRIE is probably one of the most difficult forms of IE to diagnose. Clinical presentation is frequent misleading, with fever frequently blunted and predominant pulmonary or rheumatologic manifestations. It must be suspected in the presence of prolonged or unexplained fever in a patient with a CIED. The Duke criteria and their modifications (i.e., including local signs of infection and pulmonary embolism as major criteria) have been used to diagnose IE in suspected pacemaker/ICD endocarditis [21].

In another form of IE, blood culture and echocardiography are the cornerstone of diagnosis.

However, blood cultures are more frequently negative than in native IE. Blood cultures can be positive with and without lead or valve vegetations or can be negative despite intracardiac vegetations. A single positive blood culture, without other clinical evidence of infection, should not result in CIED system removal. However, when positive cultures are obtained on different days (persistent bacteremia) – even when there is no clear source of the positive culture in the heart, on the leads, or from another part of the body despite a complete echocardiographic evaluation (suspected occult infection) – transvenous lead extraction should be strongly considered. Thus, echocardiography plays a key role in CDRIE and is helpful both for diagnosing lead vegetation and tricuspid involvement, vegetation sizing, and follow-up after lead extraction. Whenever a pacemaker lead infection is suspected, TEE is indicated because of the poor sensitivity of TTE and because this examination makes a major contribution to lesion diagnosis and precise characterization [21]. Comparative performances of TTE and TEE have been assessed by different groups [22, 23]. Vilacosta et al. [24] were the first to confirm the superiority of TEE in a single-plane technology in ten patients with suspected lead infection. More recently, the generalization of multiplane technology has significantly improved exploration quality [25]. In addition, few other imaging techniques are available. MRI is contraindicated in pacemaker carriers. CT has not been evaluated. Positive diagnosis with indium-labelled leucocyte scanning is anecdotal and not routinely performed.

Any patient suspected of having CDRIE by clinical criteria should be screened by TTE. When images are of good quality and prove to be negative, and there is only a low clinical suspicion of IE, endocarditis is unlikely, and other diagnoses have to be considered. If suspicion of IE is high, TEE should be performed in all TTE-negative cases and if TTE is positive but complications are suspected. Although TEE has superior sensitivity and specificity than TTE and is cost effective, both TTE and TEE must be systematically performed in suspected CDRIE [21]. If TEE remains negative and there is still suspicion, it should be repeated within 1 week. A repeatedly negative study should virtually exclude the diagnosis. These class I recommendations are based on level B evidence. However, both TTE and TEE may be falsely negative (i.e., occult infection). In our experience, ICE examination may be useful for accurate intraluminal scanning of the right cardiac chambers and great venous vessels, increasing echocardiographic sensibility and specificity (Fig. 7.7).

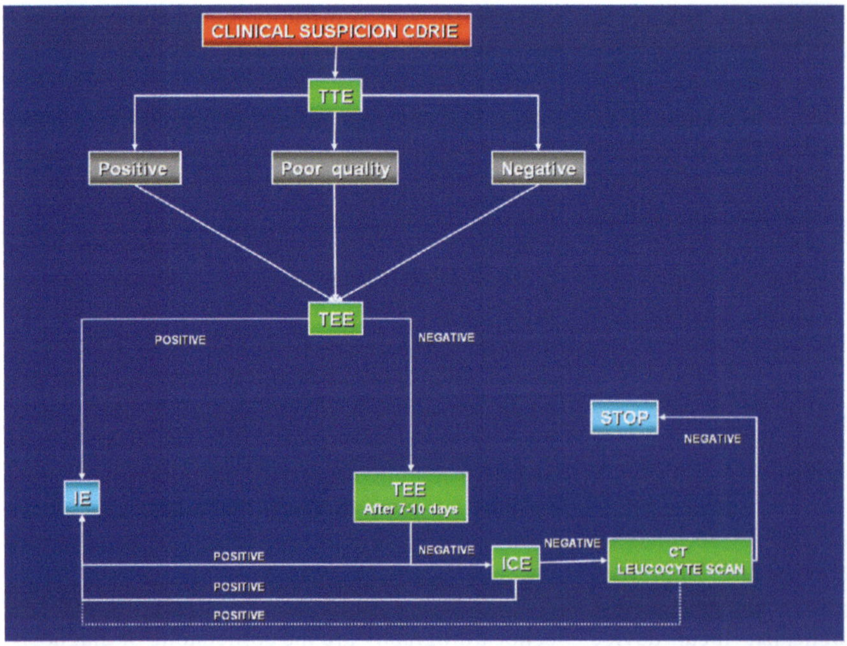

Fig. 7.7 Diagnostic strategy in suspected cardiac-device-related infective endocarditis (CDRIE). *CT*, computed tomography; *ICE*, intracardiac echocardiography; *IE*, infective endocarditis; *TEE*, transoesophageal echocardiography, *TTE*, transthoracic echocardiography

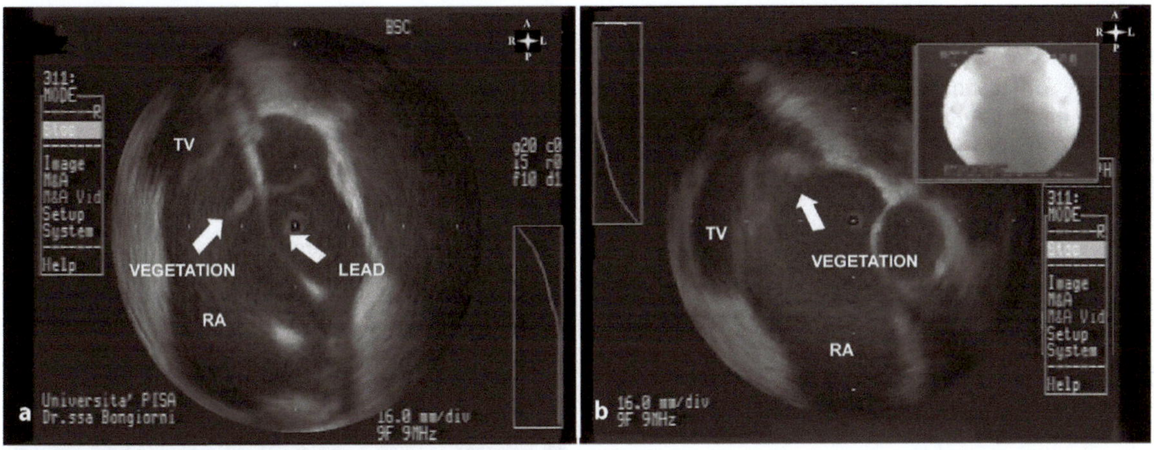

Fig. 7.8 Intracardiac echocardiography (ICE) showing pacing-lead-related vegetation (a). After lead removal, postprocedural full ICE interrogation shows remnant vegetation attached to the tricuspid valve. (b) *RA*, right atrium, *RV*, right ventricle

Regardless of the technique used, echocardiographic findings considered to be major criteria in the diagnosis of CDRIE is documentation of a mobile, echodense mass attached to the valvular or to the mural endocardium/vessel wall or to implanted leads [21] (Figs. 7.6 and 7.8). As a rule, if voluminous vegetation images do not constitute a diagnostic difficulty, such is not the case with other aspects, where discriminating between infectious lesions, thrombosis, or fibrin deposits is not easy. Dumont et al. [26] reported on three patients who exhibited isolated atypical echographic images in the form of microfilaments. Systematically performing TEE in a group of chronically implanted patients without any sign of infection elicited images of that type in high proportions of up to 29% in Victor et al.'s series [23]. In literature, Klug et al. did not describe any microfilament structure but reported a sheath-like aspect surrounding the leads, most often in combination with one or several vegetations. In their classification, the atypical aspect was considered as a minor clinical criterion [27]. Whereas strands are commonly observed by TEE on prosthetic heart valves, especially mitral valves, their significance remains unknown in patients with endovascular leads [28]. In addition, these strands are not always detected during successive examinations of the same patient, which makes their evaluation all the more difficult [29]. Lastly, although they are associated with a risk of peripheral embolism, their exact nature (fibrin, thrombus, pannus, etc.) is still unknown and the exact significance is still a matter of debate. Whether pacemaker-lead-associated strands promote infection remains hypothetical.

Additionally, the maximum vegetation size is important prior to intervention, as many vegetations may embolize and break up into the pulmonary circulation during transvenous lead removal. With regard to vegetation size, the optimal approach is still a matter of discussion. In a consecutive series of 52 patients, Klug et al. reported the results of pacemaker lead removal. The choice of technique was based on vegetation size and presence of alteration of the tricuspid valve [27]. In their study, vegetations >1 cm, verified by TEE, were surgically removed using extracorporeal circulation. Surgical extraction may be preferred for patients with larger vegetations; however, mortality rates up to 12.5% have been reported after surgical lead extraction [3]. A limited number of reports describe successful transvenous lead extraction with larger vegetations. If septic embolism occurred or infection was complicated by large vegetations, the ideal therapeutic strategy (either transvenous or using extracorporeal circulation) is not clear but probably depends on vegetation size [20]. Therefore, vegetations with a high probability of obstructing a main stem of the pulmonary artery – which means that a vegetation >2-cm diameter might be of borderline size – ought to be removed by open heart surgery. However, we had several patients with vegetations >2 cm who underwent successful transvenous lead removal, especially patients with high perioperative risk and prior complex cardiac operations, without major adverse events such as severe pulmonary embolism. Vegetation size, shape, and friability; presence or absence of a patent foramen ovale, atrial septal defect (ASD), or ventricular septal defect (VSD); and other surgical indications and goals all need to be considered when making this decision. The largest vegetation size that can be safely removed nonsurgically remains to be defined [29].

7.3.2.2 Intraprocedural Assessment: Complication Monitoring

During lead removal, echocardiography may be used as a complementary imaging tool in addition to fluoroscopy. TTE imaging (acquired from a chest or subcostal window) is discouraged because it may increase the risk of infection, is logistically difficult during fluoroscopy, and inadequately displays far-field structures. Multiplanar TEE imaging overcomes some of these drawbacks. The probe is placed to show the midesophageal four-chamber view, and the image depth is adjusted to include the tricuspid annulus and RV apex. The purpose is to monitor wall invagination during traction/dilatation and pericardial effusion after tip detachment. However, the procedure has poor patient acceptance and requires general anesthesia with endotracheal intubation [30].

In our daily practice, performing lead removal under local anesthesia and mild sedation, we prefer ICE monitoring. This approach has both advantages and disadvantages. The probe may be positioned below the dilatation site to monitor sheath advancement and scar dissection, avoid vessel torsion (sheath rotation control at vessel planes) (Fig. 7.9), and may then be withdrawn at the TV plane, to control myocardial wall invagination and pericardial effusion (Fig. 7.10). Pericardial effusion is a common serious complications associated with transvenous lead extraction. It may occur immediately following lead removal due to perforation of RV free wall. ICE monitoring may provide early detection and accurate diagnosis of pericardial effusion prior to arterial blood pressure and hemodynamic changes. Where the fluid collects probably depends on how the pericardium can expand and where the perforation/damage is located. A pericardial effusion that increases to a moderately large amount can be detected anterolateral to the RV. In patients with large effusion, fluid totally surrounds the heart and the heart seems to settle or drop posteriorly within the fluid, and accumulation of pericardial fluid becomes primarily anterior (Fig. 7.10). In patients with cardiac tamponade, the most popular and reliable echocardiographic sign is collapse of the cardiac chambers in diastole, especially with diastolic invagination of the RV and/or right atrial wall during diastole. The dynamic wall motion of the RA and its appendage and the RV can be evaluated with ICE imaging, and its invagination during diastole may be easily detected when cardiac tamponade occurs. The main limitation is that ICE removal is required when a crossover from venous entry site approach to a femoral/transjugular approach is necessary [19].

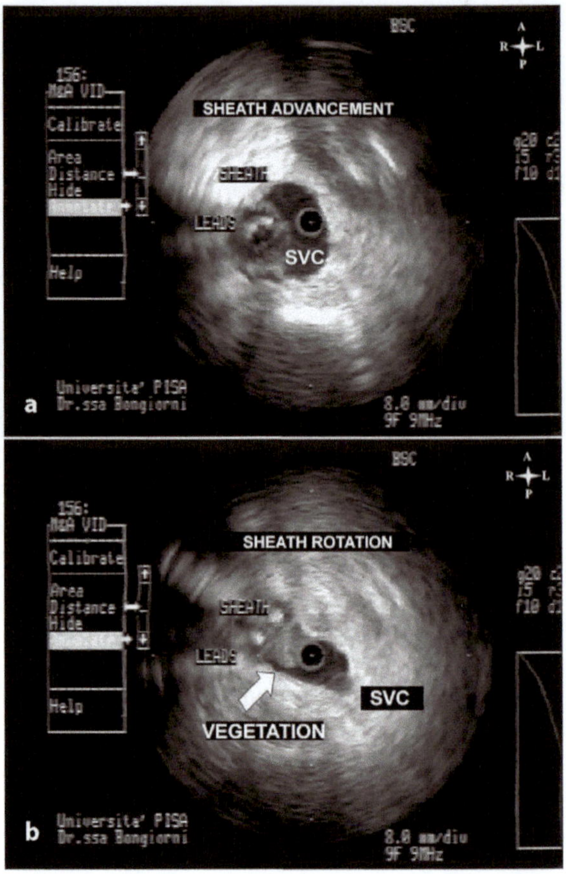

Fig. 7.9 Intracardiac echocardiography (ICE) showing sheath rotation and counterrotation on the lead at the SVC plane (**a**). Note vessel torsion during sheath rotation (**b**). *SVC*, superior vena cava

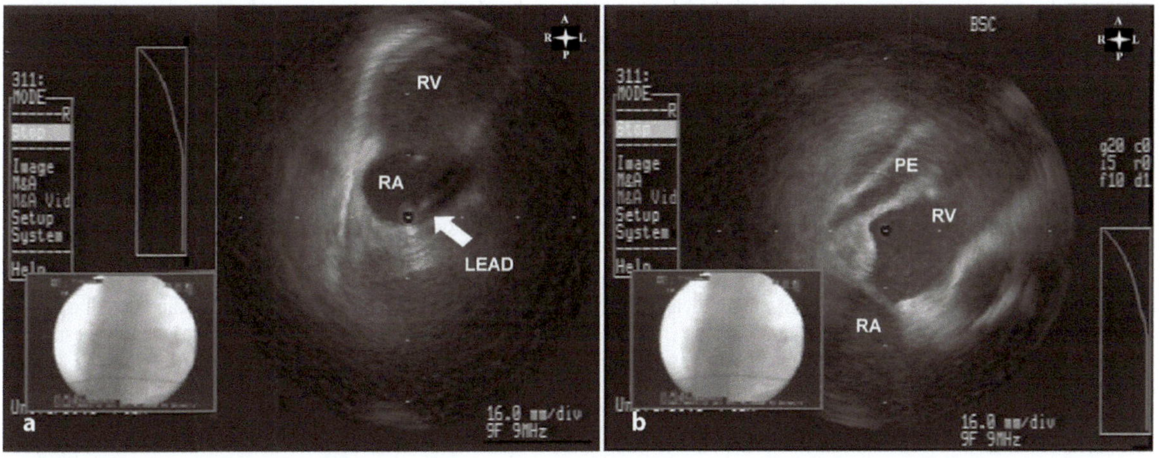

Fig. 7.10 Intracardiac echocardiography (ICE) view at the tricuspid valve level before (**a**) and after (**b**) ventricular lead removal. ICE was useful in the early assessment of pericardial effusion and the following cardiac tamponade. *PE*, pericardial effusion; *RA*, right atrium, *RV*, right ventricle

7.3.2.3 Postprocedural Assessment: Reimplantation Timing

Timing of reimplantation is subject to debate. Whereas some authors recommend delaying reimplantation for as long as 6 weeks in cases of CDRIE [31], others recommend that a new device be inserted when patients are no longer bacteremic [32]. Based on retrospective analysis and review of published literature, the Mayo Clinic proposed guidelines for cardioverter–defibrillator infections to assist clinicians in patient management [33]. In our practice, we decide to reimplant on the basis of clinical and echocardiographic findings (see Chapter 9). In presence of remnant vegetations ≤2 cm (Fig. 7.8), device reimplantation is performed after 48 h without fever. If vegetation ≥2 cm persists and the patient is not PM dependent, we wait for some days before reimplanting.

7.4 Other Imaging Techniques

Application of modified Duke's criteria determines a variable percentage (about 15–20%) of patients with possible diagnosis, despite correct diagnostic process, strictly not indicated to aggressive therapy. In the context of lead extraction, an inconclusive classification of suspected CDRIE based only in blood culture and echocardiography can lead to dangerous delay in correct treatment. Although the role of additional techniques, such as CT and radiolabeled leucocyte scans, is not well defined, in selected cases, they may be useful. The main application field is identification of CDRIE patients with a suspected infective process but without a definite diagnosis (Fig. 7.7) Although there are no guidelines or standardized consensus about the use of such techniques, CT and radiolabeled leucocyte scans may be useful in identifying cardiac and extracardiac infective foci in suspected occult infections. By collecting about 40 ml of blood, the process leads to the labelling of concentrated granulocytes with ^{99}Tc-hexamethylpropyleneamine oxime (^{99}Tc-HMPAO) or ^{111}in-oxine, which are therefore reinjected in a peripheral vein. Early and late planar and tomographic scans, fused with CT images, may allow identification of infective sites, determination of the extent of infection along the device, implantation site, heart structures, and potential sites of distal embolization. It must be noted that the use of this technique is, at the moment, not proposed for routine use.

References

1. Mond HG, Irwin M, Ector H, Proclemer A (2008) The world survey of cardiac pacing and cardioverter-defibrillators: calendar year 2005 an International Cardiac Pacing and Electrophysiology Society (ICPES) project. Pacing Clin Electrophysiol 31(9):1202–1212

2. Epstein AE, Dimarco JP, Ellenbogen KA et al (2008) ACC/AHA/HRS 2008 Guidelines for device-based therapy of cardiac rhythm abnormalities. J Am Coll Cardiol 51:1–62
3. del Rio A, Anguera I, Miro JM et al (2003) Surgical treatment of pacemaker and defibrillator lead endocarditis: the impact of electrode lead extraction on outcome. Chest 124:1451–1459
4. Frame R, Brodman RF, Furman S et al (1993) Surgical removal of infected transvenous pacemaker leads. Pacing Clin Electrophysiol 16:2343–2348
5. Verma A, Wilkoff BL (2004) Intravascular pacemaker and defibrillator lead extraction: a state-of-the-art review. Heart Rhythm 1(6):739–745
6. Smith MC, Love CJ (2008) Extraction of transvenous pacing and ICD leads. Pacing Clin Electrophysiol 31(6):736–752
7. Bongiorni MG, Giannola G, Arena G et al (2005) Pacing and implantable cardioverter-defibrillator transvenous lead extraction. Ital Heart J 6(3):261–266
8. Balter S (1999) Radiation safety in the cardiac catheterization laboratory: basic principles. Catheter Cardiovasc Interv 47(2):229–236
9. Bongiorni MG, Soldati E, Zucchelli G et al (2008) Transvenous removal of pacing and implantable cardiac defibrillating leads using single sheath mechanical dilatation and multiple venous approaches: high success rate and safety in more than 2000 leads. Eur Heart J 29(23):2886–2893
10. Byrd CL (2007) Managing device related complications and transvenous lead extraction. In: Ellenbogen KA, Kay GN, Lau CP, Wilkoff BL (Eds.) Clinical cardiac pacing, defibrillation and resynchronization therapy, 3rd edn. Saunders Elsevier, Philadelphia pp 883–902
11. Kennergren C (2008) A European perspective on lead extraction: part I. Heart Rhythm. 5(1):160–162
12. Kennergren C (2008) European perspective on lead extraction: part II. Heart Rhythm. 5(2):320–323
13. Wong PS, Otto CM (2002) Echocardiographic views of the right heart. In: Otto CM, ed. Practice of clinical echocardiography. W.B. Saunders, London, pp 742–751
14. Shanewise JS, Cheung AT, Aronson S et al (1999) ASE/SCA guidelines for performing a comprehensive intraoperative multiplane transesophageal echocardiography examination: recommendations of the American Society of Echocardiography Council for Intraoperative Echocardiography and the Society of Cardiovascular Anesthesiologists Task Force for Certification in Perioperative Transesophageal Echocardiography. J Am Soc Echocardiogr 12(10):884–900
15. Schwartz SL, Gillam LD,Weintraub AR et al (1993) Intracardiac echocardiography in humans using a smallsized (6F), low frequency (12.5 MHz) ultrasound catheter. J Am Coll Cardiol 21:189–198
16. Bruce CJ, Packer DL, Belohlavek M et al (2000) Intracardiac echocardiography: newest technology. J Am Soc Echocardiogr 13:788–795
17. Nanda NC, Miller AP (2005) Principles of intracardiac echocardiography. J Interv Card Electrophysiol 13(Suppl 1):S7–S10
18. Zanchetta M, Rigatelli G, Pedon L et al (2002) Intracardiac echocardiography during catheter-based procedures: ultrasound system, examination technique, and image presentation. Echocardiography 19:501–507
19. Bongiorni MG, Di Cori A, Soldati E et al (2008) Intracardiac echocardiography in patients with pacing and defibrillating leads: a feasibility study. Echocardiography 25(6):632–638
20. Wilkoff BL, Love CJ, Byrd CL et al (2009) Transvenous lead extraction: Heart Rhythm Society expert consensus on facilities, training, indications, and patient management. Heart Rhythm 7:1085–1104
21. Horstkotte D, Follath F, Gutschik E et al (2004) Task Force Members on Infective Endocarditis of the European Society of Cardiology; ESC Committee for Practice Guidelines (CPG); Document Reviewers. Guidelines on prevention, diagnosis and treatment of infective endocarditis executive summary; the task force on infective endocarditis of the European society of cardiology. Eur Heart J 25(3):267–276
22. Choo MH, Holmes DR Jr, Gursh BJ et al (1981) Permanent pace maker infections: characterizations and management. Am J Cardiol 48:559–564
23. Victor F, De Place C, Camus C et al (1999) Pacemaker lead infection: echocardiographic features, mannagement and outcome. Heart 81:82–87
24. Vilacosta I, Sarria C, San Roman JA et al (1994) Usefulness of transesophageal echocardiography for diagnosis of infected transvenous permanent pacemakers. Circulation 89:2684–2687
25. Tighe DA, Tejada LA, Kirchoffer JB et al (1996) Pacemaker infection: detection by multiplane transesophageal echocardiography. Am Heart 131:616–618
26. Dumont E, Camus C, Victor F et al (2003) Suspected pacemaker or defibrillator transvenous lead infection. Prospective assessment of a TEE-guided therapeutic strategy. Eur Heart J 24(19):1779–1787
27. Klug D, Lacroix D, Savoye C et al (1997) Systemic infection related to endocarditis on pacemaker leads. Clinical presentation and management. Circulation 95:2098–2107
28. Orsinelli DA, Pearson AC (1995) Detection of prosthetic valve strands by transesophageal echocardiography: clinical significance in patients with suspected cardiac source of embolism. J Am Coll Cardiol 26:1713–1718
29. Ruttmann E, Hangler HB, Kilo J et al (2006) Transvenous pacemaker lead removal is safe and effective even in large vegetations: an analysis of 53 cases of pacemaker lead endocarditis. Pacing Clin Electrophysiol 29(3):231–236
30. Endo Y, O'Mara JE, Weiner S et al (2008) Clinical utility of intraprocedural transesophageal echocardiography during transvenous lead extraction. J Am Soc Echocardiogr 21(7):861–867
31. Darouiche RO (2004) Treatment of infections associated with surgical implants. N Engl J Med 350(14):1422–1429
32. Baddour LM, Bettmann MA, Bolger AF et al (2003) Nonvalvular cardiovascular device-related infections. Circulation 108(16):2015–2031
33. Sohail MR, Uslan DZ, Khan AH et al (2007) Management and outcome of permanent pacemaker and implantable cardioverter-defibrillator infections. J Am Coll Cardiol 49(18):1851–1859

Prevention and Treatment of Lead Extraction Complications

8

Pier Giorgio Golzio, Melissa Vinci, Elisa Pelissero and Maria Grazia Bongiorni

8.1 Definition and Classification of Complications

Lead extraction, performed with the previously described tools and techniques, is not yet free from severe risks of injuries and death. Possible complications of this procedure can be defined by the time of their onset from the moment of intervention and by their grade of severity [1, 2]. Essentially, complications can be described as:

1. Intraprocedural: any event related to the performance of a procedure that occurs or becomes evident from the time the patient enters the operating room until the time the patient leaves the operating room. This includes complications related to patient preparation, anesthesia delivery, opening and closing, and throughout the intervening time period.
2. Post procedural: any event related to the procedure that occurs or becomes evident within the 30-day period following the procedure.

Events are classified as major or minor according to severity:

1. Major complications: those that create a life-threatening situation or require a major intervention for their resolution.
2. Minor complications: not life-threatening, but require an intervention, such as medication, for their resolution.

Examples of classifications that use these definitions are shown in Table 8.1.

8.2 Incidence and Predicting Factors

Since the first publications on this subject, many studies evaluating the complication rate related to lead extraction procedures have been performed, but at this point, the complication rate has not changed significantly, being reported at nearly 2% [3]. Among the various published studies, procedural death related to device extraction has been remarkably consistent, ranging from 0.4% to 0.8% [4, 5].

The exponential growth device implantation for cardiac stimulation has brought about a parallel increase in lead extractions due to the previously described causes. Although the success rate of this procedure has increased over recent years – thanks to the introduction of new tools such as powered sheaths and a series of new techniques and approaches proposed by different operators – the numbers of adverse events have not been significantly reduced. This situation can be explained through evaluation of operator experience, as development of their ability requires quite a long training period, and a major number of complications occur in the period following the adoption of a new technique. This is particularly true when considering the first use of powered sheaths, as described by several studies [4–7]. A recent US study reported a complication rate of 4.2% over the entire 6-year experience of a single operator. This rate decreased to 1.5% when the first 3 years of the operator's experience were excluded [8].

There are many variations on how extraction can be performed utilizing established techniques. Consequently, lead extraction should not be performed without an experienced operator, a full set of tools, and plans in place to deal with complica-

P.G. Golzio (✉)
Cardiology Division, Department of Internal Medicine AOU Molinette San Giovanni Battista Hospital, Turin, Italy

M. G. Bongiorni (Ed.), *Transvenous Lead Extraction*.

Table 8.1 Classification of complications of LEAD Extraction [2]

Classification	Examples	Classification	Examples
Major complications	1. Death 2. Cardiac avulsion or tear requiring thoracotomy, pericardiocentesis, chest tube, or surgical repair 3. Vascular avulsion or tear (requiring thoracotomy, pericardiocentesis, chest tube, or surgical repair) 4. Pulmonary embolism requiring surgical intervention 5. Respiratory arrest or anesthesia related complication leading to prolongation of hospitalization 6. Stroke 7. Pacing system related infection of a previously noninfected site	Minor complications	1. Pericardial effusion not requiring pericardiocentesis or surgical intervention 2. Hemothorax not requiring a chest tube 3. Hematoma at the surgical site requiring reoperation for drainage 4. Arm swelling or thrombosis of implant veins resulting in medical intervention 5. Vascular repair near the implant site or venous entry site 6. Hemodynamically significant air embolism 7. Migrated lead fragment without sequelae 8. Blood transfusion related to blood loss during surgery 9. Pneumothorax requiring a chest tube 10. Pulmonary embolism not requiring surgical intervention

tions. Effective and safe lead removal is influenced by several factors, including implant duration. Leads in place longer are more difficult to remove. Indeed, there is a linear relationship between the increase in difficulty and the risks of intracardiac and vascular injuries over time. Moreover, multiple leads will become bound together by fibrous tissue, making removal even more difficult. A 3.5-fold increase in the risk of complication has been reported with every incremental right ventricular (RV) lead explanted. First, the higher number of the leads explanted, the higher the cumulative risk [9]. It is also plausible that the higher number of explanted leads also results in a longer dwell time and thus fibrosis of the oldest lead. Ventricular leads are more difficult to extract than are atrial leads due to their longer length. Tined and other nonisodiametric leads are also more difficult to extract, although this is not supported by data [9].

Independent predictors of major complications also include an elevated white blood count at the time of the procedure. This is usually associated with the presence of infection but may also indicate the presence of systemic inflammation. Some studies have associated the presence of infection with a greater ease of extracting chronic leads [10] without the need for powered sheaths. The presumed mechanism of this association is that the presence of infection interferes with collagen deposition and fibrosis, thereby leading to looser adhesion between the lead and the vasculature or the heart, thus resulting in greater ease of extraction. However, when examined in a multivariate model [11], the presence of infection was not an independent predictor of ease of extraction, and higher white cell count predicted a higher risk of major complications. This may reflect a heightened state of systemic inflammation rather than infection, which may also portend a worse prognosis. This assumption deserves further testing in future studies.

Worldwide experiences are reported in the literature, and the centers with the highest number of patients undergoing lead extraction provide the means for a direct and complete analysis of this issue. The Pacing Lead Extraction with the Excimer Sheath (PLEXES) trial first showed that the addition of a laser sheath significantly improves the efficiency of transvenous lead extraction with respect to telescoping stainless steel and polymer sheaths, but at the same time, the complication rate increases. Although there were no complications directly related to the application of laser energy, there were significant complications in five patients randomized to laser use and in two patients randomized to nonlaser (p = NS) [4]. In 2002, Byrd et al. reported data relative to all extractions powered with the Excimer laser from 1995 to 1999 in the United States. In total, 2,561 pacing and defibrillator leads were treated in 1,684 patients at 89 sites, with three sizes of laser sheath. Major complications were observed in 1.9% of patients, minor in 1.4%, and in-hospital death in 0.8% of cases. Multivariate analysis showed that implant duration was the only preoperative independent predictor of failure; female gender was the only multivariate predictor of complications. Success and complications were not dependent on laser sheath size. At follow-up, various extraction-related complications were observed in 2% of patients. The learning curve showed a trend toward fewer complications with greater experience [5]. European centers reported a success rate from 93% to 98%, with a complication rate ranging from 1% to 2.5%. In the Pacing Lead Surveillance Study in Europe (PLESSE), early models of transvenous implantable cardioverter–defibrillator (ICD) leads carried a 12% risk of major complication, which was more than ten times the 1% risk of major complication associated with pacing lead extraction. It is important to note that the highest risk is associated with early dual-coil ICD leads because of the risk for laceration of the superior vena cava (SVC), with subsequent mediastinal bleeding and death. In that study, patient risk for a serious complication associated with pacing lead extraction, which involved a learning curve at 14 specialized centers, was 1.7% [7]. Considering Italian centers, the most important study in terms of number of treated patients is represented by that of the Arrhythmology Unit, Cardiac and Thoracic Department, Pisa, where between January 1997 and June 2007, 1,193 patients underwent lead extraction. Perioperative complications were observed in 98 patients. Major complications were observed in eight patients (0.7%): five were successfully treated, and three died (0.3%). Minor complications, requiring no intervention, were observed in 86 patients (7.2%). No complications directly related to the femoral or jugular venous access were observed [12].

8.3 Prevention

8.3.1 Prevention at the Time of Implant

It is reasonable to implant a lead with the awareness that lead extraction may one day be necessary. Thus, it is important to consider lead implantation techniques and hardware that will allow easier extractions. The use of single-coil ICD leads instead of dual-coil leads may decrease the risk and difficulty of possible future lead extraction [13]. Medial subclavian vein approaches should be avoided because of the risk of crush, which would then require subsequent – and likely difficult – extraction. Isodiametric leads with active fixation are likely to be more easily and completely removed. As the DF-4 standard becomes widely available for ICD leads, this will make dissection easier. This quadpolar in-line connector requires a smaller ICD header, and the lead is shorter, because no yoke is needed. Even if some concerns about DF-4 malfunctioning leads still remain (impossible addiction of subcutaneous arrays and pace-sense leads), smaller pocket volume, and shorter and simplified lead design should reduce adhesions [14–16]. ICD leads with Gore-Tex™ coating or with a backfilled flat coil design will facilitate easier and safer extraction procedures [17–19]. Particular attention should be paid to the leads. Breaks and cuts in the lead insulation should be carefully avoided. As for fixation sleeves, these should not be tied too firmly, as this results in angulation and distortion of the lead axis, which could predispose to subsequent damage.

Anything that could increase the risk of infection must be avoided. Patient hemostasis should be perfect to avoid a pocket hematoma. The subcutaneous suprafascial location of the pocket should be created in the cleavage plane between the pectoralis fascia and the subcutaneous adipose tissue. Location of the pocket within the subcutaneous adipose tissue may give rise to a risk of subsequent adipose necrosis, with thinning of skin and increased risk of ulceration. For the pocket hematoma, observation should be preferred, and

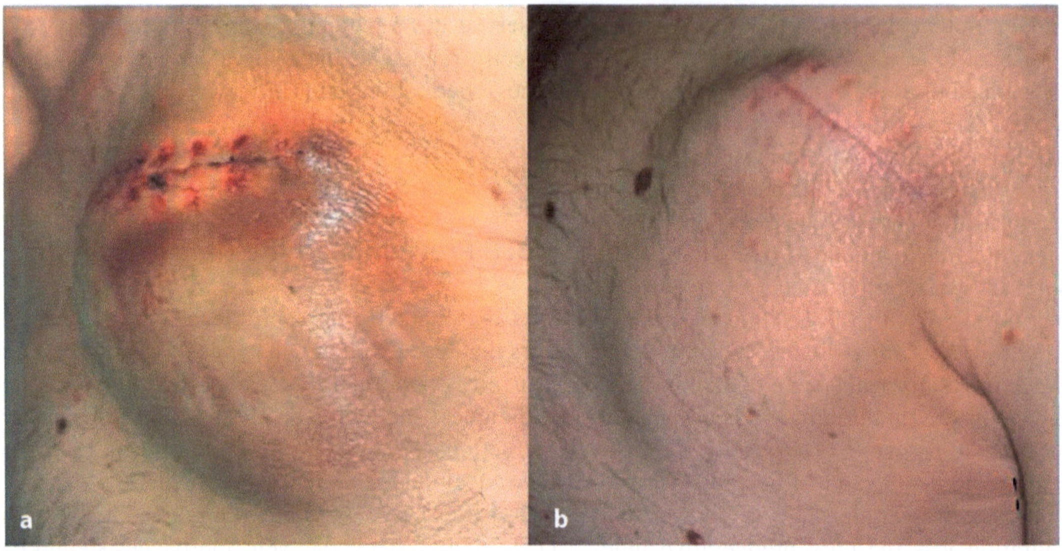

Fig. 8.1 Nonpainful, considerable hematoma after elective implantable cardioverter–defibrillator (ICD) replacement in a patient with mechanical aortic valve prosthesis (**a**). ICD pocket of the same patient after 1 month without surgical intervention for hematoma drainage (**b**)

puncture with a needle should be avoided. An adequate course of antibiotics should be administered (Fig. 8.1) [20]. In the cases of a pocket hematoma, opening the pocket may be less risky than transcutaneous puncture with regard to subsequent development of infection.

In cases of local reparative interventions with pulse-generator removal, the importance of leaving the leads intact must be emphasized. Leads must be capped (thus avoiding fibrous obliteration of the inner lumen by blood clots, which in turn prevents further stylet insertion) and secured firmly and safely to fibrous tissue (muscular fascia) with non-absorbable suture thread to avoid lead migration, which is also possible in the intravascular space [21]. The leads must maintain their original full length to allow easier anchorage during extraction: an extravascular lead fragment shorter than 3–5 cm in the subclavian region may preclude extraction maneuvers.

8.3.2 Physician Qualifications

Physicians wishing to perform this procedure should be properly trained in the technique. The simple act of watching an instructional video demonstration or observing an operator performing the procedure is not adequate. With regard to this issue, we are obliged to emphasize these five aspects:

1. Physicians being trained in this technique should extract a minimum of 40 leads as primary operator under the close surveillance of a skilled one.
2. Analysis of lead extraction outcomes suggests that the frequency of procedural (radiographic) failure drops dramatically after the first 10–20 procedures have been performed [22, 23].
3. Lower complication rates are associated with prior experience of 30 procedures; however, complication rates continue to decline up to 400 cases.
4. Performing a specific number of procedures does not guarantee proficiency, competency, or patient safety; outcome data are necessary to assess performance.
5. Training should be obtained at centers with adequate volume, experience, and expertise.

It is recommended that physicians being trained in this technique perform a *minimum* of 20 lead extractions as the primary operator under the direct supervision of a qualified training physician. Exposure to the venous entry site, as well as femoral retrieval techniques, should be included. The supervisor should have performed 75 lead extractions with an efficacy and safety record that is consistent with published data.

8.3.3 Minimum Facility Requirements for the Performance of Lead Extraction

As the possibility of vascular catastrophe is very real, both the physician and the institution must be capable of responding immediately and appropriately to any problems that arise. To achieve this level of preparedness, the hospital must have the following services on site and immediately available during the lead extraction procedure:

1. Temporary pacing and defibrillation/cardioversion equipment in the procedure room.
2. Monitoring equipment for invasive arterial pressure and oxygen saturation.
3. High quality fluoroscopy: a high-quality fluoroscopy system is a mainstay for lead extraction. Visualization of small lead components (such as stretched conductor coils, screws and embolized lead fragments) is fundamental to the safe performance of lead extraction. The equipment may be a fixed fluoroscopic system or a mobile "high quality" C-arm. Personnel specifically able to operate and troubleshoot this equipment are also required.
4. Extraction tools: essential tools are described in the appropriate chapter. The choice of a specific tool will depend on the physician's preferences and experience.
5. Cardiovascular implantable electronic devices (CIED) implantation tools: all of the usual implantation tools should be available. Different stylets (with different lengths, stiffness, and caliper) are mandatory, as are different introducer sheaths and guide wires. Traction must never be started without a guidewire or stylet inserted into the coil. The thickest stylets allowing advancement to the tip must be used to provide the highest tensile and distortion strength; however, these should be not thinner than 0.014 in. and should be longer than the lead. Angiography catheters (pig tails, multipurpose) should be immediately available.
6. Transthoracic ultrasound (TTE) and transesophageal ultrasound (TEE) capability must be immediately available: transthoracic echocardiography equipment in working order should always be at hand in or next to the operating room, and physicians capable of performing and interpreting echocardiographic procedures must be on hand. In some centers, intracardiac echocardiography (ICE) is performed immediately before the extraction procedure. This is generally to preoperatively evaluate presence and dimensions of lead vegetations prior to the extraction procedure in order to guide further therapeutic strategy.
7. Pericardiocentesis tray available in the procedure room, as well as personnel trained in the technique of pericardiocentesis.
8. Anesthesiological support.
9. A cardiothoracic surgeon on site and capable of promptly initiating an emergency procedure: the surgeon must be well familiarized with all potential complications of lead extraction and reimplantation and with the different surgical approaches for managing complications. For instance, surgical approaches used to treat an SVC tear, a right atrial or ventricular perforation, or a coronary sinus tear are quite different.
10. Thoracotomy tray immediately available: all instrumentation necessary to perform thoracotomy, sternotomy, and vascular repair should be immediately available and in perfect working order.

8.4 Treatment

8.4.1 Recognition of Vascular Collapse

Continuous monitoring of arterial pressure is *mandatory* in any extraction procedure in order to quickly detect changes in hemodynamics and pro-

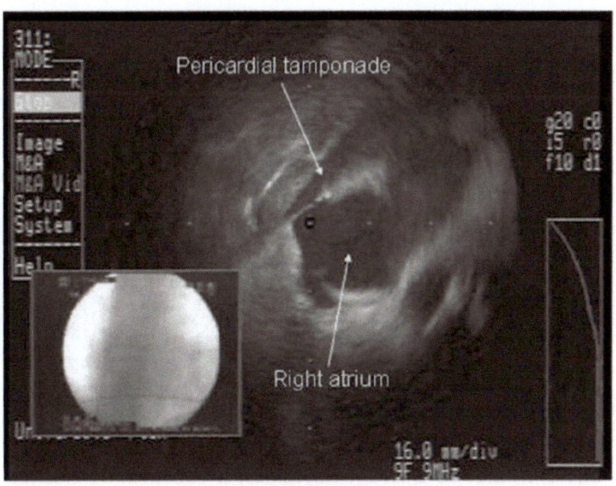

Fig. 8.2 Visualization of a cardiac tamponade by intracardiac echocardiography soon after lead extraction

vide efficacy in complication management. A delay in diagnosis of tamponade may have very serious consequences. If cardiac tamponade is suspected, TTE or ICE is mandatory to confirm diagnosis and quickly begin management (Fig. 8.2). Bleeding into the mediastinum or pleural space has a slower presentation and may have a delayed diagnosis because hemodynamic changes initially respond to fluid administration. The need to support hemodynamics with continuous fluid administration requires prompt, careful evaluation for pleural or mediastinal hemorrhage.

8.4.2 Management of Vascular Complications

Prompt recognition of complication is the most important determinant of good outcome. Iatrogenic bleeding that complicates routine catheterization and electrophysiological procedures is successfully treated in the majority of cases with pericardiocentesis (Fig. 8.3). In case of tamponade, pericardiocentesis should be less effective, perhaps because of differences in the size and nature of the laceration or perforation. If pericardiocentesis is ineffective in restoring blood pressure and there is evidence of significant continued bleeding, surgery must be rapidly performed. Any physician involved with lead extraction should be capable of performing emergency pericardiocentesis, and all equipment necessary for this procedure should be immediately available at the time of extraction (Fig. 8.4) [24].

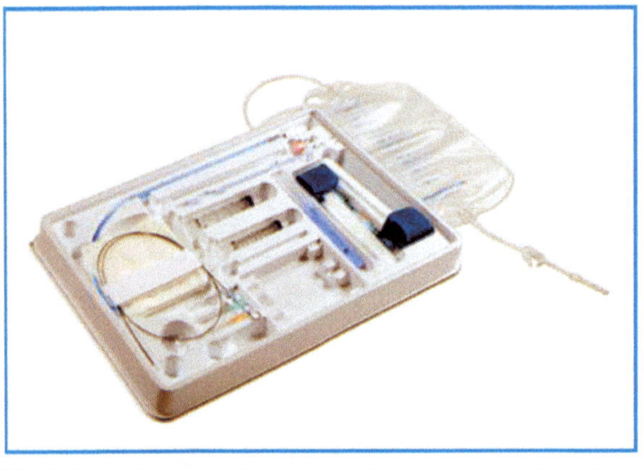

Fig. 8.3 Kit for pericardiocentesis: Usually contains high-flow pigtail or straight catheter; dilator; three-way stopcock; guide wire double-ended (J & straight); different kinds of needles; different kinds of Luer-lock syringes; a bag with connecting tube; gauzes; fenestrated drape; absorbent barrier; a double-ended alligator-clip cable

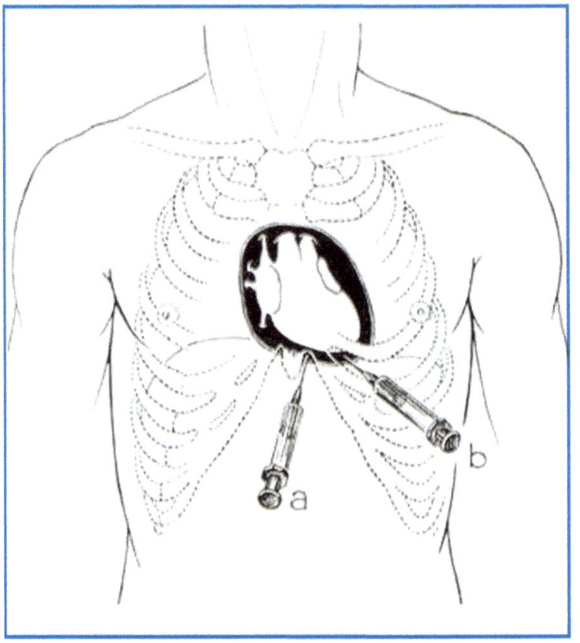

Fig. 8.4 Apical and paraxiphoid areas are the most common sites of needle insertion for pericardiocentesis

The pericardiocentesis technique can be described as follows: needle drainage of pericardial fluid requires the physician to detect a point on the patient's thorax or epigastric area in which to insert the needle. Most common sites of access are illustrated in Fig. 8.3. The needle inserted at a 15° angle to bypass the costal margin and advanced slowly until the pericardium is pierced and blood is aspirated. To ensure that blood comes out of the pericardial space, it is possible to advance the wire under fluoroscopy to verify its reflection at the top of the pericardial space. For prolonged drainage, a guide wire passed through the sheath will facilitate the introduction of a pigtail angiographic catheter.

8.4.3 Superior Vena Cava Tear

Superior vena cava tear is a dramatic event with high mortality rates and is most frequently associated with laser dilation and double-coil ICD leads [25].

Some operators have utilized a large balloon to tamponade a bleed from the SVC. In this manner, it is possible to temporarily prevent bleeding while awaiting surgical assistance. A guidewire should be positioned in the subclavian or internal jugular vein via the femoral vein before the beginning of the procedure, and a 30- or 40-ml balloon can be placed over a guidewire into the SVC in the event of tearing. This initiative should be shared with a surgical team because, theoretically, it can cause enlargement of the tear, creating disaster.

8.4.4 Traumatic Tricuspid Regurgitation

Traumatic tricuspid regurgitation (TTR) is not uncommon after lead extraction, being observed by transthoracic echocardiography in almost 9% of cases. Independent risk factors include the use of additional tools, beyond simple traction (mainly laser sheaths and lassos), and female gender. TTR may be severe, requiring surgical repair of the tricuspid valve. In the long term, right-sided heart failure may develop, requiring intensive medical therapy [26].

8.4.5 Embolization of Lead Fragments

Embolization of lead fragments has been described [27–29]. Because of the possibility of late complication due to retained fragments, attempts should be made to retrieve foreign material migrated into distal segments of the pulmonary arterial tree. This emphasizes the importance of having different retrieval tools (lassos, catcher, goose-neck snares) immediately available. Sometimes, hemodynamic angiographic catheters (multipurpose, pigtail, and so on) may be useful [30].

8.4.6 Venous Thrombosis/Disseminated Intravascular Coagulation

Patients with important comorbidities undergoing extraction often experienced venous thrombosis and embolism. The extraction process itself may result in a prothrombotic state, and in addition, patients are not routinely placed on anticoagulation therapy following extraction due to bleeding risk. Moreover, the systemic infectious process may predispose to disseminated intravascular coagulation, particularly after opening of the infected pocket, when a great bacterial charge may enter the freed venous access.

8.4.7 Other Complications

Other less frequent complications of lead extraction include arteriovenous fistulas that present either acutely or in the days following the procedure. Pericardial tamponade could be clinically evident several hours after the procedure. Patients undergoing lead extraction should be monitored for at least 24 h in the intensive care unit, with echocardiography performed electively immediately after the procedure and 6 h later to evaluate the pericardial space and tricuspid valve integrity. Life-threatening arrhythmias such as ventricular tachycardia, torsade de pointes, and ventricular fibrillation are rare but possible complications.

References

1. Love CJ, Wilkoff BL, Byrd CL et al (2000) Recommendations for extraction of chronically implanted transvenous pacing and defibrillator leads: indications, facilities, training. North American Society of Pacing and Electrophysiology Lead Extraction Conference Faculty. Pacing Clin Electrophysiol 23:544–551
2. Wilkoff BL, Love CJ, Byrd CL et al (2009) Transvenous lead extraction: Heart Rhythm Society. expert consensus on facilities, training, indications, and patient management. Heart Rhythm 6:1085–1104
3. Kutalek SP (2004) Pacemaker and defibrillator lead extraction. Curr Opin Cardiol 19:19–22
4. Wilkoff BL, Byrd CL, Love CJ et al (1999) Pacemaker lead extraction with the laser sheath: results of the pacing lead extraction with the excimer sheath (PLEXES) trial. J Am Coll Cardiol 33:1671–1676
5. Byrd CL, Wilkoff BL, Love CJ et al (2002) Clinical study of the laser sheath for lead extraction: the total experience in the United States. Pacing Clin Electrophysiol 25:804–808
6. Roux JF, Page P, Dubuc M et al (2007) Laser lead extraction: predictors of success and complications. Pacing Clin Electrophysiol 30:214–220
7. Kennergren C, Bucknall CA, Butter C et al (2007) Laser assisted lead extraction: the European experience. Europace 9:651–656
8. Agarwal SK, Kamireddy S, Nemec J et al (2009) Predictors of complications of endovascular chronic lead extractions from pacemakers and defibrillators: a single-operator experience. J Cardiovasc Electrophysiol 20:171–175.

9. Byrd CL, Wilkoff BL, Love CJ et al (1999) Intravascular extraction of problematic or infected permanent pacemaker leads: 1994–1996. U.S. Extraction Database, Med Institute. Pacing Clin Electrophysiol 22:1348–1357
10. Bracke FA, Meijer A, van Gelder LM (2001) Pacemaker lead complications: When is extraction appropriate and what can we learn from published data? Heart 85:254–259
11. Jones SO IV, Eckart RE, Albert CM, Epstein LM (2008) Large, single-center, single-operator experience with transvenous lead extraction: Outcomes and changing indications. Heart Rhythm 5:520–525
12. Bongiorni MG, Soldati E, Zucchelli G et al (2008) Transvenous removal of pacing and implantable cardiac defibrillating leads using single sheath mechanical dilatation and multiple venous approaches: high success rate and safety in more than 2000 leads. Eur Heart J 29:2886–2893
13. Rinaldi CA, Simon RD, Geelen P et al (2003) A randomized prospective study of single coil versus dual coil defibrillation in patients with ventricular arrhythmias undergoing implantable cardioverter defibrillator therapy. Pacing Clin Electrophysiol 26:1684–1690
14. Haqqani HM, Mond HG (2009) The implantable cardioverter-defibrillator lead: principles, progress, and promises. Pacing Clin Electrophysiol 32:1336–1353
15. Shein MJ, Moynahan M (2008) Testing new ICD technology. N Engl J Med 359:2610
16. Hauser RG, Almquist AK (2008) Learning from our mistakes? Testing new ICD technology. N Engl J Med 359: 2517–2519]
17. Wilkoff BL, Belott PH, Love CJ et al (2005) Improved extraction of ePTFE and medical adhesive modified defibrillation leads from the coronary sinus and great cardiac vein. Pacing Clin Electrophysiol 28:205–211
18. Hackler JW, Sun Z, Lindsay BD et al (2010) Effectiveness of implantable cardioverter defibrillator lead coil treatments in facilitating ease of extraction. Heart Rhythm 7(7):890–897
19. Di Cori A, Bongiorni MG, Zucchelli G et al (2010) Transvenous extraction performance of expanded polytetrafluoroethylene covered ICD leads in comparison to traditional ICD leads in humans. Pacing Clin Electrophysiol 33:1376-1381
20. Bongiorni MG, Di Cori A, Soldati E et al (2009) Il rischio Iatrogeno connesso all'impianto di pacemaker e defibrillatori. G Ital Cardiol 10 (6):395–406
21. Golzio PG, Bongiorni MG, Chiribiri A, Franco E (2007) Extraction of the inner coil of a pacemaker lead slid into the pulmonary artery. Pacing Clin Electrophysiol 30:273–275
22. Bracke FA, Meijer A, Van Gelder B (1998) Learning curve characteristics of pacing lead extraction with a laser sheath. Pacing Clin Electrophysiol 21:2309–2313
23. Smith HJ, Fearnot NE, Byrd CL et al (1992) Intravascular extraction of chronic pacing leads: the effect of physician experience. Pacing Clin Electrophysiol 15:513 [abstract]
24. Spodick DH (2003) Acute cardiac tamponade. N Engl J Med 349:684–690
25. Hauser RG, Katsiyiannis WT, Gornick CC et al (2010) Deaths and cardiovascular injuries due to device-assisted implantable cardioverter-defibrillator and pacemaker lead extraction. Europace 12: 395–401
26. Franceschi F, Thuny F, Giorgi R et al (2009) Incidence, risk factors, and outcome of traumatic tricuspid regurgitation after percutaneous ventricular lead removal. J Am Coll Cardiol 53:2168–2174
27. Eckart RE, Hruczkowski TW, Lanzberg MJ et al (2006) Pulmonary arterial embolization of pacemaker lead electrode tip. Pacing Clin Electrophysiol 29:784–787
28. Walters MI, Kaye GC (1999) Pulmonary embolization of a pacing electrode fragment complicating lead extraction. Pacing Clin Electrophysiol 22(5):823–824
29. Calvagna GM, Evola R, Valsecchi S (2010) A complication of pacemaker lead extraction: pulmonary embolization of an electrode fragment. Europace 12(5):613
30. Golzio PG, Bongiorni MG, Giuggia M et al (2007) Retrieval of pacemaker lead tip embolized into the distal pulmonary arterial bed during extraction procedure. Pacing Clin Electrophysiol 30:1558–1561

9 The Implantation of New Leads after Extraction

Giulio Zucchelli and Ezio Soldati

9.1 Introduction

The natural consequence of lead extraction procedures is the need for a subsequent device reimplantation. For this reason, when an extraction procedure is planned, the patient should be aware of the potential risks and complications related to both procedures and should be informed of potential alternatives in case of transvenous reimplantation failure. Reimplantation is not necessary in all the patients. The need for reimplantation after lead extraction cannot be always predicted before pacing/defibrillating system removal. In previous published studies, reimplantation rate has been reported to vary from 48% to 87% of cases [1–3]; in our experience, according with other centers, reimplantation of a new device is usually not required in about 20% of patients [4, 5]. However, in all patients undergoing lead extraction, especially in case of previous infection, the ongoing need of a cardiac device should be reassessed [6].

The indication for the extraction can explain different reimplantation settings. Generally, two different scenarios can be described: patients with a cardiovascular implantable electronic device (CIED) infection and patients with a malfunctioning lead. Moreover, in the era of cardiac resynchronization therapy (CRT), a specific skill in biventricular device reimplantation is required in large-volume centers and will be described separately.

G. Zucchelli (✉)
2nd Cardiovascular Department AOUP, Santa Chiara University Hospital, Pisa, Italy

M. G. Bongiorni (Ed.), *Transvenous Lead Extraction.*

9.2 Reimplantation After a Cardiac Device Infection

Usually, CIED infections can be classified as follows [5]: (1) nonbacteremic local infection with negative blood cultures and absence of vegetations at echocardiography; (2) bacteremic infection without endocarditis (negative echocardiography); (3) endocarditis (vegetations at echocardiography and diagnosis according to Duke's criteria). Bacteremia is considered significant if two separate positive blood cultures yielding the same microorganism is associated with fever or other signs of systemic inflammatory response syndrome. Lead/valve vegetations are diagnosed with transthoracic (TTE), transesophageal (TEE), or intracardiac echocardiography (ICE). Particularly, ICE is always performed in case of fever or bacteremia in order to exclude endocarditis [7]. Removing infected pacing/defibrillating leads is done after at least 2 weeks of antibiotic therapy; particular attention is dedicated to patients with endocarditis, in whom more than 3 weeks of preoperative antibiotic therapy is considered necessary for safe extraction and reimplantation. Independent of the strategy used in managing infected patients, the risk of relapse is relatively high (2–3%) [8].

Timing of a new device reimplantation after extraction of an infected one remains a subject of debate and is influenced by the causative agent and clinical presentation of CIED infections. Current guidelines consider that a new CIED system can be implanted into patients who have no valvular- or lead-associated vegetations even when they have positive preoperative blood cultures, as long as there is no further clinical evidence of systemic infection and blood cultures drawn within 24 h of CIED system removal remain negative for at least

72 hours (indication: class IIa; level of evidence: C). Reimplantation is still considered safe in case of positive lead-tip cultures or preoperative sepsis if there are no further signs of infection and postoperative blood cultures are negative after 72 h (indication: class IIa; level of evidence: C). In some experienced centers, reimplantation is considered safe when performed at a remote anatomical site longer than 36 h after extraction in patients who are apyretic, without cellulites, and have documented negative blood cultures [9]. We usually wait at least 48 h after removal if no signs of infection are evident. In patients with bacteremic infection without endocarditis (negative echocardiography) and without signs of local infection, ipsilateral reimplantation can be performed only in selected cases (e.g., in CRT patients, after at least 14 days of postextraction antibiotic therapy, and absolutely changing the pocket site). However, this kind of recommendation is not shared by all experts, and the guidelines suggest avoiding an ipsilateral replacement device implantation.

Some authors recommend contralateral reimplantation as early as 36 h after extraction in patients with local symptoms only of device-related infection [10]. In some instances, it is considered safe to perform a contralateral same-day reimplantation [11]. The reasons for a same-day reimplantation are usually pacemaker (PM) dependency or hemodynamic need for CRT in case of biventricular pacing. In fact, the risk of subsequent CIED infections and venous thrombosis increases while maintaining a transvenous temporary device, and for this reason, it cannot be used indefinitely [12]. Same-day reimplantation is considered safe if the patient is clinically proven not to have active systemic bacteremia or infection by blood culture at the time of extraction and there is a lack of transesophageal echocardiographic evidence for endocarditis and the presence of a normal white blood cell count.

In our experience, the presence of vegetations does not usually preclude early reimplantation. We think that a robust antibiotic therapy before extrac-

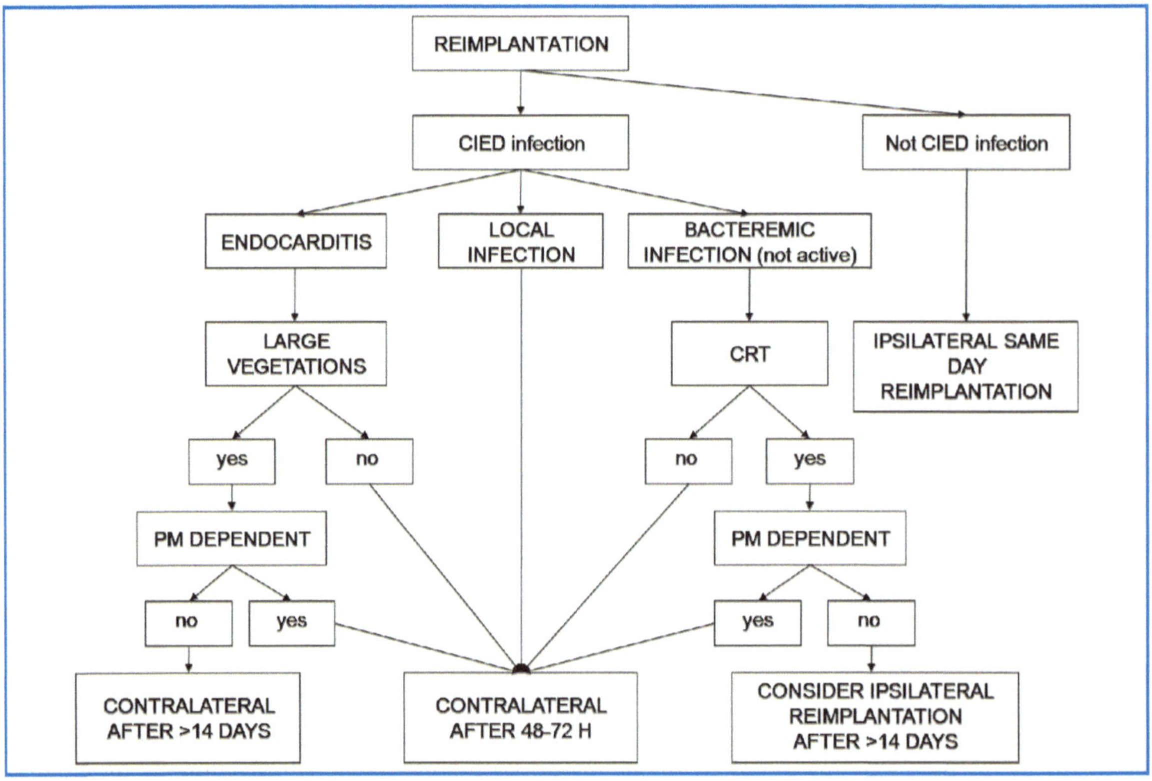

Fig. 9.1 Timing of reimplantation in presence/absence of cardiovascular implantable electronic device (CIED) infection. Reimplantation must be always delayed in the presence of cellulites, fever, or active bacteremia

tion is the key to preventing new relapse after reimplantation. However, current guidelines suggest delaying reimplantation for at least 14 days after removal in patients with valvular- or lead-associated vegetations. Alternative options to reduce this delay include vegetation debridement and epicardial lead implantation (Fig. 9.1). Some consideration must be given to particular cases: (1) large vegetations; (2) patients undergoing extraction with contralateral site not appropriate for use; (3) CRT recipients.

9.2.1 Large Vegetations

Vegetation is considered large when it is >2 cm. In this situation, our strategies differ according to whether or not the patient is PM dependent. In the former case, if the patient is apyretic and the preoperative cultures are negative, we perform an early reimplantation usually after 48 h; in the latter, we prefer to implant the new device in the contralateral site after at least 1 week of postextraction antibiotic therapy. Here we point out that correct duration of preoperative antibiotic therapy represents – in our opinion – the key factor predicting a safe reimplantation procedure, and this also in case of endocarditis. In particular cases (very large vegetations without PM dependency or primary prevention in implantable cardioverter defibrillator (ICD) recipients), we do not perform reimplantation during the same hospitalization but, instead, plan ICE evaluation after at least 1 month of antibiotics and anticoagulants to demonstrate reduced vegetation dimensions. In some cases, persistence of the mass inside the right chamber is not necessarily associated with continued illness, as confirmed by resolution of fever, normal white blood cell count, and labeled leukocyte imaging that is repeatedly negative for infection. In such cases, reimplantation is still considered safe; if the venous system is patent, sometimes we prefer to use the ipsilateral site when changing the pocket.

9.2.2 Contralateral Site Not Available

In some situations, we remove leads from one side when the contralateral site has been previously used or is not available (as in the case of arteriovenous fistula). In the former case, we performed venography at the contralateral site at the time of reimplantation, and if the venous system is patent, we use it. If a significant venous obstruction is found or the contralateral site is not available, we evaluate each case individually. In case of bacteremia without endocarditis and pocket cellulites, we generally use the site of removal of the infected device, waiting at least 10 days and changing the pocket site (e.g., from a prepectoral to a subpectoral position). If at the time of extraction we encounter pocket cellulites but cannot wait to reimplant (PM dependency or hemodynamic need for CRT), we refer the patient to the surgeon for epicardial pacing. Epicardial pacing after lead extraction is described in 5% of patients. We do not use the femoral vein approach, even if it offers a less invasive option and probably a lower risk of morbidity [13]. Regardless, there is very limited literature on femoral pacing, although this technique has been used since the early 1980s. Permanent pacing via the femoral vein is currently performed in a limited number of centers worldwide. The underutilization of this approach may be due to the fear of possible thrombotic or infective complications of transfemoral pacing. The most data available are from series in which temporary femoral pacing was used. The largest series in transfemoral definitive pacing was published by Ellestad and French in 1989, which included 90 patients who had 95 PMs implanted [14]. Atrial lead displacement was the major complication and occurred in 21% of implanted leads. This occurred despite the use of long active fixation atrial leads (85 cm).

9.2.3 CRT after Lead Extraction

When biventricular device reimplantation is necessary, we usually follow the same rules that we use in other pacing settings. Particular attention must be paid to patients with a hemodynamic dependency (to evaluate for same-day contralateral reimplantation) [15]. It is also very important to reassess the real need for CRT in patients undergoing coronary sinus (CS) lead extraction; in particular, nonresponders will not be candidates to reimplantation if the previous site of pacing is considered correct, spontaneous QRS complex is narrow,

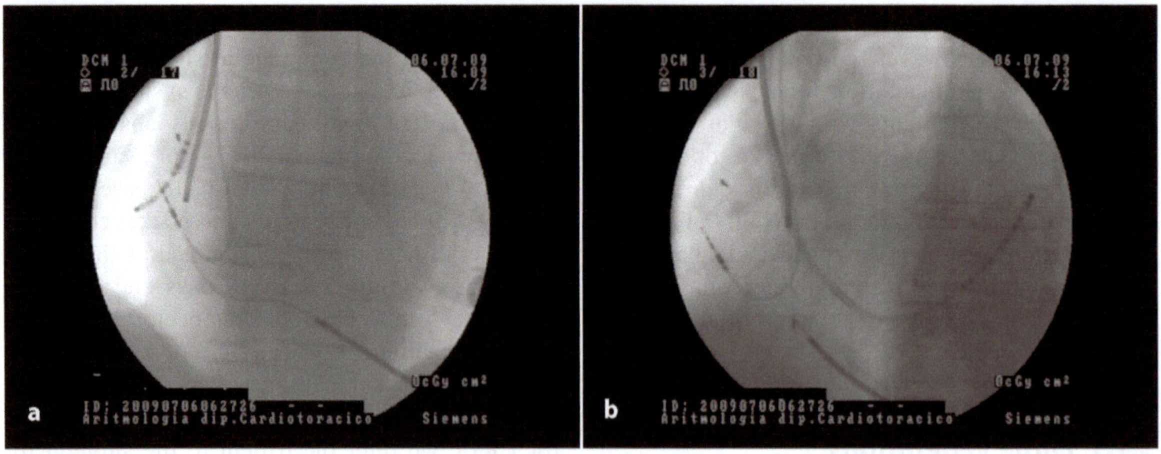

Fig. 9.2 Using a right-sided approach, the electrophysiological catheter is directed to the lateral wall of the right atrium (**a**); successful cannulation of the coronary sinus in the same patient (**b**)

and/or the patient is not PM dependent. However, it is necessary to identify patients who neither had clinical improvement after CRT nor clinical worsening (false non responders); the condition of these patients could abruptly aggravate after lead extraction if biventricular pacing is abandoned. We usually store the radiological positions of leads before extraction for accurate lead visualization and post hoc strategy delineation. Also, the availability of previous CS venography is always considered useful, especially when the lead is implanted outside the posterolateral region, in order to evaluate before reimplantation whether or not there is a potential alternative to the site previously chosen. Left ventricular (LV) lead reimplantation can be challenging due to the need for a right-sided approach and the lack of target vessels. CS cannulation can be time consuming for anatomical reasons: (1) from the right side, there is a natural predilection of the electrophysiological catheter and the LV-lead delivery system used for cannulation to be addressed to the lateral wall of the atrium (Fig. 9.2); (2) the CS ostium can be injured or occluded because of previous extraction. In a recent study, postextraction venograms demonstrated complete occlusion of the vein from which the lead was extracted in 50% of patients. Vein occlusions were present in patients with leads indwelling for >3 months and were independent of extraction method. The larger caliber CS-branch vessel was more likely to remain patent postextraction and allowed for reimplantation of a new LV lead. Failure to reimplant the LV lead transvenously was due to total occlusion of all target branches or the main CS [15, 16]. In our experience, a significant stenosis in the CS branch at the LV site of previous pacing can be demonstrated in the majority of cases (Figs. 9.3 and 9.4). However, LV lead reimplantation is usually effective and safe, and success and complication rates are comparable with first LV implant procedures, although in a large number of cases, a right-sided approach is necessary [17]. The main difference is that the LV posterolateral region is easier to reach in patients attending CRT for the first time, and sometimes reimplantation attempts require a balloon angioplasty because of narrowing or partial thrombosis of CS branches (Fig. 9.5) [18–21]. In case of lack of target vessels, we refer the patient to the surgeon for epicardial pacing (Fig. 9.6).

9.3 Reimplantation in Absence of Infection

The typical indication to reimplantation in absence of infection is PM/defibrillator lead malfunction. Other possible causes are reimplantation after extraction due to a superior vena cava (SVC) syndrome or need for new lead implantation in case of venous occlusion.

In case of malfunctioning leads, we follow one of two different strategies: we can abandon the nonfunctioning lead, or we can remove the old lead

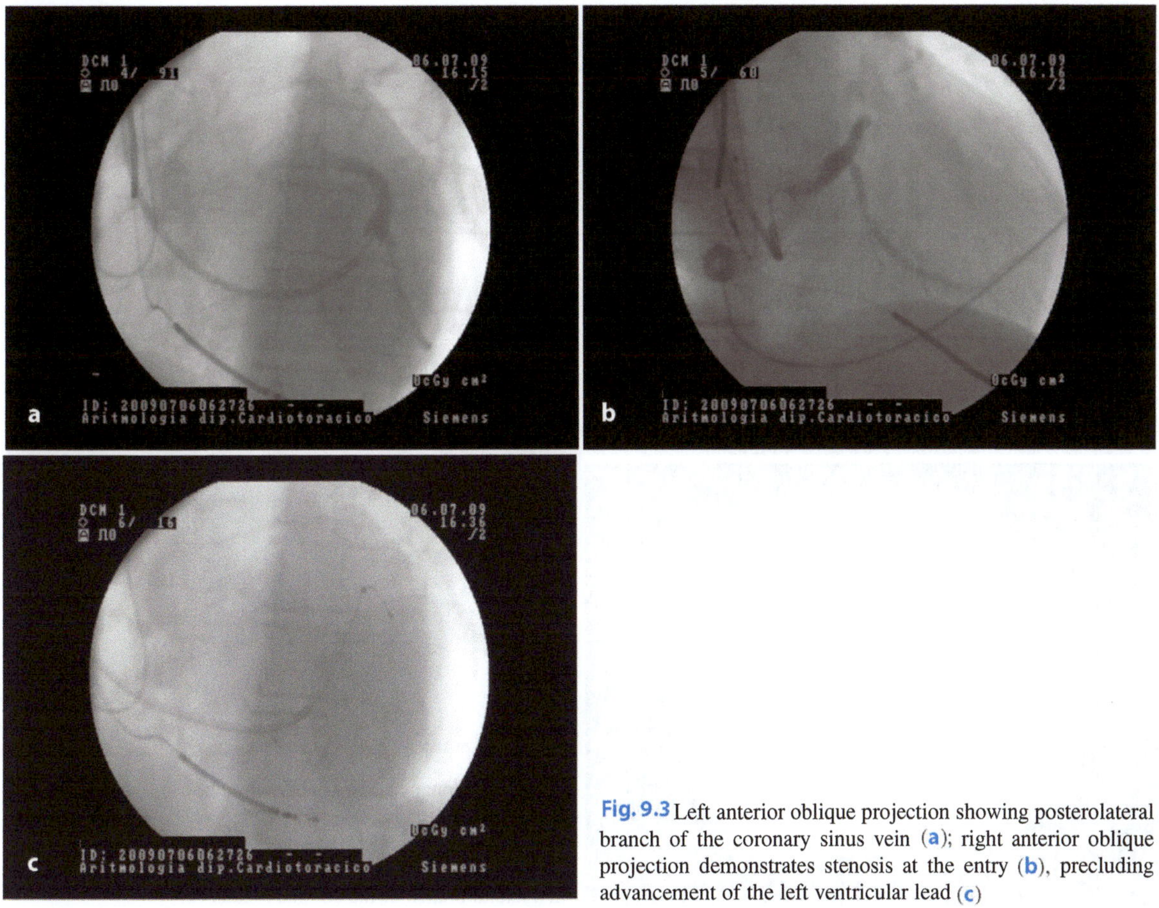

Fig. 9.3 Left anterior oblique projection showing posterolateral branch of the coronary sinus vein (a); right anterior oblique projection demonstrates stenosis at the entry (b), precluding advancement of the left ventricular lead (c)

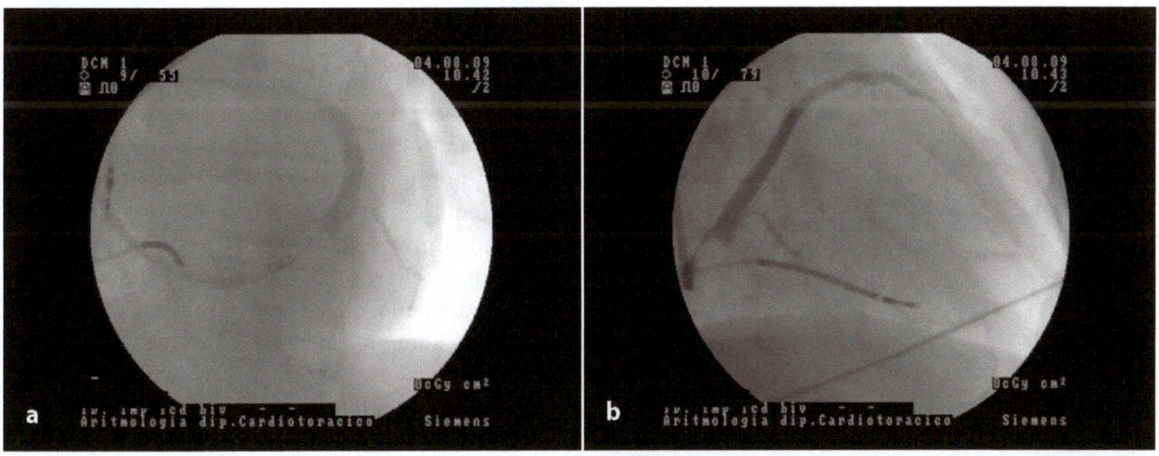

Fig. 9.4 Left (a) and right (b) anterior oblique projections showing stenosis of the posterolateral branch of the coronary sinus vein

and implant a new one. The first approach, although technically feasible and often with few short-term complications, even in pediatric patients [22], is a palliative procedure that we

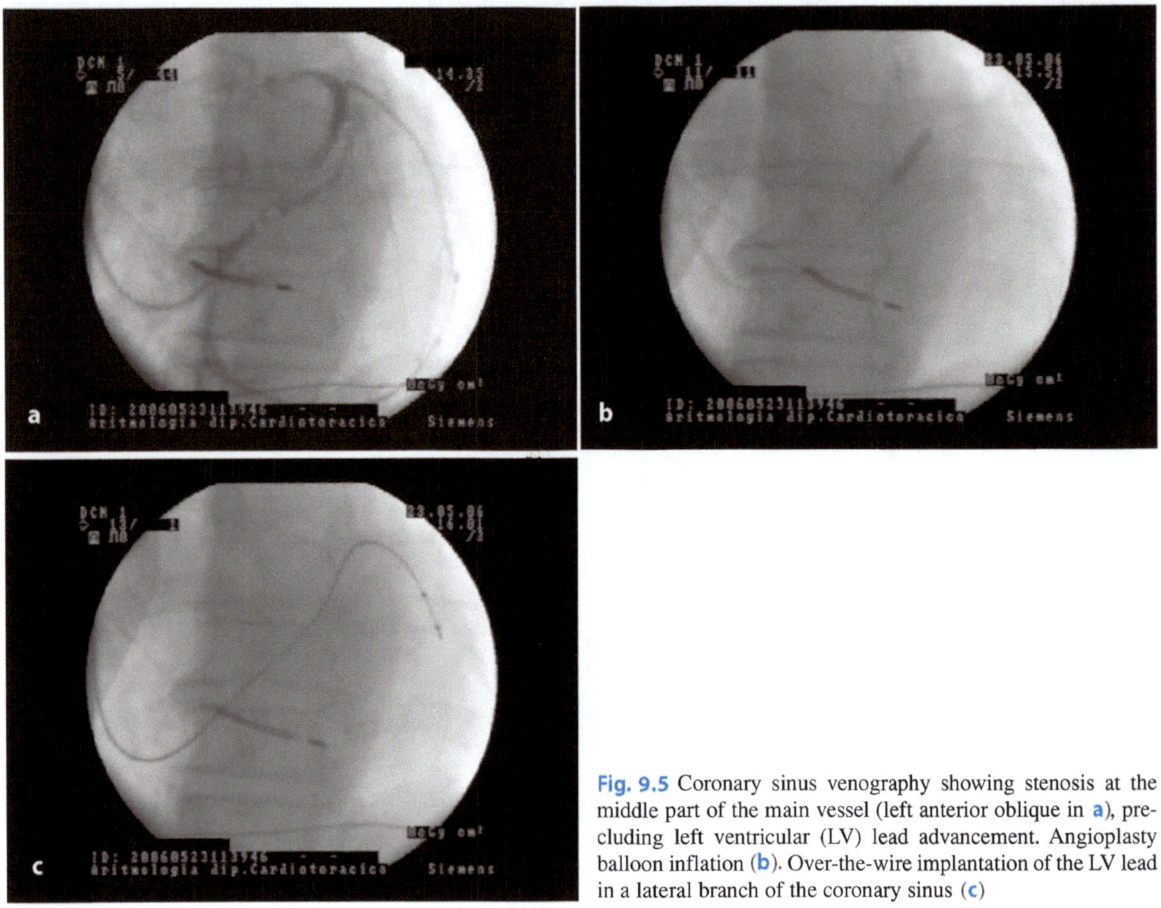

Fig. 9.5 Coronary sinus venography showing stenosis at the middle part of the main vessel (left anterior oblique in **a**), precluding left ventricular (LV) lead advancement. Angioplasty balloon inflation (**b**). Over-the-wire implantation of the LV lead in a lateral branch of the coronary sinus (**c**)

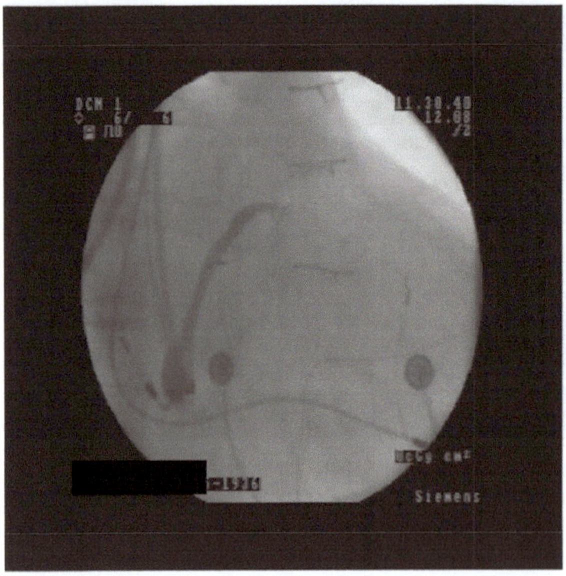

Fig. 9.6 Right anterior oblique projection showing the absence of coronary sinus branches at venography

think should be avoided in young people, particularly if more than three leads are already implanted and/or more than one abandoned lead is present [23]. Current guidelines consider it reasonable (indication: class IIa; level of evidence: C) to remove nonfunctional leads if an implantation would require more than four leads on one side or five leads through the SVC. The results of several studies have shown that complications due to noninfected abandoned leads may not be as rare as was previously thought and could produce significant morbidity and cost burden [24]. However, it is very difficult to calculate the risk-to-benefit ratio of lead extraction in these patients. The site of reimplantation in the absence of infection is usually ipsilateral, and the procedure is performed immediately after extraction. Causes of malfunctioning can be various, but the more typical is lead fracture at the venous entry site. In this case, we avoid using a retaining guide wire advanced through the extraction sheath because the placement of a new lead at the same venous entry site may result in failure of the new system. We usually do not remove leads next to the fractured one, even if these are placed via the same venous insertion site and same technique as the fractured lead and potentially are under the same forces. However, these nonfractured leads are at very high risk for failure, particularly if a single puncture of the subclavian vein ("single stick") with retained guide wire technique was used to place the two leads. If the venous system is patent at the beginning of the procedure, we usually obtain the new venous access prior to extracting the old lead, as venous occlusion or tears are not uncommon during extraction. We prefer to approach the "extrathoracic" subclavian vein to prevent the incidence of crush syndrome. Several methods are currently described to minimize complications and improve success rates of this technique [25]. The cephalic vein is a possible alternative if it was not used in the previous implant.

The occurrence of venous stenosis or thrombosis is not so rare in cardiac pacing, and despite 50 years of experience, we are unable to identify clear risk factors that lead to venous stenosis. Neither the hardware (lead size and material) nor the choice of access site (cephalic cutdown, subclavian or axillary puncture) appears to affect the rate of venous complications. A few factors were proposed as predictors of severe venous stenosis/occlusion: presence of multiple PM leads (compared with a single lead), use of hormone therapy, personal history of venous thrombosis, presence of temporary wire before implantation, previous presence of a PM (ICD as an upgrade), and use of dual-coil leads. Anticoagulant therapy seems to have protective antithrombotic effect. In the presence of venous occlusion, introduction of a new lead may be permitted through the channel created by extraction sheaths [26]. Moreover, if a guide wire can be passed through the occlusion, a passage may be created with venoplasty alone or in combination with stent placement. Particular attention is necessary during the placement of a new lead system on the side contralateral to an occluded vein, as subsequent bilateral subclavian vein occlusion could represent a dangerous situation for the patient. In some case, the stenosis can induce SVC syndrome; although venous occlusions are relatively common, true SVC syndrome is rare, with a reported incidence between 1:250 and 1:3,000 implants. The only therapy for this condition is represented by lead extraction with reconstruction of the venous wall or angioplasty with or without stenting placement. In the former case, reimplantation is performed via an epicardial path; in the latter, after vessel recanalization with balloon dilation and stent implantation, a transvenous pacing lead can be implanted successfully through the stent immediately or 6–8 weeks later [27]. If a stent is placed, it is critical that any leads be extracted prior to stent deployment so that incarceration of the leads between the stent and the vein do not occur (indication: class I; level of evidence: C) [6].

9.4 Reimplantation with Extraction in Mind

It is crucial to perform reimplantation with the understanding that extraction of that lead could be necessary in the future [28]. We try to avoid lead implantation techniques and hardware potentially associated with more difficult extraction. For these reasons, intrathoracic subclavian vein puncture is discouraged in our center due to the risk of crush requiring subsequent and probably difficult extraction. The cephalic vein is always the first choice in a contralateral implant (virgin site). As recent studies have documented that the proximal coil usually does not lower the defibrillation threshold significantly, we usually prefer to implant single-coil ICD leads at reimplantation to decrease the risk and difficulty of possible future lead extraction [29]. We emphasize also that a large percentage of patients undergoing reimplantation are approached from the right side, and in this setting, the caval coils are unlikely to be useful. The use of ICD leads with coils backfilled with medical adhesive or covered with Gore-TexTM can reduce the number of adhesions and make extraction easier and safer [30, 31]. Use of leads that are correctly sized (52 cm for atrial leads; 58 cm for ventricular leads), as well as IS-4/SJ-4 connectors for ICD leads, can reduce the amount and the volume of the proximal part of the lead present in the pocket, which may favor tissue ischemia and subsequent infection. At the time of reimplantation, we prefer to use isodiametric leads with active fixation, especially for atrial leads, for several reasons: first is that they are likely to be more easily and completely removed, if necessary; this is particularly true when the single-sheath dilatation technique is used [32]. Moreover, often when using a right-sided approach, active fixation allows the lead to be screwed out of the appendage; in fact, the appendage, which is more difficult to reach from the right side, is not a safe site of screwing after a previous extraction. The atrial lead with a passive fixation is sometime used from the left side in older patients, but this is not the rule. We use the passive fixation ventricular lead from the right side also in an ICD system with very large ventricular chambers, when we think that alternative sites out of the apex could be associated with high defibrillation threshold. It is very important to determine the previous pacing site by X-ray of the thorax or images stored at the time of extraction. Particular attention is necessary when placing the electrode in a region very close to the old pacing site, especially the apex, in order to avoid wall perforation. We believe that screwing ventricular leads to the apex should be avoided. We actually discourage the use of CS pacing leads with active fixation, considering the difficulty of removing them in case of chronic implantation [33]. Finally, we prefer to implant as little hardware as possible. For this reason, atrial single-chamber pacing is preferred when a sinus node dysfunction without history of atrial fibrillation was previously diagnosed, whereas VDD leads are favored in case of atrioventricular block.

9.5 Conclusions

Reimplantation of a new lead after extraction is a procedure requiring physician experience, skill, and often patience, particularly when it is not possible to perform an early reimplantation. The indication for the previous extraction can explain different reimplantation settings. Timing of reimplantation of a new device system after extraction of an infected device remains a subject of debate and correct duration of antibiotic therapy is considered necessary for a safe procedure. In our experience, the presence of vegetations does not usually preclude early reimplantation, but we believe appropriate antibiotic coverage before extraction is the key to preventing new infection relapse after reimplantation. Some consideration must be given to particular cases: large vegetations, patients undergoing extraction with the contralateral site unavailable for reimplantation, and CRT recipients. Finally, it is crucial to perform an "extraction-conscious reimplantation," approaching device implantation with the awareness that extraction may one day be necessary for leads currently being implanted.

References

1. Bohm A, Banyai F, Preda I et al (1996) The treatment of septicemia in pacemaker patients. Pacing Clin Electrophysiol 19:1105–1011
2. Dy Chua J, Wilkoff BL, Lee I et al (2000) Diagnosis and management of infections involving implantable electrophysiologic cardiac devices. Ann Intern Med 133:604–608
3. Cacoub P, Leprince P, Nataf P et al (1998) Pacemaker infective endocarditis. Am J Cardiol 82:480–484
4. Sohail MR, Uslan DZ, Khan AH et al (2007) Management and outcome of permanent pacemaker and implantable cardioverter-defibrillator infections. J Am Coll Cardiol 49:1851–1859
5. Tascini C, Bongiorni MG, Gemignani G et al (2006) Management of cardiac device infections: a retrospective survey of a non surgical approach combining antibiotic therapy with transvenous removal. J Chem 18(2):157–163
6. Wilkoff BL, Love CJ, Byrd CL et al (2009) Transvenous lead extraction: Heart Rhythm Society expert consensus on facilities, training, indications, and patient management. Heart Rhythm 6(7):1085–1104
7. Bongiorni MG, Di Cori A, Soldati E et al (2008) Intracardiac echocardiography in patients with pacing and defibrillating leads: a feasibility study. Echocardiography 25:632–638
8. Tarakji KG, Chan EJ, Cantillon DJ et al (2010) Cardiac implantable electronic device infections: Presentation, management, and patient outcomes. Heart Rhythm 7(8):104–1047
9. Borek PP, Wilkoff BL (2008) Pacemaker and ICD leads: Strategies for long-term management. J Interv Card Electrophysiol 23(1):59–72
10. Byrd C (2000) Management of implant complications. In: Ellenbogen K, Kay G, Wilkoff BL, eds. Clinical cardiac pacing, 2nd edn. WB Saunders, Philadelphia, pp 669–694
11. Nandyala R, Parsonnet V (2006) One stage side-to-side replacement of infected pulse generators and leads. Pacing Clin Electrophysiol 29:393–396
12. Klug D, Balde M, Pavin D et al (2007) Risk factors related to infections of implanted pacemakers and cardioverter-defibrillators results of a large prospective study. Circulation 116:1349–1355
13. Mathur G, Stables RH, Heaven D et al (2001) Permanent pacemaker implantation via the femoral vein: an alternative in cases with contraindications to the pectoral approach. Europace 3:56–59

14. Ellestad MH, French J (1989) Iliac vein approach to permanent pacemaker implantation. Pacing Clin Electrophysiol 12:1030–1033
15. Burke MC, Stobie P, Tierney SP et al (2003) Time to reimplantation after device system extraction, pocket excision and primary closure in localized pocket infection. Pacing Clin Electrophysiol 26:36 [abstract]
16. De Voogt G, Ruiter JH (2006) Occlusion of the coronary sinus: a complication of resynchronization therapy for severe heart failure. Europace 8:456–458
17. Zucchelli G, Solarino S, Soldati E et al (2009) Cardiac resynchronization therapy after left ventricular lead extraction: feasibility and outcome of conventional transvenous approach. Heart Rhythm 6:S256[abstract]
18. Zucchelli G, Soldati E, Segreti L et al (2008) Cardiac resynchronization after left ventricular lead extraction: usefulness of angioplasty in coronary sinus stenosis. Pacing Clin Electrophysiol 31:908–911
19. Kowalski O, Lenarczyk R, Prokopczuk J et al (2006) Effect of percutaneous interventions within the coronary sinus on the success rate of the implantations of resynchronization pacemakers. Pacing Clin Electrophysiol 26:1075–1080
20. Worley SJ, Gohn DC, Pulliam RW (2008) Focused force coronary venoplasty to eliminate a refractory stenosis preventing LV lead placement in two patients. Pacing Clin Electrophysiol 31(11):1503–1505
21. Worley SJ, Gohn DC, Pulliam RW (2008) Coronary vein rupture during venoplasty for LV lead placement. Pacing Clin Electrophysiol 31(7):904–907
22. Silvetti MS, Drago F (2008) Outcome of young patients with abandoned, nonfunctional endocardial leads. Pacing Clin Electrophysiol 31:473–479
23. Suga C, Hayes DL, Hyberger LK et al (2000) Is there an adverse outcome from abandoned pacing leads? J Interv Card Electrophysiol 4:493–499
24. Bohm A, Pinter A, Duray G et al (2001) Complications due to abandoned not infected pacemaker leads. Pacing Clin Electrophysiol 24:1721–1724
25. Harada Y, Katsume A, Kimata M et al (2005) Placement of pacemaker leads via the extrathoracic subclavian vein guided by fluoroscopy and venography in the oblique projection. Heart Vessels 20(1):19–22
26. Pace JN, Maquilan M, Hessen SE et al (1997) Extraction and replacement of permanent pacemaker leads through occluded vessels: use of extraction sheaths as conduits- balloon venoplasty as an adjunct. J Interv Card Electrophysiol 1:271–279
27. Ing FF, Mullins CE, Grifka RG et al (1998) Stent dilation of superior vena cava and innominate vein obstructions permits transvenous pacing lead implantation. Pacing Clin Electrophysiol 21(8):1517–1530
28. Smith MC, Love CJ (2008) Extraction of transvenous pacing and ICD leads. Pacing Clin Electrophysiol 31:736–752
29. Rinaldi CA, Simon RD, Geelen P et al (2003) A randomized prospective study of single coil versus dual coil defibrillation in patients with ventricular arrhythmias undergoing implantable cardioverter defibrillator therapy. Pacing Clin Electrophysiol 26:1684–1690
30. Wilkoff BL, Belott PH, Love CJ et al (2005) Improved extraction of ePTFE and medical adhesive modified defibrillation leads from the coronary sinus and great cardiac vein. Pacing Clin Electrophysiol 28:205–211
31. Hackler JW, Sun Z, Lindsay BD et al (2010) Effectiveness of implantable cardioverter defibrillator lead coil treatments in facilitating ease of extraction. Heart Rhythm 7(7):890–897
32. Bongiorni MG, Soldati E, Zucchelli G et al (2008) Transvenous removal of pacing and implantable cardiac defibrillating leads using single sheath mechanical dilatation and multiple venous approaches: high success rate and safety in more than 2000 leads. Eur Heart J 29:2886–2893
33. Bongiorni MG, Di Cori A, Zucchelli G et al (2010) A modified transvenous single mechanical dilatation technique to remove a chronically implanted active-fixation coronary sinus pacing lead. Pacing Clin Electrophysiol [Epub ahead of print]

10 Problem-Solving in Lead Extraction

Maria Grazia Bongiorni and Ezio Soldati

10.1 Introduction

Transvenous lead removal is a complex technique. Many conditions play a role in lead extraction procedures and may affect technique, approaches, and results. In each case, lead design, lead damage, and patient anatomy may be significantly different, regardless of the removal technique. The description of any technique for transvenous lead extraction is always theoretical, exemplifying the most common situation; it must be emphasized that it is impossible to analyze and elucidate all possible conditions present in clinical practice [1–3]. The operator must plan the extraction procedure, and during the actual procedure, tailor techniques and tools to the individual circumstances in order to succeed and avoid complications [4, 5]. The fact that each case will have different conditions increases the importance of the extractor's experience. Nevertheless, the number of different factors affecting the procedure may outweigh the operator's experience, thus demanding that the operator develop an individual solution for each case. The aim of this chapter is to identify some of the most common conditions that make transvenous lead extraction difficult and to describe possible solutions in order to achieve successful extraction and reduce complications. Before discussing difficult situations during transvenous lead extraction, some basic principles are described.

First, the operator must define a strategy for the procedure, including all possible alternative approaches in case problems or difficulties arise. Planning a strategy always includes identifying an exit strategy. One of the most important points is that with any manoeuvre or approach the possibility of reversal must be considered. Whenever an interventional approach is chosen, the possibility of having to return to the initial situation if the first approach is unsuccessful must be accurately considered every time. The second point is that extraction techniques and related tools are primarily designed for "normal" leads. Every modification of lead conditions or damage due to lead characteristics or failure (free-floating leads, subclavian crush, loss of insulation, wire protrusion) or previous ineffective attempts at removal are likely to require unconventional approaches to overcome unique obstacles.

All the following critical points during pacing and implantable cardioverter–defibrillator (ICD) transvenous lead removal and their solutions are summarized in Table 10.1.

10.2 Free-Floating Leads

The intravascular position of the leads or lead fragments is relatively common in patients undergoing transvenous lead extraction. Lead to remove can be free floating either as (1) the result of lead fracture in its intravascular course or (2) the result of an intervention.

1. Spontaneous fracture of a lead is not common, and the most frequent cause is subclavian crush (Fig. 10.1).
2. Changing an exposed into free-floating lead is more common. Most of these leads are malfunctioning or infected; at the time of abandonment,

M.G. Bongiorni (✉)
2nd Cardiovascular Department AOUP, Santa Chiara University Hospital, Pisa, Italy

M. G. Bongiorni (Ed.), *Transvenous Lead Extraction*.

Table 10.1 Critical points during pacing and implantable cardioverter–defibrillator (ICD) transvenous lead removal

Critical points	Problems	Standard approach limitations	Solutions
Free-floating leads	Venous entry site approach impossible for unexposed intravascular leads	Binding-site dilatation with the transfemoral workstation is often ineffective, particularly in the ventricle	Transjugular approach
Lead damage	Coil is lengthened or any stylet cannot be inserted	Dilating sheath with high-energy dilatation may induce venous tears or complete lead fracture	Transjugular approach
Loss of insulation	The coil is in direct contact with tissue	Advancement of dilators may fracture the coil; traction may induce coil lengthening or tissue tears	Use a catheter with lumen to fill the role of lacking insulation
Narrow space between clavicle and first rib	Difficult sheath advancement	Use of large sheaths often precluded	Transjugular approach
Tight or calcified binding sites	Binding sites fibrous and stiff, often calcified, difficult dilatation	Aggressive dilatation from the venous entry site; mechanical dilation required. Mechanical or powered dilatation ineffective on calcified adhesions	Transjugular approach
Hard turns in lead course	Force or energy of dilatation is not applied to the binding site but directly to the venous wall	Dilators apply excessive dilating force, increasing the risk of vein damage	Transjugular Approach
Tight binding sites into the coronary sinus	Difficult dilatation into the coronary sinus, difficult C-shaped lead course	Dilators cannot be advanced into the coronary sinus; dilatation cannot be advanced to the binding site	Transjugular approach; reverse Pisa approach; dilatation from the femoral vein
Tight binding sites in the right ventricular outflow tract	Difficult dilatation into the outflow tract; difficult C-shaped lead course	Dilatation cannot be advanced to binding sites or tip; high risk of tears	Transjugular approach; reverse Pisa approach; dilatation from the femoral vein

the connector and a portion of the lead were cut as far as possible from the generator's pocket ("cut and leave") and then left either with no fixation or inadequately fixed to the tissue, thus allowing subsequent lead slippage into the insertion vein. Rarely free-floating lead fragments are the result of an unsuccessful attempt at removal (Figs. 10.2 and 10.3).

In the presence of free-floating leads, the first issue is how to grasp the lead. The key points in these cases are fragment length, position, and binding sites to the vascular and/or cardiac walls. For the purpose of transvenous extraction, the basic issue is whether there is a site where the course of the free-floating lead is free from binding sites and consequently can be caught. If it is impossible to catch the lead, transvenous techniques are not applicable. Removal strategy is then dependent on grasping site. If the lead can be grasped near the tip (in case the tip is not fixed) or at the proximal end of the intravascular portion, the most reliable approach is to use a loop retriever in order to firmly hold the lead. At this point, the condition of the tip is the most important issue. In the presence of free-floating leads with free tips, traction may result in sliding the lead through the

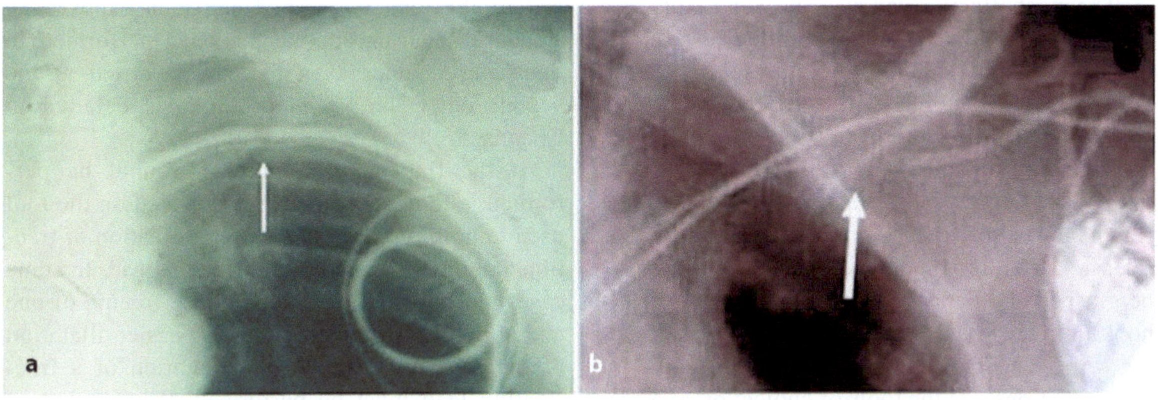

Fig. 10.1 (a) X-Ray of the costoclavicular region in two pacemaker patients. (b) Note the spontaneous fracture of leads in this region due to subclavian crush (*arrows*)

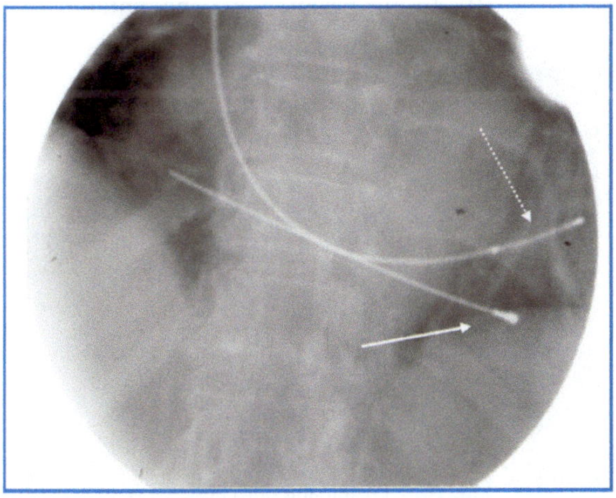

Fig. 10.2 Preprocedural fluoroscopic posteroanterior view of patient referred to our center for lead extraction. Note the free-floating, fractured, old unipolar lead (*solid arrow*) with the proximal end in the atrial region as a result of a previous, unsuccessful attempt of removal. The temporal pacing lead is placed in the right ventricle (*dashed arrow*)

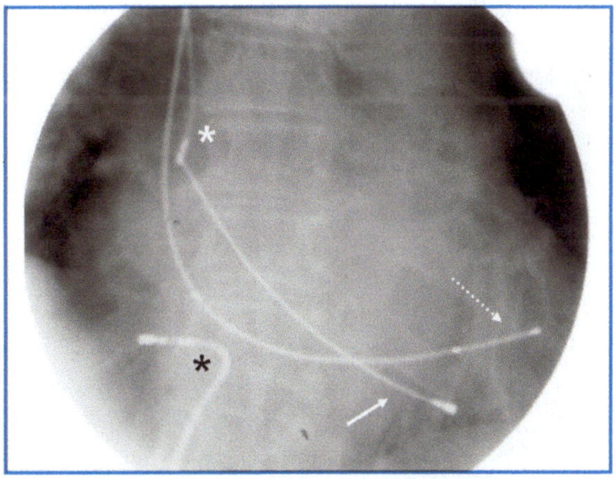

Fig. 10.3 Preprocedural fluoroscopic posteroanterior view of patient just seen in Figure 10.2. Note the free-floating lead (*solid arrow*) with the proximal end captured by a lasso catheter (*white star*) inserted through the internal jugular vein. Deflecting catheter (*black star*) was used to move the free-floating lead and to facilitate its end capture by the lasso. Temporal pacing lead was placed in the right ventricle (*dashed arrow*)

binding sites and finally in removal. The transfemoral approach is preferred in these conditions. In presence of free-floating leads with anchored tips (i.e., lead migration into the venous system, with the proximal end inaccessible in the pacemaker pocket and the tip fixed in the heart), dilatation is required. Whenever dilatation is necessary, the fragment length and position play a key role in deciding which approach to use. If the lead fragment is long enough to expose the proximal end at a vascular insertion of the loop retriever, it can be exposed and submitted to a standard dilatation procedure for exposed leads using the transjugular approach [2, 6, 7].

The most effective venous approach in this case is the right internal jugular vein, due to both the highest proximity and the straightest lead course to the heart. A second choice is the subclavian vein. If the fragment is too short to expose the proximal end with any possible venous approach, the lasso, or loop retriever, is used as an extension of the fragment to allow access to the fragment and thus release it from the binding sites. If the lead cannot be grasped at an end, tools that allow the use of a hook in order to hold the lead, such as tip-deflecting wires and catchers designed specifically for such situations, are the tools of choice; or, as a second choice, deflectable electrophysiology (EP) catheters or pigtail catheters [2] (Fig. 10.4). The operator must always check for the possibility of releasing the lead from capture in case of failed removal. Once the lead is caught, two possible solutions may be attempted. First, traction can result in freeing one of the ends of the fragment, thus allowing one of the previously described approaches to be performed. Traction must be applied very carefully to avoid further damage to the lead, entanglement of the lead in the tool, or difficult disruption at a binding site that may induce tears in venous and cardiac walls. If traction is not effective, dilation is required. A transjugular approach is then performed [2]. The right internal jugular vein is percutaneously cannulated using a large introducer (usually 11 F); then a lasso is advanced via the jugular vein and the proximal end of the lead is grasped and then exposed. A standard superior approach is then performed in the same manner as with leads exposed at the venous entry site. The technique is detailed in Chapter 5.

If the transjugular approach cannot be performed, a long sheath can be advanced on the tool used to hold the lead, and the combination of traction and pressure are used to free the lead. In some cases, the force applied may induce freeing of one end of the lead fragment, allowing easier dilatation of the other end. Whenever dilatation of a free-floating lead must be performed, the position of the lead and binding sites must be considered. Some authors report that using the transfemoral approach is the best way to remove free-floating leads [8–10]. In our practice, we encountered sig-

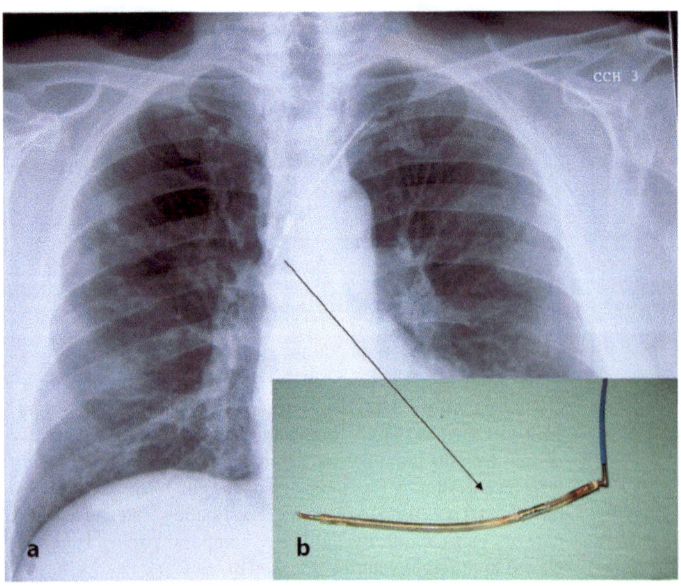

Fig. 10.4 Posteroanterior chest X-ray of a patient who underwent an unsuccessful attempt at lead removal. (**a**) Note the two pacing-lead pieces embedded into a binding site at the superior vena cava level. (**b**) The fragmented leads were removed by catching their distal end with a lasso inserted through the transfemoral approach

nificant difficulty removing free-floating leads that are adherent to the ventricular wall. The advancement of the femoral sheath into the ventricle and adherence dilatation to the tip was often impossible. Long Teflon sheaths (designed for the femoral approach) are commonly too soft to perform effective dilatation, and rotational movements are impossible using these tools. Research for alternative solutions to these problems led us to introduce the transjugular approach [2, 7].

10.3 Lead Damage

As mentioned, extraction techniques and related tools are mainly designed for leads in normal condition. Any damage to the lead, due to its characteristics or failure (subclavian crush, loss of insulation, wire protrusion) or to previous ineffective attempts at removal, may heavily impact the transvenous removal procedure, often requiring unconventional approaches. In the following paragraphs the most common situations are addressed.

10.3.1 Failure to Advance a Stylet into the Coil Lumen

The use of a locking stylet during transvenous removal can be due to the decision to use a traction device (as the main extraction tool or in combination with sheaths). Obviously, if the stylet cannot be inserted or if it stops very early in the coil lumen, traction cannot be performed. Regardless of the use of traction devices, the presence of a stylet into the lead is helpful during any dilatation technique. Either mechanical or powered sheaths, while advancing over the lead and freeing it from binding sites, induce mechanical stress on the lead body. The stiffer the lead, the more effective and safe is dilatation.

First, failure to advance a stylet can be due to damage or fracture of the coil or to turns in the course of the lead. If advancement stops in the proximal tract of the lead, the operator must check to see whether the obstacle can be overcome by cutting the lead and advancing the stylet along the undamaged portion. In some ways, obstacles can be removed when the course of the lead is modified by the effects of dilatation, and subsequent attempts to advance the stylet at the different steps of the procedure may finally result in the advancement to the tip. In the absence of a stylet into the lead, the lead is unable to support mechanical stress induced by dilatation, mainly in the proximity of binding sites. Dilatation must be performed very carefully in the presence of hard turns of the lead body due to the risk of lead damage. On the other hand, excessive traction can result in lead damage, thus affecting removal effectiveness and safety. In this situation, we suggest checking for the possibility of crossing to a different venous approach. If the freed part of the lead is long enough, or if the lead can be slipped through binding sites, the use of a transjugular approach can minimize the difficulty of dilatation in the absence of the stylet. The straight course of the lead can address most dilatation force at the interface between lead and fibrous tissue. The absence of turns in the course of the lead decreases the risk of lead damage or complications.

10.3.2 Insulation Loss

The outer insulation of pacing and implantable cardioverter–defibrillator (ICD) leads is relatively slippery in order to facilitate lead movement and implantation. This characteristic also plays a role in transvenous lead removal; the presence of intact insulation makes sliding dilators over the lead easier. In the absence of insulation or when the insulation is damaged, removal may be challenging.

1. When the insulation is absent in a small part of the lead (i.e., leads damaged by subclavian crush), the obstacle can be overcome by careful dilatation of this portion. Whenever a dilating sheath is advanced over an insulation break, the free edge of the broken insulation may cause a serious obstacle to progression due to the different size of the inner and outer part of the lead. In these cases, the problem can be overcome by using a dilator closer in size to the lead size when close to the break, then advancing a larger, outer telescopic sheath over the smaller one. If the break is near the venous entry site, it is possible that, after portion of the lead is freed, traction may slide the break outside the venous entry site, thus allowing the distal part of the insulation to be grasped.

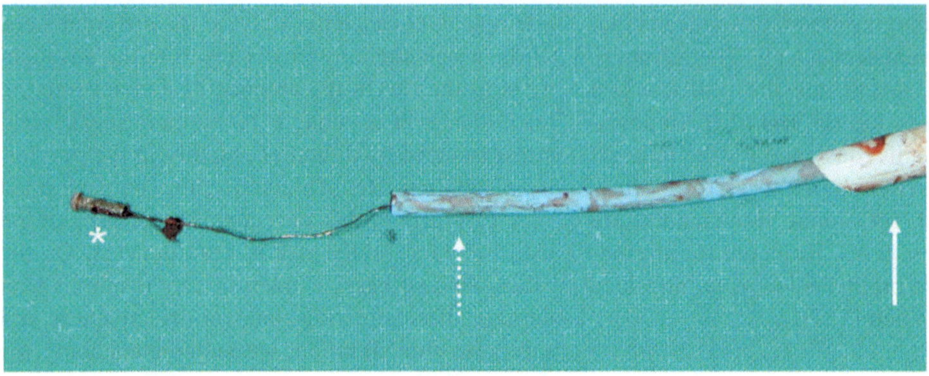

Fig. 10.5 New insulation may be provided for a damaged lead by using a piece of multipurpose catheter (*dashed arrow*), advancing it over the lead (*white star*) as far as possible then sliding the sheath over the catheter (*solid arrow*). This could be useful for leads that have lost insulation for a lengthy tract, or over its entire length due to, for example, a previous removal attempt

2. When insulation is absent for a long portion or for the entire length of the lead as a result of a removal attempt, the operator faces two problems. First, performing traction by holding the lead by the coil alone may induce coil lengthening and damage the cardiac structures. Second, progression of dilating sheaths over the unprotected coil is very difficult.

The possible solution may be to provide a "new" insulation. In these cases, the authors use a piece of multipurpose catheter, advancing it over the lead as far as possible, till the tip or close to the most proximal binding site (Fig. 10.5). Using this "dress" for the lead, the disadvantages induced by damage are minimized and, while the coil is held, sheath advancement and dilatation can be effectively and safely performed.

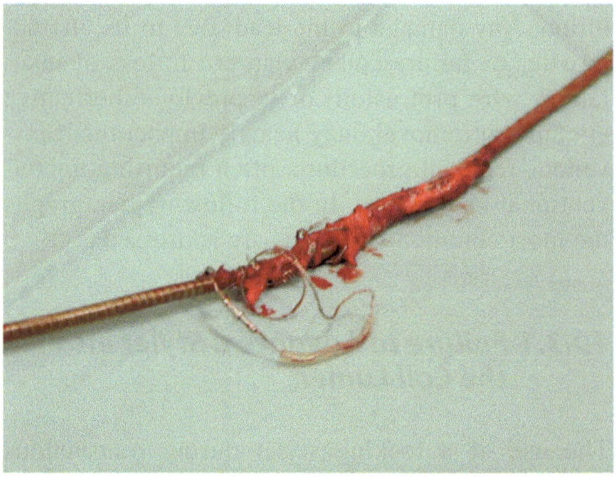

Fig. 10.6 Coil fracture induced by the dilating-sheath maneuver. This situation could be dangerous due to the risk of vessel tears or lacerations caused by disrupted metal wires

10.3.3 Coil Damage

As mentioned, coil damage or lengthening result in more complex transvenous removal procedures. The insertion of any stylet is usually impossible, so the related advantages are lost; in the same way, traction is not transmitted to the entire length of the lead and usually results in insulation fracture, changing the lead to a free-floating one. If the coil is badly damaged or fractured, transvenous removal approaching the lead from the venous entry site may be unsuccessful and potentially dangerous. If the coil is damaged, one of the most important issues is the presence of insulation at the site of the damage. Coil lengthening, as often occurs due to too much traction, may prevent advancement of the stylet; much more important is the absence of insulation. When the coil is devoid of insulation, dilating sheaths may be advanced other than over the lead body, thus inducing coil fracture. The broken conductor can thus be pushed into the venous wall, inducing tears or lacerations (Fig. 10.6). In addition, traction over the lead may cause the metallic coil to slide on the vessel wall, resulting in a serious risk of complications. An attempt can be made, but the operator must use all possible care to avoid further lead damage. If this careful attempt is ineffective, using the transjugular approach must be considered [2].

10.4 Difficult Dilator Advancement and Dilatation

Many difficult conditions in transvenous removal may be related to the patient's anatomy or be the result of physiological interaction between the patient and the implanted leads. In some cases, this particular setting may affect either the effectiveness or safety of removal procedures, thus requiring different solutions.

10.4.1 Narrow Space Between Clavicle and First Rib

In most extraction techniques, exposed leads are approached at the venous entry site, usually through the cephalic or subclavian vein. In this situation, the dilator – regardless of the energy used to free the lead from adhesions – must be advanced over the lead, crossing the space between the clavicle and the first rib. The anatomical dimensions of this site are variable: a very narrow space exists in a significant percentage of patients and may be responsible of difficulties at implant as well as lead damage induced by compression. In these patients, advancement of dilators that are necessarily larger than the lead size may make the attempt difficult or even impossible, particularly when powered sheaths are used. In such circumstances, if the leads cannot be slipped through this narrow costoclavicular space, the possible solution may be to cross to the transjugular approach.

10.4.2 Tight or Calcified Binding Sites

The physiological interaction between the patient and the implanted leads may cause very tight binding sites to develop over the time. Particularly in patients who underwent implant at a young age, adhesions may be particularly tough and stiff; calcium may collect in the fibrous tissue at these points. In these conditions, dilatation is difficult and sometimes may even be impossible, regardless of the energy used. Aggressive dilatation of tough or calcified binding sites may cause venous tears. Once again, the possible solution is not to increase the aggressiveness of dilatation but to move around the obstacle. The transjugular approach may solve most of these situations. When the lead can be slipped though the binding site, the dilation of challenging adhesions becomes unnecessary. If the difficult binding site is in the superior vena cava (SVC) or more distal, the transjugular approach is helpful, even if the lead cannot be slipped through. Grasping the lead proximally to the adhesion and exposing it at the neck usually allows the dilating sheath to be advanced in a straight course over the lead to the binding site, thus increasing the effectiveness of dilatation and reducing the risk of serious complications.

10.4.3 Hard Turns in the Lead Course

To free the lead from adhesions, the action of the dilator must be mainly applied at the interface between lead and fibrous tissue. The presence of hard turns in the course of the lead may be an important problem, because the dilating sheath is usually so stiff it cannot follow the lead, and dilating energy is then delivered to the venous wall. Even if a stylet and lead tension is applied, in order to use the lead as a guiderail for dilator advancement, sheaths are still usually unable to progress. This condition often occurs in right-sided leads, where a 90° angle between the subclavian and innominate vein is common (Fig. 10.7); in left-sided implants, the difficulty is at the junction between

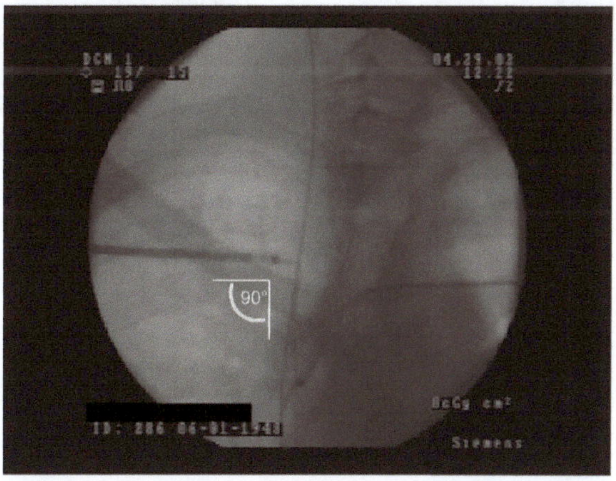

Fig. 10.7 Posteroanterior chest X-ray of a pacemaker patient. Note the 90° angle between right subclavian and innominate vein. In these cases, despite the presence of the stylet and tension on the lead (which allows using the lead as a rail), sheath advancement could be challenging or, in some cases, impossible. This condition often occurs with right-sided leads

the innominate vein and SVC. In either of these cases, both hard turns and binding sites are frequently encountered, making dilatation challenging and the risk of tears in the venous wall high.

When dilatation is ineffective or is determined to be unsafe, the operator must check the possibility of sliding the lead through the binding site and subsequently performing a transjugular approach. Even if sliding the lead is impossible, movement of the lead in another venous access (grasping it above the adherence as, explained in Chapter 5), may be helpful, allowing the operator to change the course of lead body, to reduce the degree of the angle, and finally to approach the binding site in a more effective way.

10.4.4 Tight Binding Sites into the Coronary Sinus

Most leads for left-ventricular (LV) pacing can be removed by manual traction [11–13]. When binding sites requiring dilatation are present, they are commonly located in the subclavian or innominate vein, the SVC, or at the coronary sinus [14]. Dilatation into the coronary sinus or in its branches is uncommon; when required, it may be challenging [15]. LV leads are thin, and the mechanical stress induced by sheath advancement is poorly supported. In addition, the dilator must be advanced from the subclavian vein to the coronary sinus, thus running some sort of C-shaped course. The energy of dilatation is usually wasted along that course; rotation is difficult, and the stiffness of the sheath mainly results in traction at the distal end of the lead. The risk of tears in the venous wall and subsequent bleeding is therefore increased.

Under these conditions, a possible solution is to change the venous approach in order to change the position of the proximal part of the LV lead. The straightest path into the coronary sinus is from the femoral vein. The LV lead can be made free floating by grasping it in the right atrium and then sliding it into the inferior vena cava (IVC). In some

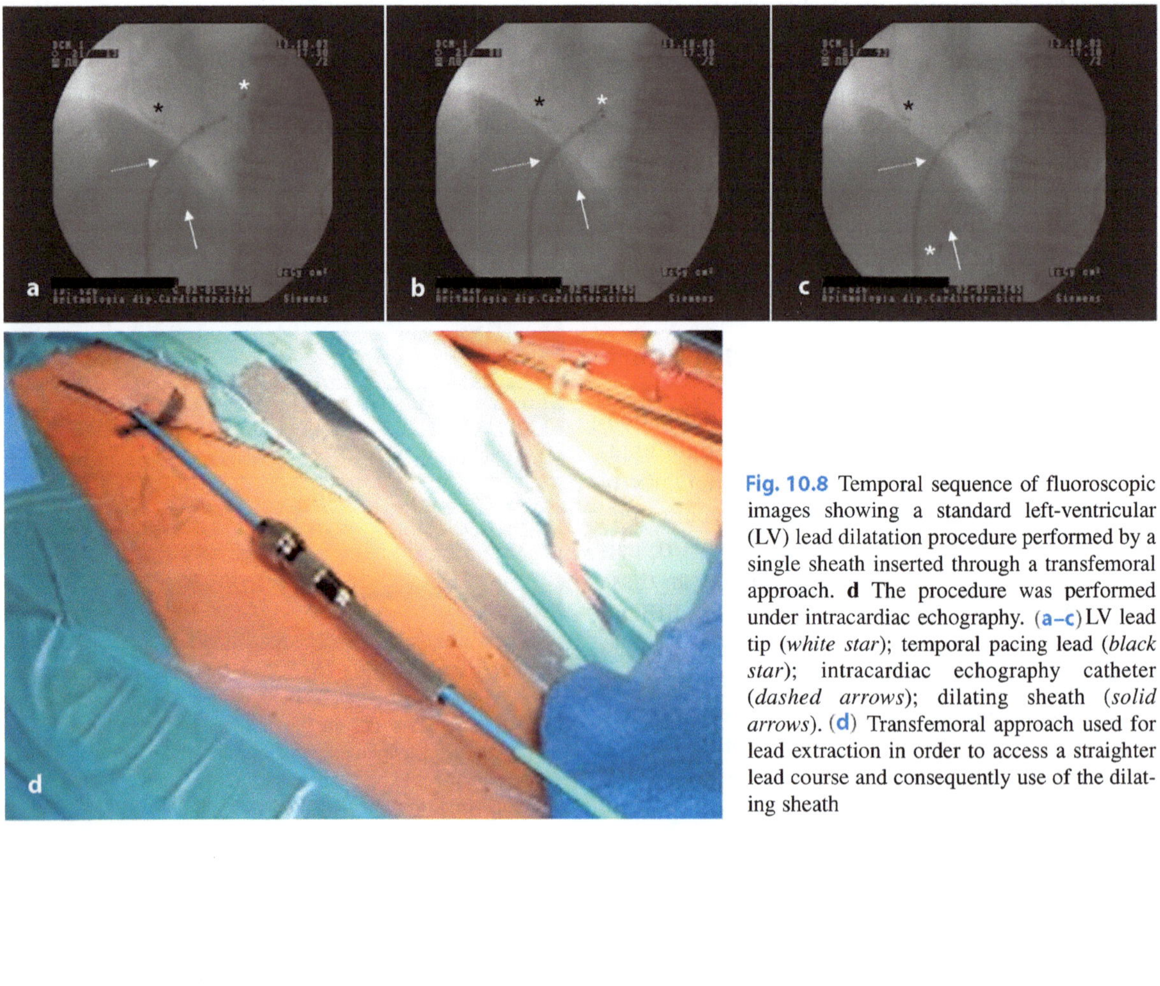

Fig. 10.8 Temporal sequence of fluoroscopic images showing a standard left-ventricular (LV) lead dilatation procedure performed by a single sheath inserted through a transfemoral approach. **d** The procedure was performed under intracardiac echography. (**a–c**) LV lead tip (*white star*); temporal pacing lead (*black star*); intracardiac echography catheter (*dashed arrows*); dilating sheath (*solid arrows*). (**d**) Transfemoral approach used for lead extraction in order to access a straighter lead course and consequently use of the dilating sheath

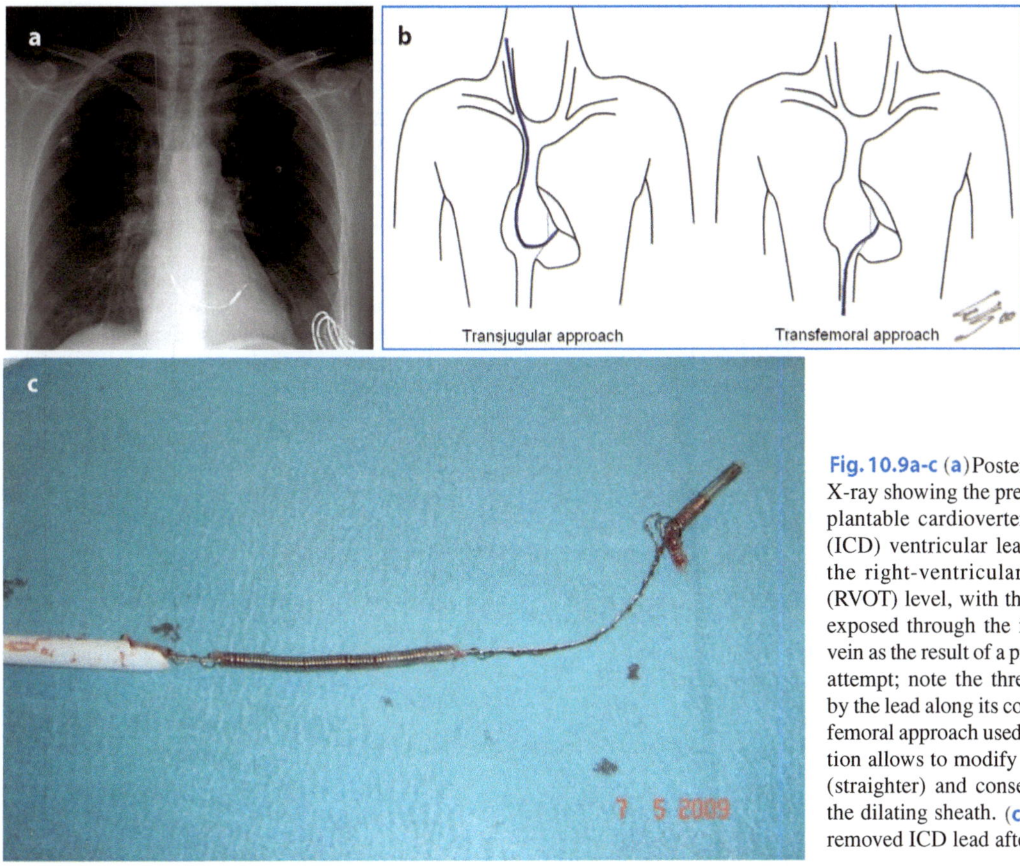

Fig. 10.9a-c (**a**) Posteroanterior chest X-ray showing the presence of an implantable cardioverter–defibrillating (ICD) ventricular lead implanted at the right-ventricular outflow tract (RVOT) level, with the proximal end exposed through the internal jugular vein as the result of a previous removal attempt; note the three angles taken by the lead along its course. (**b**) Transfemoral approach used for lead extraction allows to modify the lead course (straighter) and consequently to use the dilating sheath. (**c**) Damaged and removed ICD lead after extraction

cases, the greater length of LV leads allows for lead exposure and standard dilatation (Fig. 10.8). When the lead is not long enough for this purpose, the loop retriever to grasp the lead can be used as an extension of the lead itself. In this situation, the dilating sheaths must be inserted over the shaft of the lasso catheter before its insertion in the femoral vein. Dilating sheaths longer than usual are required and should be available to the operator. We used this approach (a reverse Pisa approach) in some difficult cases of LV extraction.

10.4.5 Tight Binding Sites in the Right-Ventricular Outflow Tract

Most considerations reported in the previous paragraph can be applied to pacing or defibrillating leads implanted in the right-ventricular outflow tract. If tight binding sites requiring dilatation are present in the distal part of the lead, dilatation from the implant vein may be challenging and unsafe. The mechanical stress induced by dilatation is mainly addressed tangentially to the course of the lead, resulting in traction to the tip. As the leads implanted in this position have a screw-fixation mechanism, the ineffectiveness of dilatation is associated with a significant increase in the risk of possible serious complications. Even in this case, changing the venous approach and the lead's position can be an effective solution. As previously described, once the lead is made free floating, it can be approached through the femoral vein, allowing a straighter dilatation course (Fig. 10.9). This approach was used by the authors in a case of ICD lead removal and resulted in complete removal without complications.

References

1. Byrd CL, Schwartz SJ, Hedin NB (1991) Intravascular techniques for extraction of permanent pacemakers leads. J Thoracic Cardiovasc Surg 101:989–997

2. Bongiorni MG, Soldati E, Zucchelli G et al (2008) Transvenous removal of pacing and defibrillating leads using single sheath mechanical dilatation and multiple venous approaches: high success rate and safety in more than 2000 leads. Eur Heart J 29(23)2886–2893
3. Love CJ (2007) Lead extraction. Heart Rhythm 4(9):1238–1243
4. Smith MC, Love CJ (2008) Extraction of transvenous pacing and ICD leads. Pacing Clin Electrophysiol 31(6):736–752
5. Love CJ, Wilkoff BL, Byrd CL et al (2000) Recommendations for extraction of chronically implanted transvenous pacing and defibrillator leads: indications, facilities, training. North American Society of Pacing and Electrophysiology Lead Extraction Conference Faculty. Pacing Clin Electrophysiol 23(4 Pt. 1):544–551
6. Magney JE, Flynn DM, Parsons JA et al (1993) Anatomical mechanisms explaining damage to pacemaker leads, defibrillator leads, and failure of central venous catheters adjacent to the sternoclavicular joint. Pacing Clin Electrophysiol 16:445–457
7. Bongiorni MG, Giannola G, Soldati E et al (2005) Pacing and implantable cardioverter-defibrillator transvenous lead extraction. Ital Heart J 6:261–266
8. Jarwe M, Klug D, Beregi JP et al (1999) Single center experience with femoral extraction of permanent endocardial pacing. Pacing Clin Electrophysiol 22:1202–1209
9. Klug D, Jarwe M, Messaoudène SA et al (2002) Pacemaker lead extraction with the needle's eye snare for countertraction via a femoral approach. Pacing Clin Electrophysiol 25:1023–1028
10. Belott PH (2007) Lead extraction using the femoral vein. Heart Rhythm 4(8):1102–1107
11. De Martino G, Orazi S, Bisignani G et al (2005) Safety and feasibility of coronary sinus left ventricular pacing lead extraction: a preliminary report. J Interv Card Electrophysiol 13(1):35–38
12. Kasravi B, Tobias S, Barnes M, Messenger J (2005) Coronary sinus leads extraction in the era of cardiac resynchronization therapy: single centre experience. Pacing Clin Electrophysiol 28(1):51–53
13. Tyers GF, Clark J, Wang Y et al (2003) Coronary sinus lead extraction. Pacing Clin Electrophysiol. 26(1 Pt. 2):524–526
14. Bongiorni MG, Zucchelli G, Soldati E et al (2007) Usefulness of mechanical transvenous dilatation and location of areas of adherence in patients undergoing coronary sinus lead extraction. Europace 9:69–73
15. Bongiorni MG, Di Cori A, Zucchelli G et al (2010) A modified transvenous single mechanical dilatation technique to remove a chronically implanted active-fixation coronary sinus pacing lead. Pacing Clin Electrophysiol [Epub ahead of print]

MIX
Papier aus verantwortungsvollen Quellen
Paper from responsible sources
FSC® C105338

If you have any concerns about our products,
you can contact us on
ProductSafety@springernature.com

In case Publisher is established outside the EU,
the EU authorized representative is:
Springer Nature Customer Service Center GmbH
Europaplatz 3, 69115 Heidelberg, Germany

Printed by Libri Plureos GmbH
in Hamburg, Germany